Treatment of cardiac emergencies

Treatment of cardiac emergencies

EMANUEL GOLDBERGER, M.D., F.A.C.P.

*Assistant Clinical Professor of Medicine, Albert Einstein
College of Medicine; Attending Physician (Cardiology),
Montefiore Hospital and Medical Center; Consulting Cardiologist,
Misericordia Hospital and Lincoln Hospital, New York, New York;
Consulting Cardiologist, St. Joseph's Hospital, Yonkers, New York*

Chapter 13, Acute Dissecting Aneurysms of the Aorta, by

MYRON W. WHEAT, Jr., M.D.

*Director, Thoracic and Cardiovascular Surgery,
Department of Surgery, University of Louisville
School of Medicine, Louisville, Kentucky*

With 231 illustrations

The C. V. Mosby Company

SAINT LOUIS / 1974

Library of Congress Cataloging in Publication Data

Goldberger, Emanuel, 1913-
   Treatment of cardiac emergencies.

   "Chapter 13, Acute dissecting aneurysms of the
aorta, by Myron W. Wheat, Jr."
   1. Heart failure.   2. Medical emergencies.
I. Wheat, Myron W   1924-   II. Title.
[DNLM: 1. Heart diseases—Therapy. 2. Emergencies.
WG205 G618t 1974]
RC682.G55   616.1′2′025   73-12750
ISBN 0-8016-1850-9

VH/VH/B   9 8 7 6 5 4 3 2 1

Preface

"When you prepare for an emergency, the emergency ceases to exist."

Preparation for cardiac emergencies includes knowledge of the cardiac emergency syndromes that can occur; the supplies and equipment available for cardiac emergencies; and the pharmacology, dosage, and administration of drugs useful for cardiac emergencies.

Therefore this book is divided into three parts. Part one describes the cardiac emergency syndromes. Chapter 1 describes syncope, which may or may not presage a cardiac emergency. Also included are chapters on cardiac arrest, cardiogenic shock, the bradyarrhythmias, and the tachyarrhythmias, including descriptions of bradyarrhythmia-tachyarrhythmia syndromes and descriptions of arrhythmias associated with digitalis toxicity and with acute myocardial infarction.

Following this are chapters on acute myocardial infarction, cardiopulmonary emergencies (massive pulmonary embolism and acute pulmonary edema), hypertensive emergencies, acute dissecting aneurysms, and acute cardiac tamponade.

I have emphasized the emergency treatment of these cardiac syndromes and have described as much as possible the relative priorities of the various drugs and other treatments that can be used. I have also indicated my own preferences for treatment, in addition to describing the viewpoints of other cardiologists. For example, I believe that cardiac pacemakers are very valuable in the treatment of the Adams-Stokes syndrome, for the bradycardia-tachycardia syndrome, and at times for the "overdriving" of tachyarrhythmias. However, I believe that, with rare exceptions, they are generally not indicated in the treatment of arrhythmias complicating acute myocardial infarction.

Part two contains a discussion of the equipment and apparatus used for cardiac emergencies, including a chapter on cardiac monitoring systems, in which I have pointed out the limitations of cardiac monitor electrocardiograms. The chapter on defibrillators and cardioverters includes a discussion of the indications and contraindications for cardioversion (synchronized DC shock). There are also three chapters on cardiac pacemakers, including a description of the techniques of inserting temporary transvenous pacemakers, the characteristics of pacemaker electrocardiograms, the various types of cardiac pacemakers, the use of pacemakers for "overdriving" tachyarrhythmias, and the indications and contraindications for temporary and long-term cardiac pacing.

In Part three are described the drugs used for cardiac emergencies, in terms of their pharmacology, absorption, indications, contraindications, side effects and toxicity, interactions with other drugs, dosage and administration, and preparations available. In addition to the commonly used emergency drugs, Part three contains a discussion of drugs such as bretylium tosylate and dopamine, which are not yet commercially available.

Monitor lead electrocardiograms are used

as much as possible to illustrate the text. At the end of each chapter and at the end of the discussion of each drug in Part three, I have included a list of selected references for the interested reader.

I deeply appreciate the cooperation and encouragement I have received from many persons, including the following: Dr. Myron W. Wheat, Jr., who was kind enough to write the chapter, Acute Dissecting Aneurysms of the Aorta; my many colleagues in the Department of Medicine of the Albert Einstein College of Medicine, particularly, Drs. M. Cohen, G. Galst, H. Klein, S. Leblang, and P. Rogal, for giving me the opportunity to follow the progress of some of their patients in the CCU of the college hospital; Frances Williams and her staff of electrocardiographic technicians in the college hospital, for taking some of the tracings used in this study; Drs. J. Scheuer, S. Furman, D. Escher, J. Frieden, and J. Cooper, of the Montefiore Hospital and Medical Center, for their many courtesies to me in the cardiac catheterization lab, the pacemaker clinic, and the CCU of the hospital; Drs. S. P. Schwartz, C. D. Enselberg, and D. Bonheim, for their interest and cooperation; Harriet Glazier and Anne Solomon for the line drawings; my son, Ary, for reading the manuscript and for his many helpful suggestions; my wife, for her devotion; my good friend Herbert F. McAuliffe, for proofreading the text; and the trustees of the Dr. Louis B. and Anna H. Goldberger Memorial Foundation for Medical Research, for sponsoring this project.

Emanuel Goldberger

Contents

Part one

Cardiac emergency syndromes

1 / Syncope

Definition

Syncope, or fainting, is a transient loss of consciousness. It is most commonly due to cerebral hypoxia secondary to inadequate cerebral blood flow. Syncope is discussed here in the context of cardiac emergencies because it may be an important clue to cardiac disease, and early treatment of patients with syncope may avert future cardiac emergencies. However, it is important to recognize that most people who faint do not have underlying cardiac problems.

Differential diagnosis

Syncope must be distinguished both from conditions in which there may be weakness, faintness, or dizziness, but no loss of consciousness, and from other conditions, such as epilepsy, in which patients actually lose consciousness. The following conditions may be confused with syncope.

Vertigo. Vertigo causes the patient to experience a sense of movement. The patient feels that he is moving (subjective vertigo) or that objects are moving around him (objective vertigo). The patient may fall to the ground, but he does not lose consciousness, and his pulse and blood pressure remain normal.

Sleep. An elderly patient may doze briefly in a chair, simulating syncope, but the pallor and pulse changes of syncope are absent. However, sudden appearance of such dozing-off episodes may be a sign of syncope. *Narcolepsy* refers to paroxysmal attacks of sleep without loss of consciousness. Many patients with narcolepsy also have *cataplexy,* sudden attacks during which muscle tone is lost, and the patient may fall to the ground.

Conversion hysteria. The patient, usually a female, may have an attack of hysterical fainting. However, there is no pallor, and there are no changes in pulse or blood pressure. In addition, the fall to the ground is characteristically graceful, causing no injury.

Hyperventilation syndrome. Rarely, hyperventilation will lead to actual syncope. In most cases, the patient complains of dizziness and lightheadedness. He may also note circumoral paresthesias, numbness and tingling in the fingers and toes, sweating, palpitations, tinnitus, and tremulousness. In addition, dyspnea, feelings of fear and unreality, tightness around the chest, nausea, vomiting, diarrhea, blurred vision, and even loss of voice may occur.

Hypoglycemia. Hypoglycemia, occurring spontaneously or after an insulin overdose, may produce syncope or even coma. Milder hypoglycemia, such as postprandial hypoglycemia, may cause weakness, trembling, diaphoresis, and other symptoms that should be distinguished from syncope. Patients may have a tachycardia, but the blood pressure is normal.

Convulsive disorders. Convulsive disorders may simulate syncope because convulsions may occur during syncope if unconsciousness lasts approximately 10 sec or longer. In epileptiform attacks, however, the convulsions precede the loss of consciousness. In syncope, loss of consciousness precedes the convulsion. Tonic convulsive movements with the patient's eyes upturned are common in epileptiform attacks but are rare in syncope. However, clonic movements of the arms may occur in both conditions. Tongue biting and urinary incontinence are also common in epileptic seizures but are rare in syncope. Postictal headache, drowsiness, and mental confusion are common findings. In contrast, patients after syncopal attacks may feel weak but are mentally alert. In *petit mal* seizures, there is transient loss of consciousness, but the patient does not fall down.

Pathophysiology

Syncope can be classified in the following principal ways.

1. Simple syncope
2. Syncope of cardiac origin
3. Syncope due to postural (orthostatic) hypotension
4. Syncope due to excessive vagal reflexes
5. Syncope due to cerebral factors

Simple syncope

Simple syncope, also called vasodepressor or vasovagal syncope, is the most common type of fainting. Attacks of simple syncope are characteristically: (1) precipitated by "stress," (2) initiated when the subject is standing or sitting, and (3) terminated rapidly when the subject becomes recumbent.

Sudden pain, fright, venipuncture, the sight of blood, and so on are common causes of simple syncope. Stress, in such cases, induces a reflex vasodilatation in the muscles. However, if muscular activity is inhibited, a marked peripheral pooling of blood occurs, with a resultant decreased cardiac output, leading to syncope.

The patient may faint without warning or may experience a brief period of premonitory symptoms, including nausea, pallor, abdominal discomfort, weakness, yawning, perspiration, unsteadiness, and blurred vision. Syncope occurs when the systolic blood pressure falls below approximately 70 mm Hg. During the prodromal period there may be a tachycardia. However, during the faint the pulse usually slows to 50 or even 40 beats per min.

Consciousness returns rapidly when the patient falls to the ground. However, fainting may recur if the patient tries to sit or stand too rapidly.

Syncope of cardiac origin

Syncope of cardiac origin may occur when the patient is in any position. However, syncope occurring when the patient is in the recumbent position is almost always due to cardiac causes. In such cases, fainting is usually secondary to decreased cardiac output. The most common causes of cardiac syncope are arrhythmias (both bradyarrhythmias and tachyarrhythmias) and mechanical obstruction to cardiac blood flow.

The causes of cardiac syncope are discussed below.

Complete atrioventricular (AV) block and the Adams-Stokes syndrome. The term Adams-Stokes syndrome denotes syncope associated with complete AV block. Complete AV block does not necessarily cause syncope. Indeed, some patients do not show syncope even when the ventricular rate is below 30 per min.

Patients with permanent or transient complete AV block may faint for several reasons, including: (1) transient asystole, (2) transient ventricular tachycardia or fibrillation, (3) sudden slowing of the idioventricular pacemaker secondary to drugs, electrolyte imbalance, and so on, and (4) sudden change from sinus rhythm or partial block to complete AV block. In all cases, syncope results from a significant drop in cardiac output.

Unconsciousness occurs after approximately 5 to 10 sec of asystole. If the heart does not beat for 15 to 20 sec, cyanosis, venous distention, and twitching of the face and upper limbs develops. The pupils may become fixed, the patient may become incontinent, and positive Babinski reflexes may appear.

Multiple Adams-Stokes attacks may produce central nervous system injury, with consequent mental confusion and other signs of an organic brain syndrome.

Other bradyarrhythmias. Sinus bradycardia with sudden slowing of the ventricular rate, with transient asystole, or with sinoatrial (SA) block may also produce syncope.

Paroxysmal tachyarrhythmias (supraventricular or ventricular). When the ventricular rate becomes rapid (especially exceeding 180 per min), cardiac output may decrease markedly, with resultant syncope.

Bradycardia-tachycardia syndrome. Attacks of bradyarrhythmias with syncope alternate with supraventricular tachyarrhythmias (Chapter 8).

Aortic stenosis. Syncope with aortic stenosis has been called effort syncope. However, patients with aortic stenosis may also faint while at rest. Syncope with aortic stenosis is an ominous prognostic sign. The average period of survival after the onset of syncope in these patients is 3 years. The syncope may occur with or without angina. There may be initial pallor, weakness or lightheadedness, or no warning signs.

Syncope in these patients is probably due to inadequate flow through the stenosed aortic valve, leading to decreased coronary and cerebral perfusion. In the early phases of syncope, these patients may show sinus rhythm. However, during the later phases of syncope, supraventricular and ventricular arrhythmias appear. Sudden death may occur as a result of ventricular fibrillation or of asystole.

Patients with aortic stenosis may also faint if complete AV block suddenly develops. Of course, they may faint from noncardiac causes.

Idiopathic hypertrophic subaortic stenosis (IHSS). Fainting associated with IHSS typically occurs immediately after exertion. During exercise there is increased venous return to the heart. When the exercise stops and the venous return decreases, forceful cardiac contractions may continue. During these contractions the hypertrophied ventricular septum may actually reach the anterior mitral leaflet and may obstruct the flood of blood from the heart. Syncope may also occur as a result of transient arrhythmias in these patients.

Other valvular lesions. Syncope associated with exertion may also occur with other valvular lesions, such as mitral stenosis and pulmonary stenosis.

Acute myocardial infarction. Acute myocardial infarction is not a common cause of syncope. Syncope may occur at the onset of acute infarction or later on. The exact mechanism of syncope is unknown. Multiple factors may be involved, including vagal reflexes from the affected coronary artery or ischemic muscle, or sudden bradyarrhythmias or tachyarrhythmias. The syncope is usually not related to pain.

Acute pulmonary embolism. Increased pressure in the pulmonary circuit can cause vagally mediated bradycardia and hypotension. Massive pulmonary embolism may also be associated with a sudden drop in cardiac output due to obstruction and to tachyarrhythmias.

Dissecting aneurysm of the aorta. Syncope, mental confusion, visual disturbances, or hemiplegia may occur if the dissection of the aortic arch interferes with the flow of blood into one of the common carotid arteries.

Primary pulmonary hypertension. Syncope with exertion may occur in patients with primary pulmonary hypertension, probably because of the inability of the cardiac output to increase adequately with exercise.

Tetralogy of Fallot. Syncope associated with increased cyanosis may also occur with exertion in patients with tetralogy of Fallot. The syncope is due to increased right-to-left shunting of blood as a result of increased obstruction to pulmonary outflow or to decreased peripheral resistance. Recently, supraventricular tachycardia has been reported as a cause of cyanotic syncopal attacks in children with tetralogy of Fallot.

Quinidine syncope. Quinidine syncope is a sign of quinidine toxicity and is usually due to transient ventricular fibrillation.

Cardiac tumors or ball valve thrombus. Cardiac syncope can occur as a result of a ball valve thrombus or left atrial myxoma. Syncope can occur when the patient is in the recumbent position, when he changes position, or when he is exercising. Tumors of the right or left ventricle may also be associated with syncope.

Syncope associated with prolongation of the Q-T interval. In 1957 Jervell and Lange-Nielsen described a syndrome of congenital deafness, prolongation of the Q-T interval, syncopal attacks, and sudden death. Since that time, syncope associated with Q-T prolongation without deafness has been described. Syncope in these cases is probably due to ventricular arrhythmias.

Pacemaker syncope. Pacemaker syncope can occur in a patient with a ventricular demand pacemaker when the patient's spontaneous heart rate suddenly becomes slow and the pacemaker starts to function at a slow rate. It is not serious, and the patient should be forewarned that this may happen.

Syncope due to postural (orthostatic) hypotension

When a normal subject stands up from a supine position, there is an initial drop in blood pressure due to pooling of blood in the legs. This fall in blood pressure stimulates baroreceptors, and a sympathetically mediated vasoconstriction and tachycardia occur. Diastolic blood pressure may become slightly elevated, and systolic pressure may rise or fall slightly. If this homeostatic mechanism for maintaining blood pressure and cardiac output is disturbed, postural hypotension with syncope may result.

Postural hypotension can be classified as either *functional* or *organic,* depending on whether there is a structural impairment of vasomotor (sympathetic) reflexes.

Functional postural hypotension. Patients with normal vasomotor reflexes may faint for a number of reasons. When a normal patient stands, a tachycardia and initial rise in diastolic blood pressure occur. However, such factors as excessive venous pooling, drug effects, or inadequate circulatory volume may interfere with the normal homeostatic mechanisms. When patients with these conditions stand, cardiac output falls because of inadequate venous return. The patient may experience weakness, nausea, and pallor on standing, and syncope may occur.

Excessive venous pooling may occur in persons with extensive varicose veins in the lower extremities, or more rarely, with a venous angioma in the leg. Syncope due to venous pooling may also occur in patients after prolonged standing in hot weather, in patients recovering from febrile illnesses, or in those confined to bed for a long time, with a resultant loss of muscle tone. Syncope due to venous pooling may also occur in athletes who suddenly stand still after vigorous exertion (postexercise vasodilatation), in pregnant women, and in patients during treatment of angina with nitrites.

Functional postural hypotension can also occur in patients with a decreased circulating blood volume due to excessive diuresis, vomiting, diarrhea, hemorrhage, or Addison's disease.

Finally, certain drugs, notably ganglionic-blocking agents such as guanethidine (Ismelin), phenothiazines (particularly if used parenterally), and l-dopa, may interfere with the normal postural reflexes.

Marked postural changes may be indicated in the electrocardiograms (ECGs) of patients with functional orthostatic hypotension. A sinus tachycardia may occur. In addition, the T waves may become inverted in all the precordial leads and in leads II,

III, and aV_F. These changes disappear almost immediately when the patient lies down. (Similar postural ECG changes may appear in persons who do not have postural hypotension.)

Organic postural hypotension. Less frequently, postural hypotension is due to impaired or absent vasomotor reflexes. Patients with organic impairment of sympathetic function can be classified into two subgroups.

Idiopathic postural hypotension. Idiopathic postural hypotension is a specific syndrome that was first described by Bradbury and Eggleston. It affects men four times as frequently as women and is often associated with impotence and anhidrosis. In addition, patients with this condition may have other abnormalities, including muscular rigidity and tremor, fixed heart rate, low basal metabolic rate (BMR), mild anemia, and slight elevation of the blood urea nitrogen concentration. When these patients stand, there is no adequate sympathetic response. Consequently, both systolic and diastolic blood pressures fall precipitously, without any increase in heart rate.

Chronic postural hypotension secondary to other diseases. A number of specific diseases are associated with impaired sympathetic activity, including tabes dorsalis, intracranial tumors, multiple cerebral infarcts, Simmonds' disease, syringomyelia, Guillain-Barré syndrome, diabetic neuropathy, porphyria, Addison's disease, and amyloidosis. The ECG in patients with these conditions remains unchanged even if syncope occurs.

Syncope due to excessive vagal reflexes

The following types of vagal syncope have been described.

Carotid sinus syncope. Hypersensitivity of the carotid sinus is a relatively rare cause of syncope. Most of the patients are older men. Syncope may be precipitated by sudden turning of the head, a tight collar, or shaving the neck. Some patients may have a carotid sinus tumor or large cervical lymph glands. These patients often give a history of sudden fainting while standing.

The most common mechanism of carotid sinus syncope is reflex vagal inhibition of the heart (cardioinhibition), producing sudden sinus bradycardia, AV block, or even cardiac standstill. This type of syncope can be blocked by atropine.

In rare cases, carotid sinus stimulation can cause a reflex vasodilatation with hypotension and syncope, independent of changes in heart rate (vasodepressor reaction). This type of carotid sinus syncope is blocked by sympathomimetic agents (such as ephedrine).

A third type of carotid sinus syncope (cerebral) has been described in which unconsciousness occurs without cardiac slowing or a fall in blood pressure. Patients with this condition probably do not have carotid sinus sensitivity but have syncope due to cerebrovascular insufficiency.

Testing the carotid sinus reflex. Carotid sinus massage has been recommended as a diagnostic maneuver in patients suspected of having carotid sinus syncope. However, this procedure has definite risks, especially in older patients. Fatalities due to cardiac arrest have occurred during carotid sinus massage, and cerebrovascular accidents have also been reported. Because of these risks, *diagnostic* carotid sinus massage should be performed only in the hospital, with cardiac resuscitative drugs and equipment available.

The patient must be lying down and should be monitored with an ECG and frequent blood pressure recordings. The carotid sinus is located anterior to the sternomastoid muscle at the upper level of (or 1/2 inch above) the thyroid cartilage (Adam's apple). The examiner stands behind the patient, rhythmically massaging (*not* compressing) the area over the carotid sinus for up to 20 sec. The pulsating artery should be felt under the examiner's fingertips. The examiner should test the carotid sinus on each side *separately*.

Normally, carotid sinus massage causes the heart rate to slow less than 6 beats per min. In a sensitive patient, carotid sinus massage produces a syncopal attack within 20 sec. The ECG may show sinus bradycardia or arrhythmias such as sinus arrest, AV block, AV junctional rhythm, or even a short run of ventricular fibrillation.

A positive reaction to the test for carotid sinus syncope must result in unconsciousness. The development of dizziness, a faint feeling, bradycardia, or even asystole for a few seconds is not sufficient to confirm the diagnosis of carotid sinus syncope.

Diagnostic carotid sinus massage is contraindicated in the presence of significant coronary artery disease (old or recent myocardial infarction), left bundle branch block, complete AV block, and cerebrovascular disease (previous cerebral thrombosis, a history of transient cerebrovascular ischemic attacks, or the presence of a carotid artery bruit on either side). The sensitivity of the carotid sinus reflex is also increased by digitalis.

If diagnostic carotid sinus massage is contraindicated, the patient can be monitored with a radiotelemetry tape apparatus. A record showing syncope associated with sudden sinus bradycardia or asystole may suggest carotid sinus origin, and appropriate treatment can be tried (see section on definitive treatment).

Cough syncope. Syncope during paroxysms of violent coughing or laughter are probably due to a Valsalva effect.

Micturition syncope. Syncope occurring before, during, or after urination may be caused by vagal reflexes from the bladder.

Esophageal diverticula, esophageal spasm, and gallbladder colic. These can produce syncope due to vagal reflexes.

Glossopharyngeal neuralgia syncope. Paroxysmal attacks of throat pain are occasionally associated with syncope due to vagal reflexes.

Fainting lark. Voluntary syncope can be produced if one has the subject hyperventilate for about a minute and then manually compresses his chest. A similar type of voluntary fainting attack, probably also due to a Valsalva effect, can be produced in muscular young men who stretch their trunk muscles vigorously and maintain this position (stretch syncope).

Syncope due to cerebral factors

Cerebral factors, including metabolic derangements (such as hypoglycemia and hyperventilation alkalosis) and cerebrovascular disease, are uncommon causes of syncope. However, such factors do predispose the patient to fainting from other causes discussed in this chapter.

Syncope has been reported in diseases affecting the arteries supplying the brain, including Takayasu's disease (pulseless disease, aortic arch syndrome), the subclavian steal syndrome, and cervical spondylitis, and in young women with "basilar artery" migraine.

Carotid sinus pressure may cause syncope if the patient's contralateral carotid artery is occluded.

Rarely, patients may faint during transient ischemic attacks due to cerebrovascular disease. In such cases, syncope is associated with specific neurological signs such as paresthesias, paralysis, dysarthria, and visual disturbances.

Treatment
Emergency treatment

Regardless of the type of syncope, the following emergency treatment should be given.

1. Immediately place the patient face up on a bed or on the floor. A fallen patient should be left on the ground, face up.

2. Lift the lower extremities for 15 sec to increase cardiac blood return.

3. Loosen the patient's collar or any tight clothing.

4. Check the patient's pulse and blood pressure.

5. If consciousness does not return immediately, extend the patient's neck and raise the chin to prevent the tongue from falling backward and blocking the patient's airway (see section on cardiopulmonary resuscitation, Chapter 2).

6. When the patient regains consciousness, slowly raise him to a sitting position, and then slowly to a standing position. If the patient is raised too quickly, fainting may recur. It may take as long as 30 min before the patient is able to stand again.

Definitive treatment

Definitive treatment depends on the cause of syncope. One should always remember that multiple mechanisms of syncope can coexist. For example, postural hypotension, hyperventilation, and hypoglycemia may occur together. One of my patients with syncope due to aortic stenosis also had micturition syncope.

The patient's history is of great importance in diagnosing the cause of syncope. Syncope occurring when the patient is in the recumbent position suggests a cardiac cause. Syncope occurring when the patient stands up suggests postural hypotension.

Examination of the patient during an attack is most helpful. Normal skin color and blood pressure suggest that true syncope is not present. The pulse will indicate whether a bradyarrhythmia or tachyarrhythmia is present. An ECG will document the exact type of arrhythmia.

When the cause of repeated attacks of syncope is obscure, it may be of value to monitor the patient with a radiotelemetry tape apparatus for 12 hours or more to establish the cardiac rhythm associated with the syncopal attack. The syncope may not have a cardiac origin even though the patient has a predisposing cardiac condition. The reverse situation may also be present.

In addition to a routine physical examination, routine laboratory tests, ECG, and chest x-ray examination, the examiner may also try to reproduce an attack of syncope with hyperventilation or hypoglycemia, or by carotid sinus massage, depending on the circumstances of each patient. If he performs such provocative tests, the examiner must remember that symptoms such as weakness or dizziness by themselves are not significant. The patient must develop an exact reproduction of the spontaneous attacks. Finally, an electroencephalogram (EEG) may be valuable if epilepsy is suspected. Half or more patients with a convulsive disorder have an abnormal EEG between attacks. Patients with syncope should have a normal EEG.

In certain types of syncope, specific treatment may be indicated. For example:

The presence of *complete AV block* is an indication for the insertion of a transvenous ventricular pacemaker.

If *aortic stenosis* or *subaortic stenosis* is present, cardiac catheterization should be dons as soon as practicable. Aortic valve replacement or surgery on the hypertrophic septum may be necessary, particularly if there is a gradient of 50 mm Hg or more across the aortic valve. In cases of IHSS, propranolol* may help prevent syncopal attacks.

There is as yet no definitive treatment for the *prolonged Q-T syndrome.* Propranolol, diphenylhydantoin, and phenobarbital have been tried in adults. Recently, one patient with the adult form of this syndrome has been treated with apparent success with left cervicothoracic ganglionectomy.

Patients with *postural hypotension* may have a correctable cause of their syncope; for example, excessive diuresis or Addison's disease. Ace bandages, applied from the toes to just below the knees, full-length supportive hose, or supportive panty hose for women may also be very helpful.

Postural hypotention due to organic im-

---

*This and other drugs are described in Part three.

pairment of vasomotor reflexes is very difficult to treat. A high salt intake and a salt-retaining steroid such as 9-alpha-fluorohydrocortisone (Florinef) to expand the circulating volume can be used. In severe cases, a countercompression garment, or G-suit, such as the Jobst Pressure Gradient Support, may be required.

Carotid sinus syncope can be treated with sympathomimetic drugs such as ephedrine sulfate or hydroxyamphetamine (Paredrine) given orally. Atropine is helpful but cannot be prescribed in most instances for long-term use because of its many side effects. If drug therapy does not relieve the attacks, a demand type of transvenous ventricular pacemaker should be inserted. Pacemaker therapy can be used in any patient with recurrent syncope due to excessive vagal reflexes.

Prophylaxis

Most patients with syncope will benefit from Ace bandages or supportive hose, as mentioned above. These supports should be put on before the patient gets out of bed. (Such support may be contraindicated in patients who also have severe vascular disease of the lower extremities.)

Women should be advised not to wear elastic panty girdles. These girdles extend 6 to 10 inches along the thighs and may act like tourniquets, preventing venous return from the lower extremities and also producing edema.

Patients who suffer from any type of syncope should be advised to take showers and not to take hot baths. When one steps out of the bathtub after a hot bath, marked pooling of blood in the lower extremities may occur, leading to syncope.

REFERENCES

Adams RD, Harrison TR: Faintness, syncope and episodic weakness. In Harrison's principles of internal medicine, ed 6, New York, 1970, McGraw-Hill Book Co.

Bannister R, Ardill L, Fentem, P: Assessment of various methods of treatment of idiopathic orthostatic hypotension, Q J Med **38**:377, 1969.

Bohl OP, Ferguson TB, et al: Treatment of carotid sinus syncope with demand pacemaker, Chest **59**:262, 1972.

Bradbury S, Eggleston C: Postural hypotension, Am Heart J **1**:73, 1925.

Cohen, MV: Ventricular fibrillation precipitated by carotid sinus pressure; case report and review of the literature, Am Heart J **84**:681, 1972.

Dunn M: Orthostatic hypotension, Hosp Med, April 1971, p 119.

Easley RM, Goldstein S: Sino-atrial syncope, Am J Med **50**:166, 1971.

Friedberg CK: Syncope, Mod Concepts Cardiovasc Dis **40**, nos. 11,12, 1971.

Ira GH, Floyd WL, Orgain ES: Syncope with complete heart block; differentiation of real and simulated Adams-Stokes seizures by radiotelemetry JAMA **188**:707, 1964.

Jervell A, Lange-Nielsen F: Congenital deaf-mutism, functional heart disease with prolongation of the Q-T interval and sudden death, Am Heart J **54**:59, 1957.

Johnson RH, Lee G de J, et al: Autonomic failure with orthostatic hypotension due to intermediolateral column degeneration, Q J Med **35**:276, 1966.

Karp HR, Weissler AM, Heyman A: Vasodepressor syncope; EEG and circulatory changes, Arch Neurol **5**:106, 1961.

Khero BA, Mullins CB: Cardiac syncope due to glossopharyngeal neuralgia; treatment with a transvenous pacemaker, Arch Intern Med **128**:806, 1971.

Klein LJ, Saltzman HA, Heyman A: Syncope induced by the Valsalva maneuver, Am J Med **37**:263, 1964.

Kopald HH, Roth HP, et al: Vagovagal syncope; report of a case associated with diffuse esophageal spasm, N Engl J Med **271**:1238, 1964.

Lewis RK, Hazelrig CG, et al: Therapy of idiopathic postural hypotension, Arch Intern Med **129**:943, 1972.

Moss AJ, McDonald J: Unilateral cervicothoracic sympathetic ganglionectomy for treatment of long QT interval syndrome, N Engl J Med **285**:903, 1971.

Pomerantz B, O'Rouke RA: The Stokes-Adams syndrome, Am J Med **46**:941, 1969.

Rashtin RA, Hunt D, Russell RO Jr: Q-T interval prolongation, paroxysmal ventricular arrhythmias, and convulsive syncope, Ann Intern Med **75**:919, 1971.

Schwartz LS, Goldfischer J, Sprague GJ, Schwartz SP: Syncope and sudden death in aortic stenosis, Am J Cardiol **23**:647, 1969.

Selzer A, Wray HW: Quinidine syncope, Circulation **30**:17, 1964.

Shillingford JP: Syncope, Am J Cardiol **26**:609, 1970.

Voss DM, Mangin GE: Demand pacing and carotid sinus syncope, Am Heart J **79:**544, 1970.

Wayne HH: Syncope; physiological considerations and an analysis of the clinical characteristics in 510 patients, Am J Med **30:**418, 1961.

Wright KE Jr, McIntosh HD: Syncope; review of pathophysiological mechanisms, Prog Cardiovasc Dis **13:**580, 1971.

Young D, Elbl F: Supraventricular tachycardia as a cause of cyanotic syncopal attacks in tetralogy of Fallot, N Engl J Med **284:**1359, 1971.

2 / Cardiac arrest

Definition

Cardiac arrest is the stopping of effective cardiac contractions. The two most common causes of cardiac arrest are *ventricular fibrillation* and *asystole (cardiac standstill)*. A third cause of cardiac arrest has been termed *profound cardiovascular collapse*. This is characterized by the presence of identifiable QRS complexes in the ECG without an obtainable blood pressure and pulse. In such cases the ECG may show a slow ventricular rhythm or a marked sinus bradycardia. A tachycardia may develop following treatment with sympathomimetic drugs. However, the pulse and blood pressure may remain unobtainable. Profound cardiovascular collapse represents a type of *electromechanical dissociation*. (When any patient with an acute myocardial infarction develops electromechanical dissociation, cardiac rupture with tamponade must always be suspected. See p. 189.)

Etiology

In medical patients, conditions commonly associated with cardiac arrest include acute myocardial infarction; acute pulmonary embolism; second-degree or complete AV block; valvular heart disease, especially aortic or subaortic stenosis; cyanotic congenital heart disease; and cerebrovascular disease. Cardiac arrest can also occur as a complication of diagnostic procedures, such as cardiac catheterization or angiocardiography.

Toxic doses of drugs, such as digitalis, quinidine, procainamide, diphenylhydantoin, potassium salts, epinephrine, and isoproterenol and other sympathomimetic drugs, can also be associated with cardiac arrest usually due to ventricular fibrillation. Cardiac arrest due to asystole can be produced by acetylcholine and other parasympathomimetic drugs.

Cardiac arrest due to ventricular fibrillation can also occur with a fixed rate pacemaker (Chapter 15). It is also the cause of death in freshwater drowning, accidental electrocution, or lightning shock.

In surgical patients, hypoxia or hypercapnia (carbon dioxide retention) and respiratory acidosis may occur during the operation. The acidosis is associated with the development of acute hyperkalemia, which can quickly produce ventricular premature contractions, ventricular tachycardia, and cardiac arrest due to ventricular fibrillation. Cardiac arrest occurs most frequently during operations on the throat, neck, mediastinum, and heart, and during eye surgery, urological surgery, and operations done with the patient hypothermic particularly if his internal temperature falls below 86 F (30 C).

In both medical and surgical patients, excessive vagal reflexes may precipitate cardiac arrest; for example, with carotid sinus massage, for diagnosis, or for treatment of a tachyarrhythmia; in the respiratory tract, including the nasopharynx and trachea, during passage of an endotracheal tube, bronchoscope, and so on; in the gastrointestinal tract, during passage of an esophagoscope or gastroscope; during a rectal examination or even straining at the stool (Valsalva effect); in the urinary tract, during passage of a urethral catheter, and so on; during surgery on the eyes or while one is applying pressure on the eyes; and during abdominal surgery, cutting the vagus nerves, or traction on the peritoneum.

Pathophysiology

The neurons of the cerebral cortex undergo irreversible changes approximately 3 min after cardiac arrest. (However, the centers that control corneal and pupillary reflexes can survive 10 min, and the neurons of the medulla may survive 20 or more min.) Cardiac arrest is followed within a few seconds by respiratory arrest. Occasionally, respiratory arrest occurs first. If this happens, the heart may continue to beat as long as 30 min.

Diagnosis

One should not waste time making an absolute diagnosis of cardiac arrest before starting treatment, because irreversible changes in the brain occur after approximately 3 min. If the following signs are present, immediate therapy for cardiac arrest is justified: loss of consciousness that does not respond rapidly when the patient is placed in the supine position; absent pulsations in a major artery, such as the carotid, brachial, or femoral artery, where pulsations had been previously present; absent or gasping respirations; or dilated pupils. Pupillary dilatation begins approximately 45 sec after cerebral blood flow stops and is maximal in approximately 1 min and 45 sec. Therefore, maximally dilated pupils indicate that about one half of the period for potential reversibility of cerebral damage has already passed. Confirmation of cardiac arrest by finding absent heart sounds, electrocardiographic evidence of asystole, or ventricular fibrillation is not necessary at this time.

Treatment

During cardiopulmonary resuscitation, there are often so many rescuers and so many procedures done simultaneously (external cardiac compression, intracardiac and intravenous injections, intubation, defibrillation, and so on) that it is very difficult and sometimes impossible to determine what has been effective if the patient has survived or what might have been done if the patient died. In my experience, one physician should be assigned to order medications and procedures. One nurse should be assigned to see that the orders are carried out. The time of each procedure and medication should be noted on a flow chart. Continuous ECGs should be taken, preferably with one lead, such as lead II; and as drugs are administered or defibrillation is performed, the electrocardiographic technician should note the procedure or drug and the time on the ECG.

Emergency treatment

The question is often asked whether restoration of the circulation or administration of artificial ventilation should be the first step in resuscitation. Actually, it is necessary to restore *both* the circulation and the respiration of the patient, simultaneously if possible. Therefore, the term cardiopulmonary resuscitation (CPR) is preferable to cardiac resuscitation.

I prefer to give the following emergency treatment to restore the circulation, in addition to the standard method of resuscitation.

1. Immediately place the patient in a supine position (horizontal, face up). If he or she is in a semirecumbent or sitting position in bed, immediately lower the head of the bed. If the patient is lying on a pillow, remove it at once. When unconsciousness and cardiac arrest occur, the tongue falls backward and tends to block the airway with the epiglottis (Fig. 2-3, *A*) particularly if the patient's neck is flexed. Lift the neck

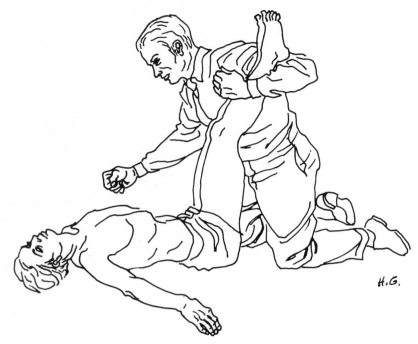

Fig. 2-1. First step in cardiopulmonary resuscitation. The rescuer lifts the patient's legs vertically and gives one thump with the folded fist to the lower sternum.

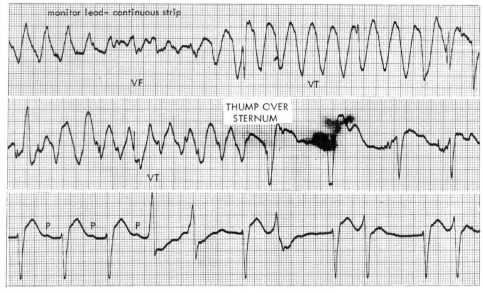

Fig. 2-2. Thump over sternum with the closed fist (thump version) restored sinus rhythm in a patient with ventricular fibrillation and ventricular tachycardia.

and tilt the head backward (Fig. 2-3, *A*).

2. Raise both lower extremities to a vertical position and keep them elevated for 5 to 15 sec (Fig. 2-1). This increases the venous return to the heart even as much as 1,000 ml. (A contraindication to leg raising is a fracture of a long bone of a lower extremity.)

If only one rescuer is present, start **CPR** (see below) after 5 sec of leg raising. If there are two or more rescuers present, start CPR immediately, but keep the legs elevated the full 15 sec. Then lower the legs, but keep them slightly elevated at an angle of approximately 15°. You can then wrap the lower extremities with Ace bandages from toes to thighs. (A contraindication to bandaging the lower extremities is the presence of severe peripheral vascular disease.)

3. Simultaneously (while raising the legs) sharply thump the patient's lower sternum with the ulnar surface of the folded fist *(thump version)* (Fig. 2-1). This may restore the heartbeat (Fig. 2-2). Rhythmic thumping of the lower sternum can keep the heart beating for hours, particularly in patients with complete AV block who develop asystole. However, when cardiac arrest occurs, the first thump may stop a ventricular tachycardia or a ventricular fibrillation, but the next thump may produce ventricular standstill. Therefore, if the patient does not respond to the first thump, external cardiac compression (see below) should be started.

These three simple maneuvers will frequently restore spontaneous heartbeats.

While performing these emergency procedures, call for help and for resuscitative supplies and equipment.

Technic of cardiopulmonary resuscitation

The National Academy of Sciences–National Research Council recommends that the following technic be done as quickly as possible and in the order shown:

A. Airway opened
B. Breathing restored
C. Circulation restored
D. Definitive therapy

Airway opened. Opening the airway is easily and quickly accomplished by tilting the patient's head backward as much as possible, as described above. However, when a trained rescuer is present, the following can be done to open the airway.

With the patient supine, place one hand behind the patient's neck and the other hand on the patient's forehead. Then lift the neck and tilt the head backward (Fig. 2-3, *A*). This stretches the neck and lifts the tongue away from the back of the throat and thus removes the mechanical blockage of the airway. Maintain the head in this position at all times. In addition, with your fingers or by suction immediately remove obvious foreign material in the mouth or throat.

Breathing restored. If the patient does not resume spontaneous breathing after his head has been tilted backward, immediately begin artificial ventilation by either the mouth-to-mouth or the mouth-to-nose method. The first blowing effort will determine whether there is any obstruction in the airway.

When using *mouth-to-mouth ventilation,* maintain the patient's head in a position of maximum backward tilt, with one of your hands behind the neck. In the unconscious patient, this usually allows the mouth to drop open. Then pinch the patient's nostrils together with the thumb and index finger of your other hand. Open your mouth widely. Take a deep breath, make a tight seal with your mouth around the patient's mouth, and blow in about twice the amount the patient normally breathes (Fig. 2-3, *B*). (About 500 ml air enters the lungs with an average breath. Therefore, you will breathe into the patient about 1,000 ml air with each breath.)

You can place a clean gauze or folded handkerchief over the patient's mouth and

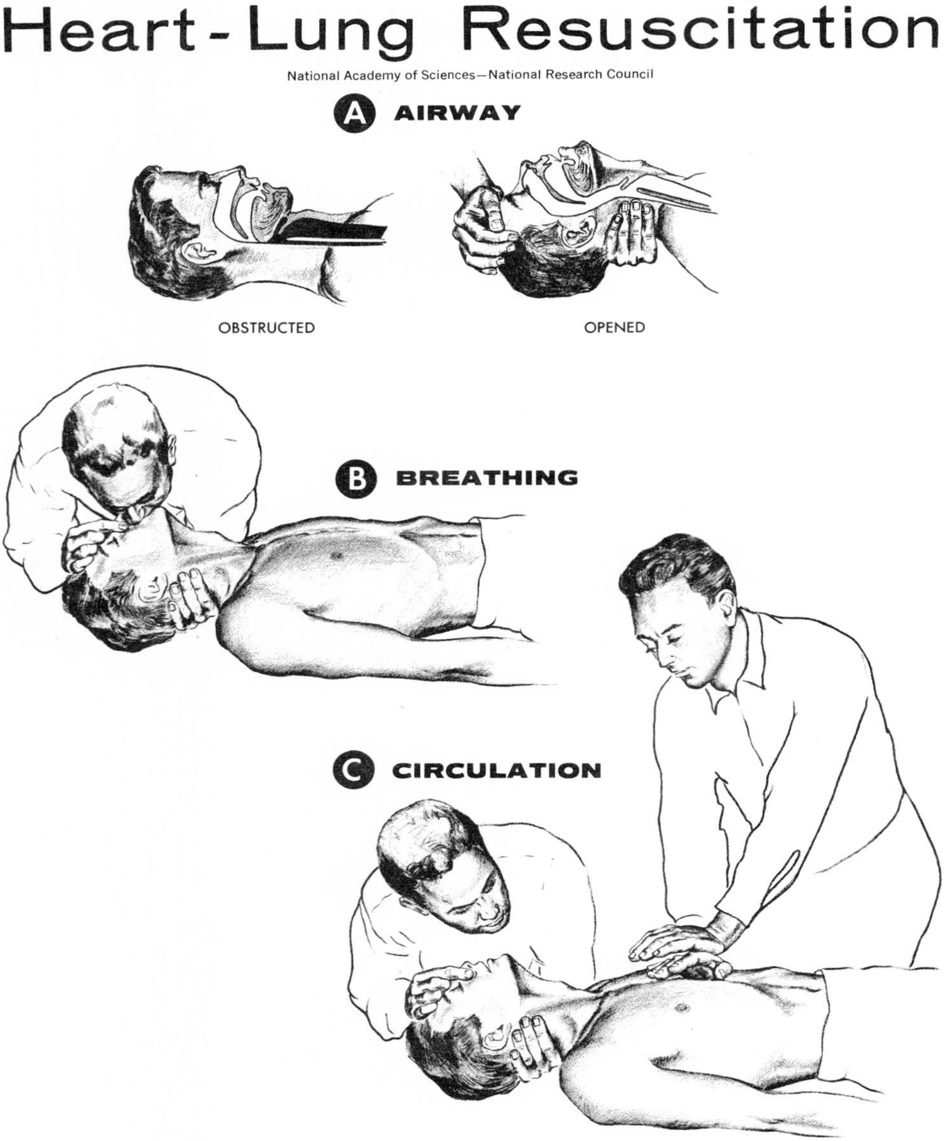

Heart-Lung Resuscitation

National Academy of Sciences—National Research Council

Ⓐ AIRWAY

OBSTRUCTED   OPENED

Ⓑ BREATHING

Ⓒ CIRCULATION

Fig. 2-3. A, Obstructed airway when the patient is supine. The airway is opened when the patient's neck is lifted and the head is tilted backward. **B,** Mouth-to-mouth breathing. Notice that the rescuer has lifted the patient's neck and pinched the nostrils while doing the mouth-to-mouth breathing. **C,** External cardiac compression by one rescuer while the other rescuer is performing mouth-to-mouth breathing. (From Cardiopulmonary Resuscitation Conference Proceedings, Publication 1494, Division of Medical Sciences, National Academy of Sciences–National Research Council, Washington, D.C., 1967.)

nose. (Tuberculosis can be contracted from mouth-to-mouth breathing if the patient has active tuberculosis.) Do *not* use a facial tissue to cover the patient's mouth. The tissue will get wet and mat quickly. Then remove your mouth and allow the patient to exhale passively. Repeat this cycle approximately 12 times per min.

Adequate ventilation is ensured on every breath if you (1) see the chest rise and fall, (2) feel resistance of the lungs as they expand, and (3) hear the air escape during exhalation.

You can use *mouth-to-nose ventilation* if it is impossible to open the patient's mouth. This frequently occurs before unconsciousness becomes complete. You should also use mouth-to-nose ventilation if the patient's mouth is seriously injured, if it is difficult to achieve a tight seal, or if you prefer the nasal route.

Keep the patient's head tilted back with one hand, and use the other hand to push the patient's lower jaw closed and to seal the patient's lips. Then take a deep breath, seal your lips around the patient's nose, and blow in until the patient's chest rises. Remove your mouth, allowing the patient to exhale passively. Repeat this cycle approximately 12 times per min. When mouth-to-nose ventilation is used, it may be necessary to open the patient's mouth during exhalation, if this can be done, to allow the air to escape.

Occasionally, the air passages may not be completely opened even when the patient's head is properly tilted backward. If this occurs, you can achieve further opening of the air passages by displacing the patient's jaw forward so that the lower teeth are in front of the upper teeth and by simultaneously holding the patient's mouth open. This can be accomplished by grasping the jaw between your thumb and index finger and lifting it or by placing your fingers behind the angles of the lower jaw and pushing it forward.

You should strongly suspect the presence of a foreign body if you are unable to inflate the lungs after the patient's head has been properly tilted backward and the jaw displaced forward. The first blowing effort will determine whether any airway obstruction exists. If obstruction is present, quickly roll the patient onto his side and deliver firm blows over the spine between the shoulder blades to dislodge the obstruction. You should then sweep your fingers through the patient's mouth to remove any obstructing material. Then resume artificial ventilation. Sometimes you can use slow, forceful breaths to bypass a partial airway obstruction.

Mouth-to-mouth or mouth-to-nose breathing may cause distention of the patient's stomach. Slight gastric distention can be disregarded. However, marked distention may be deleterious because it reduces lung volume by elevating the diaphragm. Gastric dilatation may stimulate vagal reflexes, and it can cause regurgitation of food and aspiration into the lungs.

Gastric dilatation can be avoided during artificial ventilation, particularly if a second rescuer is present and if one of the rescuers exerts moderate pressure with a hand over the patient's epigastrium between the umbilicus and the rib cage. Signs of gastric dilatation are marked distention of the abdomen and tympany. In addition, the patient may vomit easily and frequently.

If gastric dilatation or vomiting occurs, turn the patient onto his side, with the head lower than the trunk, if possible. Exert moderately firm pressure over the epigastrium. This may produce a large amount of air and vomitus. Then return the patient to the supine position for further CPR. To prevent further distention of the stomach, one rescuer should maintain moderately firm pressure on the epigastrium during the CPR.

Gastric dilatation can also be treated by intubation of the stomach with a Levin tube. In addition, suction apparatus should be available in case aspiration occurs.

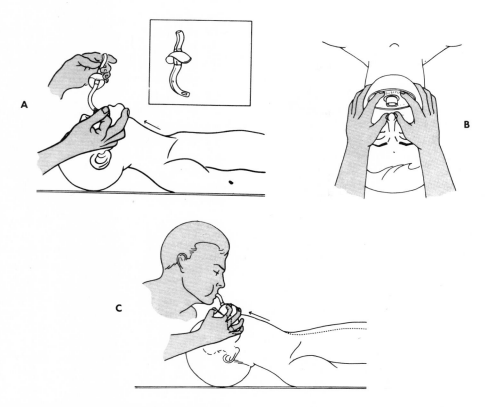

Fig. 2-4. Mouth-to-airway resuscitation, using an S-shaped airway (Resusitube). **A,** The rescuer is at the top of the patient's head. The patient's neck is lifted and the head is tilted backward. The Resusitube is inserted over the tongue until the flange rests on the patient's lips. If the mouth is tightly closed, it should be wedged open with an index finger inserted between the patient's cheek and teeth (behind the wisdom teeth). The tongue must not be pushed back into the throat. If necessary, the tongue should be held forward with the fingers while the tube is being inserted. Insert shows the Resusitube. Notice that (in an adult) the *long* end of the tube is inserted into the patient's mouth. **B,** The Resusitube is inserted into the mouth until the flange rests securely over the patient's lips. The flange is pressed over the lips with the index fingers to prevent air leakage. The patient's chin is kept up and is never allowed to sag. **C,** The rescuer takes a deep breath and blows forcibly (for resuscitating an adult) into the mouthpiece of the tube. The rescuer watches patient's chest; when it moves, the rescuer takes his mouth off the tube and lets the patient exhale passively. When the exhalation is finished the rescuer blows in the next deep breath. The first few breaths he blows must be deep and at a rapid rate. Thereafter, about one breath every 5 sec is adequate. If the patient's chest does not move, the chin-up position should be increased, the position of the rescuer's fingers on the flange of the Resusitube checked, and more forceful blows made. If the chest still does not move, the position of the Resusitube airway must be readjusted. It may have been inserted too deeply or not deeply enough. The flange must rest firmly on the patient's lips. If the patient is breathing shallow natural breaths, the rescuer must blow in at the moment the patient inhales. The rescuer takes his mouth off quickly when exhalation occurs. (Courtesy the Johnson & Johnson Co.)

Artificial airways. Attempts to reoxygenate the lungs by exhaled air methods or by means of a mask should always be made before endotracheal intubation is attempted. Various airways and masks are available and can be very helpful when properly employed in CPR.

An S-shaped oropharyngeal plastic airway with a cupped flange (Resusitube) is very helpful as an aid to mouth-to-mouth ventilation because it brings the base of the tongue forward and also prevents the patient's teeth and lips from obstructing respiration. Insert the S-shaped plastic airway over the tongue (Fig. 2-4). Even when using the airway, you must keep the patient's head tilted backward. To prevent laryngospasm or vomiting, do not use force in inserting the airway.

Once the S-shaped airway is in place, ventilate the patient, using mouth-to-airway ventilation; or you can use a self-refilling bag and mask, such as the Ambu (automatic manual breathing unit) bag or the PMR (Puritan Manual Resuscitator) bag, with either oxygen or room air.

The highest possible inhaled oxygen concentration should be provided as soon as possible. When an Ambu type of bag unit is used, an inhaled oxygen concentration of over 50% can be attained only by attaching to the intake valve a reservoir tube with a capacity equal to the tidal volume and an oxygen inflow rate of at least the patient's minute volume. When a demand valve is attached to the bag intake, 100% oxygen concentration can be obtained.

If trismus is present, use a plastic nasopharyngeal tube. It should be well lubricated and inserted parallel to the palate. (A clenched jaw or struggling is a sign that some degree of consciousness is still present.)

In the early stages of CPR do not intubate the patient with a cuffed endotracheal tube, because it wastes valuable time. Artificial ventilation has to be stopped while the patient is being intubated; if intubation is difficult, lethal hypoxia may develop. However, an anesthetist or another trained rescuer can intubate the patient after the patient has been ventilated with an S-shaped airway and an Ambu type of bag unit.

Intubation requires that the patient's head be shifted to a new position. The patient should by lying supine in bed, with his shoulders and head touching the mattress. Place a folded towel under the patient's head, and then rotate the head backward to bring the pharynx and trachea into a straight line. (When the patient is intubated and is receiving oxygen by mask or respirator, it may be difficult to determine if consciousness has returned, particularly if the patient is struggling. However, you can ask the patient to perform a simple task, such as blinking the eyes.)

Circulation restored—external cardiac compression. Restoration of circulation is done by external cardiac compression (*external cardiac massage*), which must always be accompanied by artificial ventilation. After three to five effective lung inflations, check the patient's carotid artery pulse. While keeping the patient's head tilted backward, gently locate the larynx, and after sliding laterally with the fingers flat, palpate the carotid artery area. (The carotid artery lies in a hollow between the thyroid cartilage and the anterior border of the sternomastoid muscle.) To avoid carotid sinus stimulation, feel the carotid pulse, do not compress it. If the patient is still unconscious and apneic and if there is no carotid artery pulse, start external cardiac compression immediately.

External cardiac compression consists of rhythmic pressure over the lower half of the sternum. This compresses the heart and produces a pulsatile arterial circulation because the heart lies almost in the middle of the chest between the lower sternum and the spine. When properly performed, external cardiac compression can produce a systolic blood pressure of over 100 mm Hg, with a mean blood pressure of 40 to 50 mm Hg in the carotid artery, and a carotid arterial blood flow as much as one-third normal.

For successful compression, the patient must be on a firm surface. You can place the patient on the floor, or if he is in bed, you can slide a board or tray under his upper back. Do not delay external cardiac compression to find a board.

Stand at the side of the patient and place only the heel of one hand over the lower half of the sternum (Fig. 2-3). Do *not* place your hand over the lower tip (the xiphoid process) of the sternum. Place your other hand on top of the first one (Fig. 2-3). Then rock forward to bring your shoulders almost directly above the patient's chest, keeping your arms straight. Exert adequate pressure almost vertically downward so that the lower sternum moves 1½ to 2 inches. (This requires a force of 80 to 120 lb.)

If the patient is in bed, stand on a chair or kneel on the bed to be able to exert *downward pressure* with your arms. If you stand at the side of the bed, it will be difficult to exert adequate pressure.

The rate of compression is 1 per sec (60 per min). The compression should be regular, smooth, and uninterrupted. Compression and relaxation should be of equal duration. Compression should *not* be interrupted for more than 5 sec for any reason.

While performing external cardiac compression, you must also ventilate the patient. If there is only one rescuer, follow each fifteen cardiac compressions by two quick lung inflations. If there are two rescuers, follow each five cardiac compressions by one lung inflation, without any pause in the compressions. The results of CPR are similar with either coordinated or noncoordinated compressions and ventilations.

The effects of external cardiac compression can be checked in several ways.

1. With each compression, an arterial pulse should appear. The carotid artery pulse is more meaningful than either the radial artery or femoral artery pulse.

2. The ECG also responds to the external cardiac compression. Various types of electrocardiographic artifacts may appear with each compression (Figs. 2-5 and 2-6). Occasionally, each external cardiac compression causes a recognizable QRS complex and T wave to appear (Fig. 2-5, *A*).

3. The reaction of the pupils should also be constantly checked since it is one of the best signs of the patient's condition. Pupils that constrict when exposed to light indicate that there is adequate oxygenation and adequate blood flow to the brain. Widely dilated pupils that do not react to light indicate that serious brain damage has occurred or is imminent. Dilated but reactive pupils are less ominous. One should also remember that normal pupillary reactions may be altered by the administration of atropine (which dilates the pupils) or of morphine (which constricts them).

Complications of external cardiac compression. Complications include fractures of the ribs and sternum, flail chest, laceration of the lungs or liver or other abdominal organs, pulmonary or cerebral fat emboli, laceration or rupture of the heart, herniation of the heart through the pericardium, cardiac tamponade, and hemothorax or pneumothorax. These complications can be minimized by careful attention to the details of external cardiac compression. For example:

1. Never compress over the lower tip of the sternum (over the xiphoid process), because the xiphoid process overlies the liver and when depressed can cause lethal laceration of the liver.

2. Never let your fingers touch the patient's ribs during compression. Keep the heel of your hand in the middle of the patient's chest, over the lower half of the sternum.

3. Never use sudden or jerking movements to compress the chest. The action should be smooth, regular, and uninterrupted, with one half of the cycle compression and one half of the cycle relaxation.

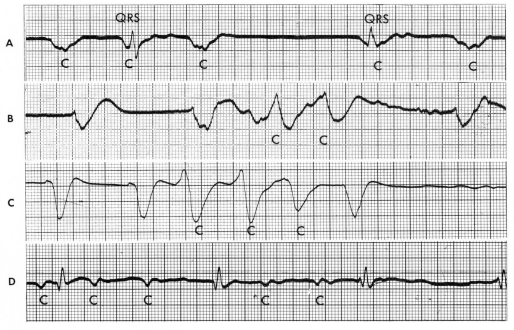

Fig. 2-5. Electrocardiographic artifacts produced by external cardiac compression. **A, B, C,** and **D** are from different patients. **C,** Electrocardiographic artifacts. **A,** A patient with ventricular stand-still. Two of the cardiac compressions were associated with QRS complexes. **B, C,** and **D,** A slow ventricular rhythm with artifacts (**C**) due to the external cardiac compression.

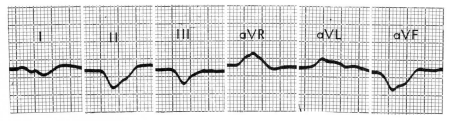

Fig. 2-6. Electrocardiographic artifacts due to external cardiac compression. The patient was in ventricular standstill. Notice that external cardiac compression characteristically produces wide, downward deflections in leads II, III, and aV_F, and an upward deflection in lead aV_R.

4. Never compress the chest and abdomen simultaneously. This can cause rupture of the liver.

5. Thomas has pointed out that when external cardiac compression is done on a patient who has had a prosthetic valve (particularly mitral or tricuspid) inserted recently, external cardiac compression may cause serious lacerations to the valve area, which would be lethal even if the patient survived the CPR. He suggests that if cardiac arrest occurs postoperatively in such patients, external cardiac compression be done for 3 to 4 min, in association with definitive treatment (see below). If resuscitation is still not successful, he suggests that the chest be opened and the heart massaged manually.

Contraindications to external cardiac compression. External cardiac compression may be ineffective in certain conditions, such as crushing injuries of the chest, internal thoracic injuries, massive air embolism or massive pulmonary embolism, tension or bilateral pneumothorax, severe emphysema, or cardiac tamponade. If cardiac arrest occurs during surgery of the neck, chest, or abdomen, it may be necessary to open the chest and compress the heart directly, in conjunction with artificial ventilation.

In addition, CPR should not be used in the following situations.

1. When cardiac arrest has lasted for more than 5 or 6 min (probably longer in cases of drowning)
2. When the patient has been in the terminal state of an incurable condition

If there is question of the exact duration of the cardiac arrest, the patient should be given the benefit of the doubt, and resuscitation should be started.

Mechanical equipment for cardiopulmonary resuscitation. Conventional pressure-cycled automatic ventilators or resuscitators are not recommended in conjunction with external cardiac compression, because the effective cardiac compressions prematurely trigger the termination of the inflation cycle. This produces shallow and insufficient ventilation. In addition, the inflation flow rates of pressure-cycled ventilators or resuscitators are usually inadequate.

Oxygen-powered, manually triggered ventilation devices are acceptable if they can provide instantaneous flow rates of 1 L/sec or more (for adults). A safety-valve release pressure of about 50 cm water should be provided. Ideally, these devices should permit the use of 100% oxygen and should permit support of airway and mask with both hands.

External cardiac compression apparatus are adjuncts that may be used when the patient requires prolonged resuscitation or transportation. They should be built in a way that allows quick application of the machine to the patient, and they should have safeguards to prevent accidental malposition of the plunger or malposition of the patient's head during use.

Definitive therapy. Definitive therapy should be started while emergency treatment is continued.

1. Start two IV infusions of 500 ml 5% dextrose in water at two sites. A venous cutdown, preferably on the greater saphenous vein, just anterior to the medial malleolus at the ankle, may be necessary to make certain that a patent vein is always available. Insertion of a venous catheter into a subclavian vein (p. 210) is also valuable in case central venous pressure monitoring has to be done or a transvenous pacemaker catheter electrode has to be inserted.

2. Treat hypotension by adding 100 mg metaraminol (Aramine)* or 8 mg levarterenol *bitartrate* (1 ampul) to one of the infusion bottles.

3. Treat metabolic acidosis with sodium bicarbonate administered IV as quickly as possible because the acidosis develops within a few minutes after the cardiac ar-

---

*This and other drugs are described in Part three.

rest. The sodium bicarbonate can be given in one of two ways.

First, a priming dose of two 50-ml ampuls of sodium bicarbonate (7.5 gm = 89.2 mEq) should be immediately injected into the IV tubing of one of the infusion bottles. Then a dose of one 50-ml ampul (3.75 gm = 44.6 mEq) should be repeated every 5 to 10 min until the circulation has been restored.

Patients with cardiac arrest often require massive doses of sodium bicarbonate (even as much as 8 to 10 ampuls) to counteract metabolic acidosis. However, the dosage of sodium bicarbonate should be monitored with serial pH determinations to prevent a metabolic alkalosis from developing. (In addition, an excessive amount of sodium bicarbonate may precipitate congestive heart failure.) The first 2 ampuls should be given immediately. The pH should then be determined, if possible. If the pH is low (7.0 or lower), an additional 2 ampuls should be given. Thereafter, 1 to 2 ampuls should be given every 5 to 10 min until the circulation is restored or until the pH rises above 7.30.

Second, sodium bicarbonate can also be given IV as a 1.5% solution. A priming dose of 100 ml should be given as quickly as possible. Then the solution should be given rapidly at a rate of 10 ml per min (approximately 150 drops per min if a regular drip bulb is used). When sodium bicarbonate is given as an IV drip, it will probably be necessary to give supplemental ampuls of sodium bicarbonate to raise the pH to above 7.30.

4. Electrical defibrillation with an unsynchronized precordial DC shock of 400 watt-seconds (ws) (Chapter 18) should be done even before an ECG is taken. If the patient has ventricular fibrillation, DC shock will often restore sinus rhythm. If the patient has ventricular standstill, the electrical shock will not do any harm.

5. As soon as the DC shock has been given, a standard ECG should be taken to determine what type of electrical activity is present in the heart. The ECG may show ventricular fibrillation, ventricular tachycardia or ventricular flutter, cardiac standstill, a slow idioventricular rhythm, or marked sinus bradycardia (rate below 50 per min). The treatment that follows depends on the ECG.

Treatment of ventricular fibrillation. If the ECG shows ventricular fibrillation (Figs. 2-8 to 2-10), the following should be done.

1. Defibrillate the patient again with an unsynchronized DC shock of 400 ws.

2. Repeat the ECG. Ventricular fibrillation may still be present. The fibrillatory waves may be fine (amplitude less than 5 mm) or coarse (amplitude greater than 5 mm) (Fig. 2-7). Fine ventricular fibrillation responds poorly to electrical defibrillation. Epinephrine increases the amplitude of the fibrillatory waves and makes the heart more responsive to the DC shock. Even when epinephrine does not change the amplitude of the fibrillatory waves, it may make the heart respond to the DC shock.

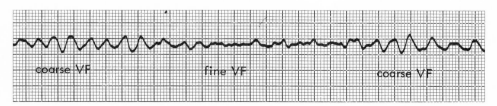

Fig. 2-7. Ventricular fibrillation. Coarse and fine fibrillatory waves are shown.

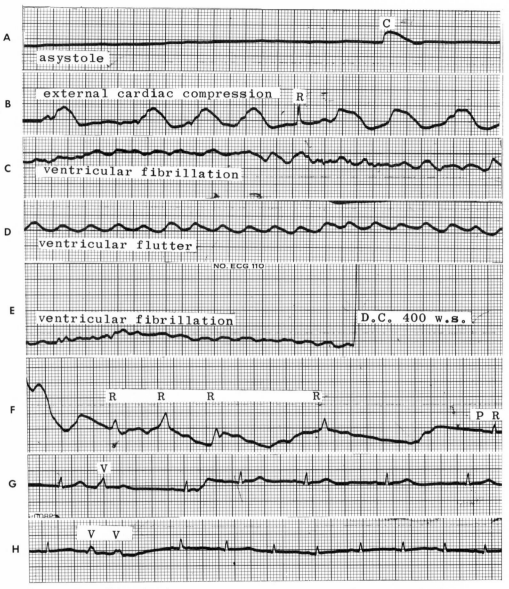

Fig. 2-8. Successful cardiopulmonary resuscitation. **A** to **H** were taken at intervals of 1 to 2 min.
A, Asystole. (C, electrocardiographic artifact due to external cardiac compression.) **B,** Asystole
with cardiac compression artifacts. (R, a QRS complex produced as a result of the cardiac compression.) **C, D, E,** Ventricular fibrillation, ventricular flutter, and ventricular fibrillation. At this
point the patient was given unsynchronized precordial DC shock. **F,** Slow, irregular ventricular
rhythm that occurred immediately after the DC shock. Notice a normal sinus beat at the end of
F. G and **H,** Sinus rhythm with occasional ventricular premature contractions (V). This often occurs
after cardiopulmonary resuscitation. It is due partly to the effect of epinephrine or isoproterenol
that has been given to the patient and partly to the release of catecholamines by the patient
resulting from the stressful episode.

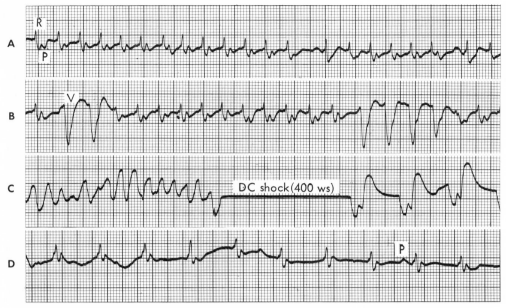

Fig. 2-9. Successful cardiopulmonary resuscitation. **A, B, C,** and **D** taken at intervals of 1 to 2 min. All show lead II. **A,** Supraventricular tachycardia, probably AV junctional. Notice the inverted P waves that follow the R waves. **B,** Ventricular premature contractions *(V)* in addition to supraventricular tachycardia. **C,** Ventricular fibrillation has developed. The patient immediately received unsynchronized precordial DC shock and developed a rapid ventricular rhythm with wide, aberrant QRS complexes. **D,** QRS complexes resemble the patient's usual pattern. A few sinus P waves *(P)* are present. Sinus rhythm returned later.

3. Inject epinephrine, 0.5 to 1 ml (1:1,000 concentration) or 5 to 10 ml (1:10,000 concentration), IV or by intracardiac injection. (A 1:10,000 solution can be prepared by taking 1 ml of the standard 1:1,000 dilution and adding it to 9 ml sterile saline.) An intracardiac injection should be made just to the left of the sternum in the fourth or fifth intercostal space, using a 3½-inch (9-cm) 22-gauge needle. (When intracardiac injections are made close to the sternum in the fourth or fifth left intercostal space, the danger of lacerating a coronary artery is minimal.) The injection should be made at a slant rather than at right angles to the surface of the heart. In this way, bleeding is less likely to occur when the needle is removed, because the intraluminal pressure of the heart will tend to close the needle hole. To avoid irritating the heart, injecting any medication into the heart muscle should be avoided. Therefore, the injection should not be made until blood is drawn into the syringe.

Continue external cardiac compression and ventilation for 1 to 2 min to allow the epinephrine to circulate through the heart.

4. Give the patient another unsynchronized DC shock of 400 ws.

5. If ventricular fibrillation persists, give the patient another IV or intracardiac dose of epinephrine. This can be repeated every 3 to 5 min as necessary.

6. Continue the external cardiac compression and the artificial ventilation.

7. In addition, give the patient an IV bolus of 75 mg lidocaine (Xylocaine). This may also make the heart more responsive to the DC shock. Injection of lidocaine can

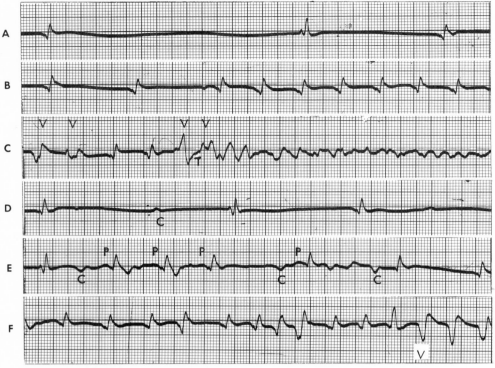

Fig. 2-10. Unsuccessful cardiopulmonary resuscitation. **A, B, C, D, E,** and **F** taken at intervals of 1 to 2 min. All show lead II. **A,** Patient had developed profound cardiovascular collapse and the heart rate had markedly slowed. Intracardiac epinephrine had been given. This increased the heart rate again, **B,** but the patient still did not have any measurable blood pressure or palpable pulse. **C,** Ventricular premature contractions (V) developed. The fourth ventricular premature contraction occurred at the apex of the preceding T wave (R on T phenomenon), and ventricular fibrillation developed. The patient immediately received unsynchronized precordial DC shock of 400 ws. **D,** Taken a few moments later. A slow AV junctional rhythm has reappeared (**C,** an artifact due to external cardiac compression). The patient was given isoproterenol IV, and external cardiac compression was continued. **E** and **F,** A supraventricular and a ventricular tachycardia that developed again. Shortly after this, the patient again developed ventricular fibrillation and died.

be repeated every 5 min, but the total dose per hour must not exceed 200 to 300 mg.

8. If lidocaine and DC shock are not effective in restoring sinus rhythm, an IV bolus of 1 mg propranolol (Inderal) can be given, followed by another DC shock.

9. If the ventricular fibrillation is due to digitalis toxicity, diphenylhydantoin (Dilantin) instead of lidocaine can be given IV. It is given in a dose of 100 mg in a period of 2 min. DC shock is then given.

If ventricular fibrillation persists, another 100 mg diphenylhydantoin is given over a 2-min period, followed again by DC shock. A total of 500 mg diphenylhydantoin can be given this way. External cardiac compression must be continued during the administration of the diphenylhydantoin.

Usually the patient will respond after two or three precordial DC shocks. However, some patients may require nine or more shocks before sinus rhythm appears.

If the patient does not respond after the third DC shock, another defibrillator should be used, if possible, because the original defibrillator may not be working properly.

When sinus rhythm is restored, lidocaine should be continued as an IV infusion at a rate not exceeding 4 mg per min, to prevent ventricular premature contractions or a recurrence of the ventricular fibrillation. If tachyarrhythmias (supraventricular or ventricular) develop after the ventricular fibrillation has been abolished, they can be treated in the usual way. The lidocaine should be continued for at least 48 to 72 hours. (If necessary, a lidocaine drip can be continued for weeks.)

If there is a possibility of a further attack of ventricular fibrillation (as in a patient with an acute myocardial infarction), procainamide or quinidine should be started orally at least 12 hours before the lidocaine is stopped.

If lidocaine is not effective in suppressing recurrent ventricular fibrillation, procainamide administered IV or IM or propranolol administered IV can be tried. When bretylium is available, it can also be used in these patients.

As soon as the condition is stable, the patient should be transferred to a cardiac care unit (CCU) where continued cardiac monitoring and treatment can be done.

Treatment of asystole. Continue treatment for hypotension and metabolic acidosis. In addition, give the following treatment.

1. Administer isoproterenol to stimulate cardiac contractions. It can be given in one of two ways: by intracardiac injection in a dose of 0.2 mg (1-ml ampul) or by IV infusion of 2 mg dissolved in 500 ml 5% dextrose in water, given at a rate to raise the ventricular rate to 60 to 70 per min. (Isoproterenol will cause vasodilation and may cause a further drop in blood pressure. Therefore, additional IV fluids may also be needed.)

2. Epinephrine can be given instead of isoproterenol by intracardiac or IV injec-

tion, just as for ventricular fibrillation (see above). (Remember that epinephrine can also precipitate ventricular fibrillation.)

3. Levarterenol can also be given by intracardiac injection instead of isoproterenol or epinephrine to initiate the heartbeat. For this purpose 0.5 to 0.75 ml of a 0.02% solution is used. (A 0.02% solution of levarterenol bitartrate is made by diluting 1 ml of the regular 0.2% solution with 9 ml isotonic saline. Each 1 ml of the resultant solution contains the equivalent of 0.1 mg of levarterenol *base*.)

4. Calcium chloride, 5 to 10 ml of a 10% solution, can be given by intracardiac or IV injection to increase the force of cardiac contractions. The dose can be repeated every 5 min.

A 10% solution of calcium gluconate can be used in place of calcium chloride. Ten to 15 ml of 10% calcium gluconate is equivalent to 5 ml of 10% calcium chloride.

5. If the above treatment is not effective, try to pace the heart electrically. An external pacemaker with electrodes on the precordium, set at a rate of 70 to 80 per min, can be tried. However, it will usually not be effective in patients with asystole. Therefore, a transvenous pacemaker catheter electrode, connected to a portable battery-operated pacemaker, should be inserted into the right ventricle. Even this may not be effective in restoring the circulation.

Emergency transthoracic pacing can also be done by passing a needle and cannula percutaneously into the right ventricle and then passing a pacing stylet through the cannula into the ventricle.

Treatment of profound cardiovascular collapse. The patient may show signs of profound cardiovascular collapse when the cardiac arrest starts, or it may develop after ventricular fibrillation or asystole have been abolished. The prognosis is grave. Usually the heart rate slows progressively. The QRS complexes widen, and asystole and death usually occur, regardless of treat-

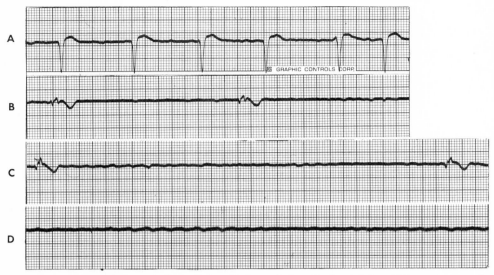

Fig. 2-11. Ventricular standstill. **A,** Taken 12 hours before **B, C,** and **D,** which were parts of a continuous strip. **A,** Atrial fibrillation with a slow ventricular rate (slightly less than 60 per min). The patient had received digitalis. **B,** Two ventricular escape beats. The base line is irregular due to the continuation of the atrial fibrillation. **C,** Further slowing of the heart. Atrial fibrillation continues. **D,** Terminal. The atrial fibrillation continues.

ment (Fig. 2-11). Treatment is essentially the same as for asystole. In addition, the following can be done.

1. Atropine in a dose of 0.4 to 1 mg can be given IV, and the dose can be repeated after 1 to 2 hours for 3 or 4 doses.

2. The central venous pressure can be measured. If it is 5 cm water or less, an infusion of 500 ml fluid should be given IV as quickly as possible (within 10 min) to expand the circulating blood volume. The type of infusion depends on the patient's history. If there are signs of blood loss, plasma or isotonic saline should be used. If there is a history of sodium loss due to excessive vomiting, diarrhea, use of diuretics, and so on, isotonic saline or 5% dextrose in isotonic saline should be infused. If the patient shows pulmonary congestion, 5% dextrose in water can be infused.

The changes in the central venous pressure or signs of pulmonary congestion can be used as a guide for further IV therapy in these patients.

Postresuscitative treatment

The patients who survive after CPR can be divided into four groups, on the basis of their subsequent neurological condition (Norris and Chandrasekar).

Group I. Immediate recovery with no sequelae.

Group II. Rapid recovery. Unconsciousness lasts for several hours. Then recovery occurs. These patients show varying emotional sequelae, such as amnesia or signs of a mild to severe organic brain syndrome with delusional thinking, confusion, difficulty in concentrating, and severe anxiety. These symptoms may last for months or longer.

Group III. Delayed recovery. These patients are unconscious for hours or days and show spasticity, aphasia, loss of vision, hemiplegia, incoordination, and other cerebellar signs. The prognosis of these patients is uncertain.

Group IV. Decerebrate state. These patients remain unresponsive and spastic and have dilated pupils. They rarely live for more than a few days or weeks.

If CPR is successful but the patient remains unconscious, the following treatment should be given.

1. Ventilate the patient with controlled ventilation, using preferably a volume-cycled respirator, such as the Engström, Puritan Bennett MAI, Emerson Postoperative, and so on.

2. The patient's internal temperature can be lowered to 89.6 to 91.4 F (32 to 33 C). If the temperature falls below this, myocardial irritability and further arrhythmias may appear. If shivering occurs, control it by IM administration of chlorpromazine (Thorazine), 25 mg every 6 hours, or promethazine (Phenergan), 12.5 to 25 mg every 6 hours, because the shivering greatly increases cerebral oxygen needs. (Both of these drugs have a hypotensive effect when given parenterally.)

When cardiac arrest occurs in a patient who has serious organic heart disease, lowering the temperature may be dangerous because it may be difficult to regulate the temperature exactly and the diseased myocardium may be excessively irritable at a low temperature.

3. Massive doses of corticosteroids can be given to reduce cerebral edema; for example, 500 mg hydrocortisone (Solu-Cortef) administered IV every 6 hours for 72 to 96 hours. The dose is then gradually reduced. Equivalent doses of other corticosteroids can also be used. However, the value of corticosteroids is questionable.

4. Limit IV fluids to approximately 1,500 ml daily to prevent water excess, hyponatremia, and further edema of the brain.

5. Urea has been used to decrease cerebral edema, which is probably present if the patient remains comatose after the circulation has been restored. It can be given IV in a dose of approximately 1.0 gm/kg body weight (40 gm in 250 ml 5% dextrose in water). The solution is given slowly over a period of 1 to 2½ hours. It can be given twice daily, if necessary. However, the usefulness of urea in overcoming postresus-citative coma has not been definitely established.

Terminating cardiopulmonary resuscitation

Termination of CPR is a medical decision and depends on an assessment of the patient's cerebral and cardiovascular status. The best criteria of adequate cerebral circulation are the reactions of the pupils, the level of consciousness, muscular movements, and spontaneous respirations. Deep unconsciousness, absence of spontaneous respirations, and fixed dilated pupils for 15 to 30 min indicate cerebral death. A flat EEG can also be used as a sign of cerebral death unless the patient has ingested a large amount of a central nervous system depressant, such as the barbiturates, or has been treated with hypothermia and has an internal temperature below 90 F (32.2 C).

One can assume that cardiac death is present when there is no return of electrocardiographic activity after 1 hour of continuous CPR. However, if there is a palpable peripheral pulse, if a systolic blood pressure of over 60 mm Hg is being maintained, if the pupils remain constricted, and if there are other signs that the body is being adequately oxygenated, CPR should be continued.

If the patient has been resuscitated and placed in a respirator, but remains in a coma, the following revised criteria of the Ad Hoc Committee of the Harvard Medical School can be used to determine death: deep unconsciousness with no responses to external stimuli or to internal needs; no movements or breathing (except artificially maintained breathing); no reflexes, with the exception of occasional spinal reflexes, such as brisk withdrawal of the lower extremities in response to painful stimuli, or an abnormal slow flexor plantar reflex that simulates a negative Babinski reflex; a flat EEG, and no changes in any of these findings after 24 hours. However, these findings are valid only if the patient is not hypothermic or if the patient has not received any central nervous system depressants, such as barbiturates.

REFERENCES

Ad Hoc Committee of the Harvard Medical School to Examine the Definition of Brain Death: A definition of irreversible coma, JAMA 205:337, 1968.

Binnie CD, et al: Electroencephalographic prediction of fatal anoxic brain damage after resuscitation from cardiac arrest, Br Med J 4:265, 1970.

Cohen LS: New therapeutic ideas and agents in the management of acute cardiac emergencies. In Eliot RS, editor: The acute cardiac emergency, Mount Kisco, N Y, 1972, Futura Publishing Co., p. 223.

Dobson M, et al: Attitudes and long-term adjustment of patients surviving cardiac arrest, Br Med J 3:207, 1971.

Don Michael TA: Precordial percussion in cardiac resuscitation, Am Heart J 69:721, 1965.

Don Michael TA, Stanford RL: Precordial percussion in cardiac asystole, Lancet 1:699, 1963.

Dreifus L: Pronouncement of death in patient with implanted cardiac pacemaker, Questions and Answers, JAMA 222:1659, 1972.

Gordon AS: Technique of cardiopulmonary resuscitation (CPR) and pitfalls in performance. In Meltzer LE, Dunning AJ, editors: Textbook of coronary care, Philadelphia, 1972, Charles Press.

Jude JR, Nagel EL: Cardiopulmonary resuscitation 1970, Mod Concepts Cardiovasc Dis 39:133, 1970.

Kouwenhoven WB, Jude JR, Knickerbocker GG: Closed-chest cardiac massage, JAMA 173:1064, 1960.

Lemire JG, Johnson AL: Is cardiac resuscitation worthwhile? A decade of experience, N Engl J Med 286:970, 1972.

Meltzer LE, Dunning AJ, editors: Textbook of coronary care, Philadelphia, 1972, Charles Press.

Messer JV: Management of emergencies; cardiac arrest, N Engl J Med 275:35, 1966.

National Academy of Sciences–National Research Council: Cardiopulmonary resuscitation, JAMA 198:372, 1966.

Norris JR, Chandrasekar S: Anoxic brain damage after cardiac resuscitation, J. Chronic Dis 24:585, 1971.

Parkhouse J: Cardiac arrest successfully treated, Br J Anaesth 34:210, 1962.

Pennington JF, Taylor J, Lown B: Chest thump for reverting ventricular tachycardia, N Engl J Med 283:1192, 1970.

Rossman PL: Gastric dilatation; a preventable complication, Consultant, January 1972, p. 59.

Safar P: Mouth to mouth airway, Anesthesiology 18:904, 1957.

Safar P: Recognition and management of airway obstruction, JAMA 208:1008, 1969.

Saphir R, Falsetti HL: The artifactual electrocardiogram recorded during closed-chest massage, JAMA 202:571, 1967.

Stephenson HE Jr: Cardiac arrest and resuscitation, ed 3, St. Louis, 1969, The CV Mosby Co.

Stephenson HE Jr: Prognosis in cerebral damage after cardiac arrest, Questions and Answers, JAMA 222:93, 1972.

Task Force on Death and Dying of the Institute of Society, Ethics, and the Life Sciences: Refinements in criteria for the determination of death; an appraisal, JAMA 221:48, 1972.

Thomas TV: Cardiac resuscitation in patients with prosthetic cardiac valves, Communication, Chest 62:652, 1972.

Weiner IH: Death criteria, Letter, JAMA 222:86, 1972.

Woodward WW: Cardiac arrest treated by elevation of the limbs for fifteen seconds, Lancet 2:1120, 1960.

Zoll PM: Rational use of drugs for cardiac arrest and after cardiac resuscitation, Am J Cardiol 27:645, 1971.

3 / Cardiogenic shock

Shock is a complex syndrome associated with inadequate perfusion of vital organ systems, especially the kidneys, brain, liver, intestines, and heart. The cardiac output may be low, normal, or even high.

Shock is usually divided into three general types.

1. Hypovolemic shock
2. Septic shock
3. Cardiogenic shock

Hypovolemic shock occurs following significant volume loss from the circulation, as in hemorrhage, trauma, burns, or severe diarrhea or intractable vomiting.

Septic shock most commonly is associated with gram-negative bacteria, such as *Escherichia coli, Klebsiella, Pseudomonas,* and *Proteus.* These bacteria produce endotoxins that injure the capillaries and cause sequestration and pooling of plasma. Therefore, septic shock is also a form of hypovolemic shock. Septic shock can also occur with infection due to gram-positive bacteria.

Cardiogenic shock characteristically occurs after acute myocardial infarction. It can also occur after massive pulmonary embolism, after open heart surgery, or with acute cardiac tamponade. This chapter emphasizes the shock associated with acute myocardial infarction.

CARDIOGENIC SHOCK ASSOCIATED WITH ACUTE MYOCARDIAL INFARCTION

Cardiogenic shock develops in 10% to 20% of patients hospitalized for acute myocardial infarction. The mortality of such patients is still approximately 80% or higher, in spite of the recent advances in coronary care. Very few patients develop shock immediately after the onset of the myocardial infarction. Instead, signs of shock usually develop hours or days afterward. About half of the patients develop shock within 24 hours, and about one sixth of the patients develop shock a week or more later.

Clinical signs

Cardiogenic shock due to acute myocardial infarction has the following characteristics.

1. The ECG shows the pattern of acute myocardial infarction or of acute coronary insufficiency (subendocardial myocardial infarction).

2. The systolic blood pressure is 80 mm Hg or less (90 mm Hg or less if the patient has been hypertensive).

3. The pulse rate is 110 per minute or faster (unless second-degree or complete AV block is present).

4. The urinary output is low, 30 ml or less per hour.

5. There are clinical signs of peripheral circulatory collapse, such as pale, mottled, clammy, cyanotic skin, with collapse of the veins of the dorsum of the hands and feet; and beads of sweat on the forehead, extending progressively to the extremities.

One should observe the skin color and skin temperature over regions such as the skin stretched over the bones of the toes and fingers which are relatively free of muscles. Palpation of the skin of the calf or forearm may be misleading because of the heat retained by the skeletal muscle circulation.

6. The patient exhibits mental changes such as restlessness and agitation at first, then apathy, lethargy, confusion, or coma.

7. The rate and depth of respirations are increased.

Differential diagnosis

Cardiogenic shock due to acute myocardial infarction must be differentiated from other conditions, including massive pulmonary embolism, acute dissecting aneurysm of the aorta, and acute cardiac tamponade.

In cases of *massive pulmonary embolism* the ECG may simulate acute myocardial infarction because signs of subendocardial injury may be present. However, these changes are usually associated with other signs, such as an S_1Q_3 pattern, sudden right or left axis deviation, acute right bundle branch block, or the development of downward T waves in precordial leads V_1 through V_5 or even V_6. Lung scan or pulmonary arteriography findings are diagnostic. (Also see Chapter 15.)

In patients with *acute dissecting aneurysm of the aorta* the pain may begin in the chest but then often spreads down the back into the abdomen or lower extremities. This is in contrast to the pain of acute myocardial infarction, which is characteristically substernal and which may spread to the shoulders, arms, or neck, or into the epigastrium or right upper quadrant of the abdomen. In addition, in acute dissecting aneurysm of the aorta, the ECG shows only nonspecific RS-T and T wave changes, which are characteristic of hypertensive heart disease but not of coronary artery disease. (Also see Chapter 13.)

Pain is not a characteristic feature in patients with *acute cardiac tamponade*. The diagnosis is suggested by the development of progressively falling blood pressure and shock, pulsus paradoxus, and markedly dis-

tended neck veins, with or without further swelling on inspiration. X-ray findings may be minimal because acute cardiac tamponade may occur when only several hundred milliliters of blood or fluid are in the pericardium. Total electrical alternans (of P waves, QRS complexes, and T waves) in the ECG, if present, is diagnostic. (Also see Chapter 14.)

Other conditions that may simulate the cardiogenic shock of acute myocardial infarction include acute hemorrhage (internal or external), acute cerebrovascular thrombosis or hemorrhage, diabetic acidosis, excessive effects of hypotensive drugs, and sepsis. A rare cause of shock associated with acute myocardial infarction is acute adrenal insufficiency due to adrenal hemorrhage in patients receiving anticoagulants.

Acute pancreatitis can be associated with the development of abnormal Q waves and abnormal RS-T segments even though acute myocardial infarction may not be found at autopsy. I have seen several such cases, and others have been reported in the literature. The mechanism causing these electrocardiographic findings is obscure because they may be present without shock. I believe that when the electrocardiographic changes of acute myocardial infarction occur in a patient with acute pancreatitis, the patient should be treated as if an acute myocardial infarct is present, in addition to being given any treatment needed for the acute pancreatitis.

Pathophysiology

When shock occurs as a result of acute myocardial infarction, the following physiological changes occur.

The decreased strength of the heart causes a reduced stroke volume and therefore a decreased minute volume of the heart (the cardiac output). This produces a fall in arterial blood pressure and underperfusion of the peripheral tissues. After a variable delay the fall in arterial blood pressure is associated with compensatory changes because of stimulation of barore-ceptors in the carotid sinus. This produces generalized sympathetic stimulation, with a secretion of norepinephrine and epineph-rine. As a result, the heart rate increases (unless AV block is present). In addition, the force of contraction of the uninvolved ventricular muscle is also increased. This raises the cardiac output toward normal. In addition, there is usually generalized constriction of the arterioles (with the ex-ception of the vessels of the heart and brain). This tends to raise the total periph-eral resistance (also see p. 34). The ar-terial blood pressure therefore tends to rise toward a normal level.

Despite these compensatory changes, the patient has a low arterial blood pressure and a low cardiac output. Urinary blood flow is decreased or may cease. Signs of gen-eralized sympathetic stimulation are pres-ent (tachycardia, peripheral pallor or cya-nosis or both, clammy skin, and so on). In addition, metabolic acidosis quickly devel-ops due to tissue hypoxia, and the blood lactate and pyruvate levels rise.

The low cardiac output and the compen-satory sympathetic stimulation are usually also associated with an increased end-dia-stolic pressure in the right ventricle and in the left ventricle (indicating congestive heart failure). The increased end-diastolic pressure in the right ventricle may be as-sociated with clinical signs of right-sided heart failure, such as increased central ven-ous pressure, and with engorgement of the liver, with a positive hepatojugular reflux. The increased end-diastolic pressure in the left ventricle may be associated with clini-cal signs of left-sided heart failure, such as rales in the lung bases, or with extensive pulmonary edema. (Cardiogenic shock with acute pulmonary edema may occur with a normal or low left ventricular end-diastolic pressure. The reason for this is discussed on p. 39.)

Theoretically, the blood volume should be normal in shock associated with acute myocardial infarction. However, in some patients it may be low, even if the patient has not been previously dehydrated by vomiting, diarrhea, or diuretics, or when hemorrhage has not occurred. The reason for this low blood volume is not known.

Pulmonary changes, with disturbances in alveolar-capillary gas exchanges, also occur in cardiogenic shock. These changes are due to pulmonary vasoconstriction, in-creased left atrial pressure, and hypoxia of the lung tissues secondary to a decreased pulmonary blood flow. As a result of these changes, the pulmonary artery oxygen pres-sure (Pa_{O_2}) may become low and may re-main abnormally low (70 mm Hg or lower) even when the patient breathes 100% ox-ygen.

In order to adequately treat a patient in cardiogenic shock, one must have objective measurements of the physiological changes that have occurred. It is possible to mea-sure the following parameters: tissue per-fusion, splanchnic blood flow, intra-arterial blood pressure, cardiac output, circulating blood volume, total peripheral resistance (systemic vascular resistance), central ven-ous pressure (CVP), left ventricular func-tion (left ventricular end-diastolic pres-sure), right ventricular function (right ven-tricular end-diastolic pressure), and pul-monary wedge pressure. Unfortunately, most of these measuremetns require special technical help, equipment, and facilities that are not available in a general hospital. The technical details of some of these mea-surements are described at the end of this chapter. Here some general statements can be made.

Tissue perfusion. Inadequate tissue per-fusion is probably the most important sign of shock. Unfortunately, there is not yet any way of directly measuring this pa-rameter. One indirect method is to mea-sure the arterial lactate concentration. (The normal range of lactic acid concen-tration in arterial blood is less than 1.5 mEq/L; that is, approximately 5 to 15 mg/

100 ml.) It has been found that when the arterial lactate concentration rises to 8 mEq/L or higher in patients with acute myocardial infarction, the mortality is 90% or higher. However, a sudden rise in arterial lactate concentration during treatment of shock is not necessarily an adverse effect. For example, lactate levels may increase after vasodilating drugs have been given. This increase is an indication that tissue perfusion has improved and that the lactic acid that has accumulated in the tissues is now being flushed into the general circulation.

Splanchnic blood flow. It would be very useful if splanchnic blood flow could be measured directly. Unfortunately, direct measurement is not possible. At the bedside, the hourly urinary output can be used to indicate splanchnic blood flow. A urinary output of more than 30 ml per hour is a sign of adequate renal and splanchnic blood flow.

Intra-arterial blood pressure. Measurement of the arterial blood pressure with a sphygmomanometer cuff may be very inaccurate when shock is present because a blood pressure reading may be unobtainable with this method, although the intra-arterial blood pressure may be adequate. In addition, intra-arterial blood pressure is often significantly higher than cuff blood pressure, particularly in patients who are markedly vasoconstricted. This discrepancy is further exaggerated when vasopressor drugs have been used.

Another difficulty of measuring blood pressure in shock is that the intra-arterial blood pressure is not the same in all arteries. For example, the intra-arterial blood pressure of the femoral or brachial artery may be different from the intra-aortic blood pressure.

Cardiac output. Patients with acute myocardial infarction show a reduced cardiac output. However, this is not the entire cause of shock, because the cardiac output values overlap between patients with myocardial infarction in shock and those not in shock. In addition, patients with severe congestive heart failure due to chronic rheumatic heart disease, for example, may have very low cardiac output and show no signs of shock.

At the bedside, cardiac output can be inferred in a general way by observation of the pulse pressure. An aneroid sphygmomanometer is better than a mercury manometer for this because the range of movement of the dial with each heartbeat indicates the pulse pressure.

Total peripheral resistance (systemic vascular resistance). The cardiac output must be studied in relation to the total peripheral resistance, which represents the resistance against which the left ventricle pumps blood. Shock is often followed by vasoconstrictor reflexes, which help conserve blood flow to vital organ systems. The degree of vasoconstriction varies from one vascular bed to another. When the peripheral resistance rises, it increases the work of the heart. This may be deleterious in a patient with cardiogenic shock.

In about one half of patients with acute myocardial infarction, with or without shock, the peripheral resistance is either normal or low. The significance of a normal or low peripheral resistance in cardiogenic shock associated with acute myocardial infarction is not yet understood. It may be due to inhibitory reflexes that originate in the infarcted ventricular muscle or in the thrombosed coronary artery.

At the bedside, it can be assumed that when the skin is cold and *clammy*, the peripheral resistance is high. However, *cold* skin may be present with a normal, low, or high total peripheral resistance.

Circulating blood volume. Since a decreased circulating blood volume may precipitate shock, measurement of the blood volume theoretically is valuable. At the bedside, the circulating blood volume is often inferred from the CVP. However, there is no absolute correlation between these two measurements. For example, a low CVP (less than 5 cm water) is an indirect sign of hypovolemia. However, a high CVP (more than 12 cm water) may or may not indicate hypervolemia and may be due to other factors (see below).

The circulating blood volume in myocardial infarction, with or without cardiogenic shock, may be low, as was mentioned above.

Central venous pressure. The CVP is the pressure in the right atrium or superior vena cava. It is the resultant of numerous factors, including the circulating blood volume, venous tone, volume of the venous return, right ventricular function, and intrathoracic pressure. Since it varies directly with the filling pressure of the right ventricle, it is a major indicator of cardiac output. However, CVP *cannot* be used as an absolute index of either the cardiac output or the circulating blood volume.

Most patients in shock due to acute myocardial infarction show a normal or elevated CVP. Therefore, if a patient with acute myocardial infarction and shock shows a low CVP, the shock may not be due primarily to the myocardial infarction but may be related to some other condition, such as a decreased circulating blood volume due to prolonged vasopressor therapy, loss of extracellular fluids due to severe vomiting, or excessive diuretic therapy.

Since the CVP reflects the right ventricular filling pressure (right ventricular end-diastolic pressure), it will be high when right-sided congestive heart failure is present. However, the CVP may be high when the right ventricular end-diastolic pressure is normal (see below).

The CVP does not accurately reflect left ventricular filling pressure (left ventricular end-diastolic pressure) and cannot be used as a sign of left-sided congestive heart failure. The CVP may be low when left-sided heart failure is present and may be high when it is absent.

The normal range of CVP is approximately 4 to 8 cm water. CVP readings in cm water can be converted to values in mm Hg by dividing the values in cm water by the constant 1.36. Similarly, CVP readings in mm Hg can be converted to cm water by multiplying by the constant 1.36.

In patients with acute myocardial infarction, the following CVP readings can be used as a guide to therapy.

A CVP reading of less than 5 cm water is a sign of hypovolemia, particularly if hypotension is also present. The hypovolemia may be due to previous use of diuretics, overconstriction due to vasoconstrictor drugs, loss of electrolytes from excessive vomiting, loss of water from the lungs due to prolonged respirator therapy, or inadequate fluid replacement.

A CVP greater than 15 to 20 cm water usually indicates right-sided heart failure. However, a high CVP reading can also occur as a result of overconstriction when vasopressor drugs are used for shock. A high CVP can also occur in massive pulmonary embolism or chronic pulmonary disease.

In patients with cardiogenic shock due to acute myocardial infarction, the CVP is usually considerably lower than the left ventricular end-diastolic pressure, whereas in patients with shock due to massive pulmonary embolism, the CVP is elevated and the left ventricular end-diastolic pressure is normal (Cohn).

CVP can be measured in the following way. A Bardic 24-inch radiopaque catheter can be inserted percutaneously through a No. 14 needle into a median basilic (or other peripheral) vein and advanced into the superior vena cava within the thorax. The tip of the catheter must be within the thorax and must lie free in the vein if one is to obtain accurate readings. Accuracy can be determined because the manometer tube will show wide excursions with each breath; it will rise when the patient strains or coughs or when the abdomen is compressed. In addition, to make certain that the catheter is patent, one should be able to aspirate blood freely from it.

With a three-way stopcock the external tip of the catheter is connected to a saline-filled manometer. The zero level should be at the halfway point on the midaxillary line, with the patient supine.

The location of the internal tip of the catheter can be ascertained by recording a unipolar lead ECG, using a catheter with a special metal tip as an exploring electrode (and a well-grounded electrocardiograph) (p. 214). A simpler method of location is to pass an appropriate length of radiopaque catheter into the vein. The position of the catheter tip can then be ascertained by x-ray examination.

Inaccurate CVP readings may occur because of the following.

1. The zero point may be inaccurate.

2. The catheter tip may not be within the thorax.

3. The catheter tip may be in the right ventricular cavity. This will cause large fluctuations of the manometer column with each heartbeat. If this occurs, the catheter should be withdrawn 3 to 5 cm. The wide fluctuations should disappear as the catheter reenters the right atrium.

4. Hyperventilation may give false low readings if the fluid level does not have time to rise to its maximum level between respirations.

5. There may be ball-valve obstruction of the catheter tip, either by a clot or by pressure of the catheter tip against a vein wall. The catheter will respond to the negative intrathoracic pressure during inspiration but will not rise during expiration.

6. If the manometer is connected to an infusion bottle by way of a three-way stopcock, one must be certain that the infusion fluid does not flow into the manometer tubing while the CVP is being measured.

7. When a patient is being ventilated with a positive pressure respirator, the CVP may rise 1 to 2 cm or more. This can be prevented by momentarily disconnecting the respirator while the CVP is measured.

Complications of CVP monitoring. CVP monitoring is necessary in patients with shock. However, the following complications can occur.

Thromboembolic complications may occur if the catheter is inserted into a small tributary vein that is then ligated. It is preferable to place the catheter percutaneously in a large vein, such as the median basilic, subclavian, or internal jugular vein.

Cardiac perforation with pericardial tamponade can be avoided by using a radiopaque catheter with a tip that is not beveled. The location of the catheter tip can be located by x-ray examination. It should be positioned in the superior vena cava, not in the right atrium. In addition, the distal end of the catheter should be securely taped to the skin to prevent movement.

Catheter tip embolism can occur when a catheter that has been inserted through the lumen of a sharp-edged veinpuncture needle is withdrawn while the needle is held firmly in the soft tissues. The sharp edge of the needle may shear the catheter tip. If this happens, the tip will float in the bloodstream and may lodge in the right heart or in one of the pulmonary arteries.

If catheter tip embolism occurs, it may be possible to snare it during cardiac catheterization. Thoracotomy is sometimes necessary. However, the tip can be left in the heart or lung unless the patient develops signs of sepsis from it.

Sepsis can occur at the point of insertion of the catheter into a vein. Sepsis can be avoided by using sterile technic. If sepsis occurs, the catheter should be removed, and the wound area and the catheter tip should be cultured. If continued CVP monitoring is indicated, a new catheter should be inserted at a distant site.

When the subclavian or internal jugular vein is used for CVP monitoring, the following additional complications may occur. *Pneumothorax* is usually not significant and disappears spontaneously. Subcutaneous emphysema, hemothorax, or chylothorax may also occur. If *puncture of the carotid or subclavian artery* occurs, manual compression over the artery for 5 min will stop the bleeding. However, subclavian or jugular vein cannulations have been safely done on patients who were receiving anticoagulants. *Air embolism* can be avoided by placing the patient in Trendelenburg's position during the insertion of the catheter and telling the patient not to breathe deeply. *Brachial plexus injury* has also been reported.

Emergency treatment

Most of the parameters for measuring cardiovascular function in cardiogenic shock cannot be readily measured in the usual hospital setting. However, the following serial measurements should be made in all cases of cardiogenic shock: CVP, blood pressure, and urinary output. In addition, the patient should be observed for clinical signs of shock.

The *first priority* in treating cardiogenic shock is to expand the circulating blood volume with IV fluids, using the CVP as a basic guide (see below). For many years, cardiogenic shock was treated primarily with sympathomimetic amines to raise the blood pressure by means of vasoconstriction. Such treatment has not been generally helpful and is now considered to be secondary to the use of IV fluids.

Initial treatment

1. Position the patient. Place the patient flat in bed. If severe dyspnea or pulmonary edema is present, the patient's head may be slightly elevated. Place Ace bandages from the toes to the groins. Do not put them on too tightly, particularly if the patient has poor arterial pulses in the lower extremities. Raise the lower extremities approximately 15° to return blood into the circulation.

2. Make certain that there is an adequate airway. An unconscious patient should be intubated. Ventilatory support with a volume-cycled respirator may be necessary if the arterial oxygen tension (Pa_{O_2}) falls below 70 mm Hg (see below).

3. Maintain adequate oxygenation. Give the patient 100% oxygen, using a tight-fitting mask at a flow rate of 8 to 15 L/min. A venturi type of mask, with its low flow rate, is generally not effective in raising the Pa_{O_2} in patients in shock.

The goal of the oxygen therapy is to maintain the Pa_{O_2} between 70 and 120 mm Hg (normal Pa_{O_2} is 100 mm Hg.) A tension lower than 70 mm Hg represents dangerous hypoxia. A tension higher than 120 mm Hg is not necessary; and if the Pa_{O_2} rises to 150 mm Hg or higher, oxygen toxicity may develop (p. 158). Fortunately, oxygen toxicity rarely occurs in acute myocardial infarction and shock because venoarterial shunting occurs in the lungs. Therefore, a relatively high concentration of oxygen can be used, if necessary.

If the Pa_{O_2} is less than 70 mm Hg in spite of the use of 100% oxygen by face mask, it may be necessary to intubate the patient and use assisted or controlled respiration with a volume-cycled respirator. Assisted or controlled respiration should be avoided if possible because the positive pressure that the respirator produces may be associated with a further drop in blood pressure and cardiac output.

4. Start an IV infusion with 5% dextrose in water, using a regular drip bulb at a minimal flow rate.

5. Insert a central venous catheter into the superior vena cava by cannulating the median basilic, brachial, internal jugular, or subclavian vein. Attach the catheter to a manometer and to an infusion bottle of 5% dextrose in water, with a three-way stopcock. Keep the IV tubing open with a microdrip bulb.

6. Draw blood for the following tests.

CBC

Serum electrolytes (Na, K, Cl, CO_2 [bicarbonate]), glucose, BUN
Arterial pH, Po_2, Pco_2 (and arterial lactate, if possible)
Serum enzymes (SGOT, LDH, CPK)
Typing and crossmatching of patient

7. Insert a Foley catheter into the urinary bladder to obtain accurate measurements of urinary output. Measure the urinary output every 15 min at first, then every ½ hour.

8. Monitor the patient continuously with an ECG. Get a rhythm strip every 15 min. Set the monitor alarm: upper limit 120 per min; lower limit, 50 per min.

9. Relieve pain. Use meperidine (Demerol)* 75 mg IM as needed every 3 hours. If it causes a decreased blood pressure or respiratory depression, withhold it. Do not give meperidine IV, because it has a vagolytic effect when given this way and may cause a tachycardia. Also, do not use morphine or a similar opiate, such as hydromorphone (Dilaudid), because opiates have a hypotensive effect and may cause a further drop in blood pressure.

10. Relieve agitation. Diphenhydramine hydrochloride (Benadryl) can be given in a dose of 50 mg orally or IM as needed 3 or 4 times a day. Barbiturates or diazepam (Valium) should not be used parenterally in shock, because they have a hypotensive effect.

11. Take portable x-ray films of the chest.

Definitive treatment

Correction of hypovolemia. Correct hypovolemia by expanding the circulating blood volume with IV fluids, using IV fluid tolerance tests, described below, to determine the volume of fluid to be infused. This is the first priority in treating cardiogenic shock.

IV infusions are needed in most cases of cardiogenic shock due to acute myocardial

---

*This and other drugs are described in Part three.

infarction for at least two reasons: (1) a low circulating blood volume, in addition to the acute infarction, may be a major cause of the shock; and (2) it has been found that mild volume overload may be beneficial to patients with acute myocardial infarction because the increased volume of blood that is returned to the infarcted left ventricle allows it to contract more adequately.

Although a single measurement of CVP does not accurately measure the circulating blood volume, serial changes in CVP, in association with changes in blood pressure, and physical signs of pulmonary congestion do correlate with changes in circulating blood volume.

IV fluid tolerance test

1. If the CVP is less than 15 cm water, give the patient an initial test volume of 200 to 300 ml IV fluids in a period of 5 to 10 min. Note the changes in CVP, blood pressure, and auscultatory signs in the lungs.

If the CVP remains unchanged or does not rise more than 2 to 3 cm water above the initial level, and the blood pressure remains stable or rises, and signs of pulmonary congestion do not appear or worsen, give an additional infusion of 200 ml fluid in a period of 10 min.

2. If the CVP continues below 15 cm water, and the blood pressure remains stable or begins to rise, and signs of pulmonary congestion do not appear or worsen, continue the IV infusion at a rate of 500 ml per hour (approximately 125 drops per min, using a regular drip bulb), until the low blood pressure and other clinical signs of shock disappear. Check the CVP, the blood pressure, and the lungs every 15 min.

The type of fluid used for the IV fluid tolerance test depends on the clinical situation. If the patient has an abnormally low CVP and there are also signs suggestive of sodium loss (low serum sodium concentration) due to prior excessive diuretic therapy, prior vasoconstrictor therapy (p. 41), vomiting, diarrhea, and so on, isotonic saline, equal amounts of isotonic saline and 5% dextrose in water, half-isotonic saline, plasma, or low molecular weight dextran (dextran 40) can be used. Otherwise, 5% dextrose in water can be infused.

Large volumes of IV fluids may be needed to reverse the signs of cardiogenic shock. Weil and Shubin have given more than 5 L IV over a period of 8 hours. One of Nixon's patients received 3,800 ml dextrose infusion on day 1, 700 ml plasma on day 2, 1,950 ml IV and oral fluids on day 3, and 2,225 ml oral fluids on day 4.

3. If the initial CVP is between 15 and 20 cm water, the IV fluid challenge should be done with 100 ml fluid during a 10-min period. Further IV fluids will depend on the rise in the CVP, changes in blood pressure, and signs of pulmonary congestion.

4. If the initial CVP is 20 cm water or higher, do not use the IV fluid tolerance test. Instead, start treatment with a vasodilator drug, such as phentolamine (Regitine) (p. 42) or isoproterenol (Isuprel) (p. 41).

A high CVP may occur in the absence of right-sided heart failure if the patient has received a vasoconstrictor drug, such as levarterenol (Levophed), dopamine, or metaraminol (Aramine) for the shock. A seemingly high CVP may occur if the catheter tip becomes lodged in a branch vein, such as the jugular vein. Other causes of a high CVP, such as tricuspid insufficiency, cannon waves occurring in complete AV block, pathological obstruction of the superior vena cava, or chronic pulmonary disease, are not contraindications to the use of IV fluids in cardiogenic shock.

5. A rise in CVP of more than 5 cm above the initial level when the IV fluid tolerance test is done suggests that an inadequate circulating blood volume is not the predominant cause of the shock and that cardiac "pump failure" is the primary problem.

If this happens, stop the infusion. When the CVP falls to its initial level, an additional IV fluid tolerance test can be given. If pulmonary edema develops when IV fluids are given, the patient should be digitalized (p. 44).

6. If the CVP is low (below 5 cm water), IV fluids can be given even when acute pulmonary edema is present in association with cardiogenic shock. Although acute pulmonary edema is usually associated with a high left ventricular end-diastolic pressure, it can occur when the circulating blood volume becomes so low that both the right and left ventricles do not receive an adequate volume of blood. The end-diastolic pressure in both the right and left ventricle is low, but the right ventricle continues to pump blood into the lungs, whereas the weakened left ventricle is unable to expel the small volume of blood it receives. The result is acute pulmonary edema. These patients characteristically show a low CVP (in addition to a low left ventricular end-diastolic pressure) in spite of the pulmonary edema and can respond most dramatically to IV fluids.

The pulmonary artery end-diastolic pressure or the pulmonary wedge pressure can also be used to monitor the IV fluid tolerance test because these measurements indicate changes in cardiovascular function better than CVP measurements (p. 46).

Regardless of what measurements are being used to monitor the treatment of a patient in cardiogenic shock (or of any patient), the physician must always be ready to modify treatment on the basis of the patient's clinical condition.

Therefore, if a patient in shock shows pulmonary edema and a low CVP (or a low pulmonary wedge pressure) and if treatment with IV fluids increases pulmonary congestion and worsens the patient's clinical condition, the IV fluids should be stopped until further measurements can be made and the patient's condition reevaluated.

Treatment of arrhythmias. If a tachyarrhythmia is present in a patient with cardiogenic shock, the tachyarrhythmia must be *immediately* stopped and sinus rhythm restored because the rapid heart rate decreases the cardiac output so much that it perpetuates the shock. If cardiogenic shock is associated with a bradyarrhythmia, the slow heart rate (below 50 per min) may also decrease the cardiac output so much that the shock persists until the heart rate becomes faster. The treatment of arrhythmias associated with acute myocardial infarction is described in Chapter 10.

Treatment of hypotension with sympathomimetic drugs. If the IV fluid challenge test has been done and the patient does not respond with a rise in blood pressure or with decreasing signs of shock within 1 hour, or if the patient's condition worsens, an attempt should be made to raise the blood pressure by use of sympathomimetic drugs. Briefly, sympathomimetic drugs can have five types of action on the cardiovascular system, depending on whether they stimulate or block the alpha or beta adrenergic receptors.

1. Alpha adrenergic receptor stimulation causes vasoconstriction and a rise in blood pressure.
2. Beta adrenergic receptor stimulation has two effects: vasodilatation (and a drop in blood pressure) and a positive inotropic effect on heart muscle, causing an increased strength of cardiac contraction.
3. Alpha adrenergic receptor blocking causes vasodilatation and a fall in blood pressure.
4. Beta adrenergic receptor blocking has a negative inotropic effect on heart muscle. (Drugs that have this effect are not used in the treatment of cardiogenic shock and should be avoided in the treatment of tachyarrhythmias associated with cardiogenic shock.)
5. Sympathomimetic drugs may also have cardiovascular actions that are not related to their effects on alpha and beta adrenergic receptors. In addition, a sympathomimetic drug, such as levarterenol or metaraminol, can have both alpha and beta adrenergic effects.

The following sympathomimetic drugs have been used in the treatment of cardiogenic shock.

1. Alpha adrenergic stimulating drugs
2. Alpha and beta adrenergic stimulating drugs
3. Beta adrenergic stimulating drugs
4. Alpha adrenergic blocking drugs
5. Drug combinations showing alpha and beta adrenergic stimulation, with alpha adrenergic blockage

Alpha adrenergic stimulating drugs. In the past, alpha adrenergic stimulating drugs, such as methoxamine (Vasoxyl) and angiotensin II, were recommended for the treatment of cardiogenic shock because it was incorrectly assumed that the primary disturbance in shock was the decreased blood pressure. These drugs have little or no direct effect on the heart. They are *no longer recommended* for the treatment of cardiogenic shock.

Alpha and beta adrenergic stimulating drugs. Alpha and beta adrenergic stimulating drugs, such as levarterenol, metaraminol, which is similar to levarterenol because it liberates norepinephrine from nerve endings, and dopamine, have a twofold effect: they stimulate the beta adrenergic receptors of the heart muscle and in this way have a positive inotropic effect, increasing the cardiac output; and they stimulate the alpha adrenergic receptors of the peripheral blood vessels and cause vasoconstriction and in this way cause the peripheral resistance and the blood pressure to rise. When they are given in moderate doses, their beta adrenergic effect on the heart muscle is greater than their vasoconstrictor effect. However, when they are given in large doses, the arterial vasoconstriction predominates, and the blood pressure and cardiac output may fall. When they are used to raise the systolic blood pressure to a level approximately 30 to 40 mm Hg less than the patient's usual blood pressure (a systolic blood pressure between 90 and 100 mm Hg), a maximal cardiac output with minimal increase in vasoconstriction is achieved.

Levarterenol or metaraminol should be used for the shortest time possible because the intense vasoconstriction that each causes is associated with capillary stasis and the transudation of fluid from the vascular system to the tissue spaces. When these conditions develop, the patient becomes unresponsive to the drug, the shock worsens, and the patient may die. (These conditions can be partly prevented if one gives levarterenol in dextrose in isotonic saline, rather than in dextrose in water, or if one gives metaraminol in dextrose and isotonic saline or in isotonic saline, rather than in dextrose in water.) If shock worsens because of excessive vasoconstriction produced by either of these drugs, the patient should receive plasma, isotonic saline, or dextran 40.

The action of levarterenol begins immediately and lasts about 2 min after the infusion is stopped. When metaraminol is given IV, its effect does not become manifest for several minutes and may last for 20 or more min after the infusion has been stopped. When catecholamine stores are depleted, as in patients previously treated with reserpine or guanethidine, metaraminol may not be very effective, whereas levarterenol will still be effective. However, if levarterenol infiltrates the skin, a slough may occur. This condition is rare with metaraminol.

Dopamine is the immediate biochemical precursor of norepinephrine (levarterenol) and has similar properties. However, unlike levarterenol, it produces active dilatation of the renal and mesenteric arteries. This decreases the peripheral resistance and helps prevent inadequate tissue perfusion through the important splanchnic organ systems. However, clinical studies have not yet indicated that dopamine has any significant advantages over levarterenol or metaraminol. It is still not available for general use.

Beta adrenergic stimulating drugs. Isoproterenol (Isuprel) is a pure beta adrenergic stimulator. By stimulating the beta adrenergic receptors of the heart it produces a positive inotropic effect (increased strength of cardiac contractions) and an increased chronotropic effect (increased heart rate). It also stimulates the beta adrenergic repectors of the peripheral vessels and causes peripheral vasodilatation, increased peripheral blood flow, and a decreased blood pressure. Therefore, when isoproterenol is used, the circulating blood volume should be increased by IV fluids, given either immediately before the isoproterenol infusion is started or simultaneously with it to prevent the circulating blood volume from falling excessively when the isoproterenol becomes effective. Otherwise, hypotension and shock will worsen.

The exact indications for isoproterenol in treatment of cardiogenic shock associated with acute myocardial infarction have not been clearly defined. It has been used in patients who have excessive vasoconstriction and an elevated total peripheral resistance, often due to prior treatment with drugs such as levarterenol, metaraminol, or dopamine. It may also be valuable when a patient with cardiogenic shock shows an abnormally high CVP. It should not be used if the CVP is abnormally low.

The increased peripheral blood flow produced by isoproterenol increases the oxygen needs of the heart. This may not be compensated by the increased coronary artery flow that occurs. As a result, the work of the heart may adversely increase. This is one of the reasons that isoproterenol is not routinely used in treating cardiogenic shock associated with acute myocardial infarction.

Epinephrine (Adrenalin) is similar to isoproterenol in many ways. It has a beta adrenergic effect on the heart, increasing the force of cardiac contraction, increasing the heart rate, and increasing the cardiac output. However, it also has an alpha adrenergic effect on the renal arterioles and causes marked vasoconstriction and decreased renal blood flow. It dilates the coronary arteries but increases the work of the heart disproportionately. For this reason, it is not generally used in treating cardiogenic shock. However, Nixon has suggested that when a patient in cardiogenic shock does not respond to one or two IV fluid challenges, a solution of 1 ml of 1/1,000 epinephrine dissolved in 500 ml 5% dextrose in water can be given slowly to raise the blood pressure.

Mephentermine (Wyamine) is also similar to isoproterenol because it has a positive inotropic effect on the heart and causes a mild vasodilatation. However, large doses cause vasoconstriction. In addition, prolonged administration leads to a state of myocardial refractoriness, possibly due to depletion of norepinephrine stores in the heart. It also causes side effects such as drowsiness, weeping, incoherence, and generalized convulsions. Therefore, it is not recommended for treating cardiogenic shock.

Alpha adrenergic blocking drugs. Excessive vasoconstriction may occur with shock and may be detrimental because it prevents adequate perfusion of vital organs such as the kidneys and liver. Similarly, the vasoconstriction produced by a drug such as levarterenol or metaraminol can aggravate the shock by decreasing the circulating blood volume. (The vasoconstriction that occurs is associated with tissue hypoxia and increased capillary permeability. As a result, plasma passes out of the vascular system into the extracellular spaces.) In the past, phenoxybenzamine (Dibenzyline) has been used experimentally to counteract this excessive vasoconstriction. However, it is no longer available. Phentolamine (Regitine), another alpha adrenergic blocking drug, is available. It not only counteracts excessive vasoconstriction but is particularly valuable when cardiogenic shock is associated with a high CVP (20 mm water or higher). Fifty mg (10 ml) phentolamine can be dissolved in 40 ml 5% dextrose in water and given in a Soluset at a rate of 0.5 to 2.0 mg per min. (Since each 1 ml of this dilution contains 1 mg, the rate of flow will be 0.5 to 2 ml per min.) Phentolamine has a rapid onset of action (2 to 5 min) and is also short acting (approximately 20 min).

The patient should be treated for an initial period of 20 to 30 min, with constant monitoring of the CVP. Additional IV fluids may be necessary when the CVP falls below 15 cm water, due to the vasodilating effect of the phentolamine. If improvement occurs (warming and drying of the skin, and so on), the phentolamine infusion can be stopped or continued as necessary. If shock worsens as a result of the phentolamine, levarterenol or metaraminol can be substituted for the phentolamine or can be given in conjunction with it (see below).

Drug combinations showing alpha and beta adrenergic stimulation, with alpha adrenergic blockage. The purpose of such drug combinations in the treatment of cardiogenic shock is to provide a beta adrenergic stimulating effect on heart muscle and to avoid excessive vasoconstriction due to alpha adrenergic stimulation of the peripheral arterioles. Several such combinations have been used.

1. Levarterenol and phentolamine. Various amounts of each drug can be used. From 0.5 to 2.0 mg phentolamine per min can be infused with 4 to 32 μg levarterenol bitartrate per min. (When 1 ampul of levarterenol bitartrate is dissolved in 1 L of fluid, each 1 ml of this dilution contains 8 μg levarterenol bitartrate [equivalent to 4 μg levarterenol base].)

2. Metaraminol and phentolamine. Various amounts of each drug can be used. From 0.5 to 2.0 mg phentolamine per min can be infused with 0.1 to 2.0 mg metaraminol per min. (When 50 mg metaraminol are dissolved in 500 ml fluid, each 1 ml of this dilution contains 0.1 mg metaraminol. When 100 mg metaraminol are dissolved in 100 ml fluid, each 1 ml of this dilution contains 1.0 mg metaraminol.)

When either levarterenol or metaraminol is given simultaneously with phentolamine, each drug should be given from individual infusion bottles connected to a Y tube so that variations in the dosage of each drug can be easily obtained.

Treatment of metabolic acidosis. Metabolic acidosis due to hypoxia and stagnation of blood flow is a common complication of shock. It should be treated with sodium bicarbonate given IV. The simplest way is to use ampuls of concentrated (7.5%) sodium bicarbonate. Each 50-ml ampul contains 44.6 mEq bicarbonate ions. The contents of an ampul can be injected directly into the infusion tubing. Although the amount of sodium bicarbonate needed is described in Part three, a patient may require less (or more) than usual. In addition, the bicarbonate level should be raised to approximately 20 mEq/L, but *not* to a normal value of 27 mEq/L. The rationale for this is discussed in Part three. The pH can also be used as a guide to sodium bicarbonate therapy. The pH should be raised above 7.30.

Treatment of electrolyte disturbances. Electrolyte disturbances, particularly hyponatremia, must be corrected. Hyponatremia may develop in many ways after acute myocardial infarction. Patients with acute myocardial infarction are often placed on a low-sodium diet; they are often too ill to eat adequately. Instead, they imbibe water, ginger ale, and other low-sodium liquids. The stress of the acute infarction is associated with an excessive secretion of ADH, the antidiuretic hormone of the posterior pituitary gland, which causes a retention of water in the body. If rales are present, the patient is often given a mercurial or another diuretic, which causes a further loss of sodium ions. Patients with acute myocardial infarction routinely have a vein kept open with an IV drip. If a microdrip bulb is not used and if the rate of flow is not kept minimal, the patient may receive more than 1 L daily of dextrose in water (the usual solution used).

The sodium loss and water excess produced in these ways can be further complicated if the patient develops shock and is given levarterenol or metaraminol in dextrose in water. This not only lowers the serum sodium concentration still further, but the vasoconstriction produced by either of these drugs is associated with excessive transudation of fluid from the vascular system into the extracellular spaces, so that the circulating blood volume falls. Since the osmotic pressure of the extracellular fluids is mainly dependent on the serum sodium concentration, a loss of sodium ions from the extracellular fluid spaces or dilution of the extracellular fluid with water will decrease the extracellular osmotic pressure. When the extracellular osmotic pressure is decreased, water passes out of the vascular system and out of the extracellular fluid spaces and into the cells. As a result, the osmotic pressure of the extracellular spaces rises, the osmotic pressure of the cells falls, and osmotic equilibrium occurs. However, when water passes out of the vascular system and into the cells, the circulating blood volume necessarily decreases, and the blood pressure and the cardiac output also fall still further.

If hyponatremia is present, the following treatment can be given.

1. If levarterenol is used, it should be given in dextrose in isotonic saline, rather than in dextrose in water. If metaraminol is used, it should be given in dextrose in isotonic saline or in isotonic saline, rather than in dextrose in water.

2. If IV fluids are needed, plasma, isotonic saline, or dextran 40, rather than dextrose in water, should be infused.

Other treatment

Digitalis. Digitalis is not helpful in cardiogenic shock unless acute pulmonary edema or right-sided heart failure with a CVP of 20 cm water or higher is present. (One must be certain that a high CVP has not been produced by the vasopressor drugs used for shock.)

Diuretics. Furosemide (Lasix) or ethacrynic acid (Edecrin) given IV has been used in patients with cardiogenic shock and acute pulmonary edema. However, diuretics are not effective, because an inadequate renal blood flow is present. But if the renal blood flow and urinary output improve, either as a result of increased cardiac output due to IV fluids or as a result of the use of levarterenol or metaraminol, phentolamine, or isoproterenol, the diuretics will become effective.

Diuretics may also not be effective, because the patient is in a sodium-depleted state because of previous diuretic therapy or any other mechanism.

Glucagon has been used experimentally in the treatment of cardiogenic shock associated with acute myocardial infarction because it has a positive inotropic effect that is not related to stimulation of beta adrenergic receptors. It has been used either as a 3- to 5-mg bolus IV or as an IV drip (dissolved in 5% dextrose in water) at a rate of 1 to 4 mg per hour. However, its effects have been inconstant and generally poor. In addition, it produces nausea and vomiting when given in adequate doses.

Corticosteroids. There is no definite evidence that large doses of parenterally administered corticosteroids are helpful in cardiogenic shock associated with acute myocardial infarction. However, they are excellent vasodilators and have been used successfully in noncoronary cardiogenic shock (see below).

Mechanical circulatory assist. When the usual medical methods of treating cardiogenic shock fail, mechanical assistance of the heart may be attempted with the use of, for example, an intra-aortic balloon or a venoarterial-phased partial bypass, in conjunction with all the other methods of treating the shock. Discussion of this is beyond the scope of this book.

TREATMENT OF CARDIOGENIC SHOCK ASSOCIATED WITH ACUTE PULMONARY EDEMA

The development of acute pulmonary edema is one of the most disheartening complications of shock. These patients usually die regardless of treatment. However, the condition is not hopeless, and the following treatment can be given.

1. Immediately digitalize the patient with a rapid-acting digitalis preparation such as digoxin (Lanoxin), deslanoside (Cedilanid-D), or ouabain, regardless of the other treatment used for the shock.

2. Do not keep the patient in a supine position; moderately prop the patient up.

3. Check the CVP. If it is low, give IV fluids in spite of the pulmonary edema (p. 39).

4. If the CVP is abnormally high (more than 20 cm water), a vasodilator, such as phentolamine or isoproterenol, can be given IV. As soon as the patient shows signs of clinical improvement, give additional IV fluids to maintain the CVP at approximately 15 cm water.

5. Do not perform a phlebotomy, because it will decrease the circulating blood volume still further.

6. Artificial ventilation, with a *volume-cycled* respirator such as the Bennett, Emerson, or Engström, may be helpful in such patients, particularly if respirations are shallow and if the arterial oxygen saturation is less than 70 mm Hg. However, prolonged artificial ventilation may result in a further decrease in cardiac output because the increased intrathoracic positive pressure produced even with a volume-cycled respirator decreases the venous return to the heart and therefore decreases the blood pressure and the cardiac output. (In addition, prolonged mechanical ventilation may produce water retention and dilutional hyponatremia, possibly due to posterior pituitary ADH secretion. This further complicates treatment.)

A *pressure-cycled* respirator should *not* be used in these patients, because the increased positive intrathoracic pressure it produces will decrease the venous return, the blood pressure, and the cardiac output more than a volume-cycled respirator.

TREATMENT OF CARDIOGENIC NONCORONARY SHOCK

Cardiogenic noncoronary shock is observed most frequently after open-heart surgery. It can also occur as a result of massive pulmonary embolism (Chapter 11), acute cardiac tamponade (Chapter 14), and after cardiac arrest (profound cardiovascular collapse, Chapter 2). In this section, the treatment of cardiogenic noncoronary shock associated with open heart surgery is discussed.

Treatment is generally similar to the treatment of cardiogenic shock associated with acute myocardial infarction. Since patients with cardiogenic noncoronary shock after open-heart surgery generally have heart failure and a high peripheral resistance, they respond to digitalis, IV fluids, and vasodilating drugs used in association with the IV fluids.

Digitalis. The patient should be digitalized IV with a rapid-acting digitalis preparation, such as digoxin, deslanoside, or ouabain. If the patient has been digitalized prior to the open-heart surgery, less than digitalizing doses may be needed.

IV fluids. Whole blood, plasma, dextran 40, or isotonic saline can be used. The amount of IV fluids can be determined by the IV fluid tolerance test, as described above for shock associated with acute myocardial infarction. However, in these patients, it is not necessary to raise the CVP to 15 cm water.

Vasodilating drugs. Several drugs have been used for this purpose; for example, massive doses of corticosteroids given IV, isoproterenol, chlorpromazine (Thorazine), or phentolamine.

Corticosteroids. Lillihei and his associates have used a single massive dose of prednisolone or dexamethasone given IV simultaneously with IV fluid replacement. The drug is given in a single IV bolus over a 3- to 5-min period. Vasodilation follows in 2 to 4 hours.

MEASUREMENT OF ABNORMAL PHYSIOLOGICAL PARAMETERS OCCURRING IN CARDIOGENIC SHOCK
Intra-arterial blood pressure

Intra-arterial blood pressure can be obtained with the use of polyethylene PE 160 or No. 7 Teflon indwelling catheter directed retrograde from the brachial or femoral artery to the central aorta. It is positioned by length rather than by guidance under fluoroscopic control. The artery can be entered percutaneously or by cutdown. The intra-arterial blood pressure can then be measured with a Statham db transducer and recorded on a multichannel recorder. The normal mean intra-arterial blood pressure in the central aorta varies from 74 to 108 mm Hg.

Cardiac output

Cardiac output is usually measured by the dye dilution method, with indocyanine green as an indicator. The indocyanine green is injected into the right atrium or pulmonary artery and sampled from the aorta or a peripheral artery near the aorta. A cuvette and densimeter are used to obtain the indicator dilution curves, which can be inscribed on an oscillographic recorder and then analyzed.

One of the disadvantages of this method is that when the cardiac output is low, recirculation of the dye through the heart may cause differences of as much as 25% in successive cardiac output values due to technical reasons rather than to changes in cardiac output. Radioactive indicators and precordial counting have also been used to measure cardiac output. However, large technical errors also occur. Unfortunately, the classic Fick method is impractical for seriously ill patients with myocardial infarction.

Recently, cardiac output has been measured with thermal indicators. Saline at room temperature is injected into the subclavian vein, and temperature changes in the pulmonary artery are recorded by a thermistor. (The thermistor is incorporated in a No. 5 French balloon double lumen vinyl catheter, which is introduced either percutaneously or by way of a peripheral vein cutdown and then advanced into the pulmonary artery.)

The normal range of the cardiac output is 4.0 to 8.0 L/min.

Cardiac index

The cardiac index can also be measured. It is the cardiac output divided by the body surface area. It is expressed as liters per minute per square meter. The normal cardiac index is 2.4 to 4.0 L/min/m².

Total peripheral resistance (systemic vascular resistance)

The resistance to blood flow cannot be measured directly. It is actually a theoretic value because resistance (r) is defined as the ratio between mean arterial blood pressure (p) and cardiac output (blood flow, f): $r = p/f$. Therefore, the numerical value for peripheral resistance is only as significant as the accuracy of the measurements of the intra-arterial blood pressure and the cardiac output. In addition, the term total peripheral resistance is misleading because it incorrectly implies that there is a uniform resistance throughout the body. This does not occur. For example, there may be large differences in constriction of the arteries in various organs. Some arteries, such as the renal arteries, may be very constricted, and other arteries, such as the cerebral and coronary arteries, may be dilated.

Total peripheral resistance (TPR) is calculated from the formula:

$$TPR = \frac{BP \ (mm \ Hg) \ - \ CVP \ (mm \ Hg)}{CO \ (L/min)}$$

where BP is the mean intra-arterial blood pressure, CVP the central venous pressure, and CO the cardiac output in liters per minute. Total peripheral resistance is expressed as pressure (mm Hg) and flow (L/min) units: mm Hg/L/min. If the cardiac index is substituted for the cardiac output, the body area (in square meters) is included: mm Hg/L/min/m².

Total peripheral resistance is also sometimes expressed as a *force per unit area;* namely, as dynes sec. cm⁻⁵. But this has no additional meaning and is simply 80 times the value in mm Hg/L/min. (The derivation of these formulas is described in the textbook of Yang and his associates.)

The normal range of the total peripheral resistance is: 116 to 225 mm Hg/L/min, or 900 to 1,800 dynes sec. cm⁻⁵.

Circulating blood volume

Circulating blood volume can be measured by injecting a known amount of a tracer such as iodinated I 131 serum albumin (RISA) or a dye such as Evans blue T 1824, waiting 10 to 20 min for mixing to take place, and then measuring the concentration of the tracer per unit volume of blood to obtain the blood volume. Tagged red blood cells can also be used.

However, when shock is present, the mixing time of the tracer is prolonged, and incorrect values are obtained. In addition, clinical observations of patients in shock have shown that the patient may need a much greater volume of fluid than the blood volume determination indicates.

Left ventricular function

Left ventricular function can be determined by puncturing the femoral artery percutaneously, passing a catheter retrograde into the left ventricular cavity, and measuring the left ventricular end-diastolic pressure, which will be elevated if left-sided heart failure is present. The normal left ventricular end-diastolic pressure is 5 to 12 mm Hg. It is measured at a point immediately preceding the rapid upstroke of the left ventricular pressure, which occurs 0.04 to 0.06 sec after the beginning of the QRS complex.

The presence of cardiogenic shock along with a left ventricular end-diastolic pressure of less than 12 mm Hg indicates that the circulating blood volume should be expanded. IV fluids can be given until the pressure rises to 18 to 20 mm Hg.

Pulmonary artery end-diastolic pressure and pulmonary wedge pressure

Measurement of the left ventricular end-diastolic pressure may be dangerous and may precipitate ventricular tachyarrhythmias. However, the left ventricular end-diastolic pressure can be determined indirectly by measuring the pulmonary artery end-diastolic pressure or the pulmonary wedge pressure, because it has been shown that if acute hypoxia and acidosis have been corrected and if acute pulmonary embolism, chronic pulmonary disease, or mitral valve disease is absent, the pulmonary artery end-diastolic pressure is similar to the left ventricular end-diastolic pressure.

Pulmonary artery end-diastolic pressure measurements can be easily made at the bedside by several technics; for example, using the Swan Ganz balloon catheter. A No. 6 Swan Ganz flow-directed balloon-tipped catheter can be inserted into a peripheral vein, either by cutdown or percutaneously, and the balloon tip can be inflated with air or carbon dioxide. The catheter is at first propelled by the bloodstream and is then advanced into the superior vena cava, right atrium, right ventricle, and into the pulmonary artery. Ventricular premature contractions often develop during the few seconds that the catheter tip is moving through the right ventricle, but ventricular tachycardia or ventricular fibrillation have not been reported. (However, resuscitative supplies and equipment should be immediately available.)

The insertion of the catheter does not require fluroscopy. Its position is determined by monitoring the intracardiac pressures via a transducer on a multichannel pen recorder. The zero reference point is 5 cm below the sternal angle. In most patients, the catheter can be wedged into one of the smaller pulmonary arteries, which is briefly occluded by inflation of the balloon at the tip of the catheter.

The pulmonary wedge pressure equals left atrial pressure (if mitral disease is absent) and is therefor a sensitive indicator of the presence of pulmonary congestion and left-sided congestive heart failure. The normal upper limit of the pulmonary wedge pressure is 12 mm Hg. Pulmonary congestion rarely occurs when the pulmonary wedge pressure is lower than 18 mm Hg. A pulmonary wedge pressure below 10 mm Hg in the presence of hypotension suggests that the hypotension or shock is due to an inadequate circulating blood volume.

Pulmonary wedge pressures are more significant than CVP measurements, particularly when cardiogenic shock is associated with pulmonary congestion, because a low pulmonary wedge pressure definitely indicates that IV fluids should be given, despite the pulmonary congestion.

One of the difficulties in using the Swan Ganz balloon is that it requires special apparatus. Complications with the procedure so far have been few —knotting of the catheter and one case of possible perforation of one of the pulmonary artery branches, in addition to the ventricular premature contractions, mentioned above.

Even in those patients where the catheter does not float into the wedge position, the pulmonary artery end-diastolic pressure can be measured (normal range 4 to 13 mm Hg, with a mean value of 9 mm Hg). This is also an index of mean left atrial and left ventricular end-diastolic pressure.

The pulmonary artery end-diastolic pressure has been found to be abnormally high in about 50% of patients with acute myocardial infarction, with or without shock.

The presence of cardiogenic shock and a pulmonary artery end-diastolic pressure greater than 15 mm Hg are generally signs that the left ventricular end-diastolic pressure is elevated (and that left-sided congestive heart failure is present). Conversely, a pulmonary artery end-diastolic pressure less than 10 mm Hg is associated with a normal left ventricular end-diastolic pressure (Scheinman and associates, 1973). This indicates that the circulating blood volume should be expanded.

When shock is present and the pulmonary artery end-diastolic pressure or the pulmonary wedge pressure is used as a guide to IV fluid therapy, the fluid can be given in a volume of 100 ml in 10 min. If the pulmonary artery end-diastolic pressure or the pulmonary artery wedge pressure does not rise more than 2 mm Hg, the IV fluid challenge should be continued until the pulmonary artery end-diastolic or wedge pressure reaches 15 or 16 mm Hg.

Right ventricular function

If right-sided heart failure is present, the right ventricular end-diastolic pressure will rise (normal range 1 to 7 mm Hg, mean value 4 mm Hg). This will also cause a rise in right atrial pressure (normal range 1 to 5 mm Hg, mean value 2.8 mm Hg) and a rise in CVP. However, as was previously pointed out, the CVP may be elevated independently, even if right-sided heart failure is not present.

REFERENCES

Allen HM, Danzig R, Swan HJC: Incidence and significance of relative hypovolemia as a cause of shock associated with acute myocardial infarction, Circulation 36 (Suppl 2):11, 1967.

Amsterdam EA, et al: Comparison of glucagon and catecholamines in congestive heart failure and coronary shock, Circulation 42 (Suppl 3):82, 1970.

Ayres SM, Mueller H, et al: The lung in shock; alveolar-capillary gas exchange in the shock syndrome, Am J Cardiol 26:588, 1970.

Botticelli JT, Tsagaris TJ, Lange RL: Mechanism of pressor amine dependence, Am J Cardiol 16 847, 1965.

Bradley EC, Wein MH: Vasodepressor and vasodilator drugs in the treatment of shock, Mod Treat 11:243, 1967.

Brinkman AJ, Costley DO: Internal jugular venipuncture, JAMA 223:182, 1973.

Cabulla OS, Jung RC, Aaronson J: Bedside percutaneous right heart catheterization, Letter, JAMA 220:1618, 1972.

Cohn JN: Central venous pressure as a guide to volume expansion, Ann Intern Med 66:1283, 1967.

Cohn, JN, Khatri IM, Hamosh P: Bedside catheterization of the left ventricle, Am J Cardiol 25:66, 1970.

Cohn JN, Luria MH, Daddario RC, et al: Studies in clinical shock and hypotension. V. Hemodynamic effects of dextran, Circulation 35:316, 1967.

Collins JV, Clark TJH, et al: Central venous pressure in acute myocardial infarction, Lancet 1:373, 1971.

Corday E, et al: Reevaluation of the treatment of shock secondary to cardiac infarction, Dis Chest 56:200, 1969.

Corday E, Swan HJC, et al: Physiologic principles in the application of circulatory assist for the failing heart; intraaortic balloon circulatory assist and venoarterial phased partial bypass, Am J Cardiol 26:595, 1970.

Dietzman RH, Lillihei RC: The treatment of cardiogenic shock. V. The use of corticosteroids in the treatment of cardiogenic shock, Am Heart J 75:274, 1968.

Ellis RJ, Gold J, et al: Computerized monitoring of cardiac output by thermal dilution, JAMA 220: 507, 1972.

Fishman AP: Shock lung; a distinctive entity, Circulation 47:921, 1973.

Forrester JS, Diamond GA, Swan HJC: Bedside diagnosis of latent cardiac complications in acutely ill patients, JAMA 222:59, 1972.

Goetz RH, Bregman D, Esrig B, Laniado S: Unidirectional intraaortic balloon pumping in cardiogenic shock and intractable left ventricular failure, Am J Cardiol 29:213, 1972.

Goldberg LI: Cardiovascular and renal actions of dopamine, Pharmacol Rev 24:1, 1972.

Goldberger E: A primer of water, electrolyte and acid base syndromes, ed 4, Philadelphia, 1971, Lea & Febiger.

Gunnar RM, Loeb HS: Use of drugs in cardiogenic shock due to acute myocardial infarction, Circulation 45:1111, 1972.

Gunnar RM, Loeb HS, Pietras RJ, Tobin JR: Hemodynamic measurements in a coronary care unit, Prog Cardiovasc Dis 11:29, 1968.

Herbert WH: Limitations of pulmonary artery end-diastolic pressure as the reflection of left ventricular end-diastolic pressure, N Y State J Med 72:229, 1972.

Homesley HD, Zelenik JS: Hazards of central venous pressure monitoring; pericardial tamponade, Am Heart J 84:135, 1972.

Khalil KG, et al: Thoracic duct injury; a complication of jugular vein catheterization, JAMA 221:908, 1972.

Levine ER: Oxygen therapy dosages and techniques, GP 26:129, 1962.

Lillehei RC: Pressor agents in cardiogenic shock, Am J Cardiol 23:903, 1969.

Loeb HS, Pietras RJ, et al: Hemodynamic responses to chlorpromazine in patients in shock, Arch Intern Med 124:354, 1969.

Loeb HS, Pietras RJ, et al: Hypovolemia in shock due to acute myocardial infarction, Circulation 40:653, 1969.

Luz P, Weil MH, et al: Response to phentolamine in patients in shock, Circulation 45,46 (Suppl, 2): 11, 1972.

MacCannell KL, Moran NC: Pharmacological basis for the use of adrenergic agonists and antagonists in cardiogenic shock and hypotension, Prog Cardiovasc Dis 10:55, 1967.

Mackensie GJ, et al: Circulatory and respiratory studies in myocardial infarction and cardiogenic shock, Lancet 2:825, 1964.

Mason DT, et al: Cardiogenic shock in acute myocardial infarction. In Eliot RS, editor: The acute cardiac emergency, Mount Kisco, N Y, 1972 Futura Publishing Co., Inc.

Morrison J, Killip T: Serial serum digitalis levels in patients with acute myocardial infarction, Clin Res 19:353, 1971.

Mueller HS, Ayres SM, Gregory JJ, Giannelli S Jr, Grace WJ: The evaluation and treatment of cardiogenic shock, Med Times 98:137, 1970.

Mueller HS, Ayres SM, et al: Effect of isoproterenol, l-norepinephrine, and intraaortic counterpulsation on hemodynamics and myocardial metabolism in shock following acute myocardial infarction, Circulation 45:335, 1972.

Nixon PGF: Pulmonary oedema with low left ventricular diastolic pressure in acute myocardial infarction, Lancet 2:146, 1968.

Nixon PGF, Ikram H, Morton S: Cardiogenic shock treated with dextrose solution, Am Heart J 73:843, 1967.

Nixon PGF, Taylor DJE, Morton SD: Left ventricular diastolic pressure in cardiogenic shock treated by dextrose infusion and adrenaline, Lancet 1:1280, 1968.

Page DL, et al: Myocardial changes associated with cardiogenic shock, N Engl J Med 285:133, 1971.

Parmley, WW, Diamond G, et al: Clinical evaluation of left ventricular pressures in myocardial infarction, Circulation 45:358, 1972.

Parmley WW, Sonnenblick EH: Glucagon; new agent in cardiac therapy, Am J Cardiol 27:298, 1971.

Perlroth MG, Harrison DC: Cardiogenic shock; a review, Clin Pharmacol Ther 10:449, 1969.

Porter CM, Karp RB, et al: Pulmonary artery pressure monitoring in cardiogenic shock, Arch Intern Med 127:304, 1971.

Rackley CE, Russell RO Jr: Left ventricular function in acute myocardial infarction and its clinical significance, Circulation 45:231, 1972.

Rapaport E, Scheinman M: Rationale and limitations of hemodynamic measurements in patients with acute myocardial infarction, Mod Concepts Cardiovasc Dis 38:55, 1969.

Ratshin RA, Rackley CE, Russell RO Jr: Hemodynamic evaluation of left ventricular function in shock complicating myocardial infarction, Circulation 45:127, 1972.

Sanders CA, et al: Mechanical circulatory assistance; current status and experience with combining circulatory assistance, emergency coronary arteriography, and acute myocardial revascularization, Circulation 45:1292, 1972.

Scheidt S, Ascheim R, Killip T III: Shock after acute myocardial infarction; a clinical and hemodynamic profile, Am J Cardiol 26:556, 1970.

Scheidt S, et al: Intraaortic balloon counterpulsation in cardiogenic shock; report of a co-operative clinical trial, N Engl J Med 288:979, 1973.

Scheinman MM, et al: Simplified direct Fick techniques for measurement of cardiac output in seriously ill patients, Am Heart J 83:61, 1972.

Scheinman MM, et al: Relationship between pulmonary artery end–diastolic pressure and left ventricular filling pressure in patients in shock, Circulation 47:317, 1973.

Shillingford JP, Thomas M: Acute myocardial infarction, hypotension and shock; their pathological physiology and therapy, Mod Concepts Cardiovas Dis 36:13, 1967.

Shoemaker WC, Brown RS: The dilemma of vasopressors and vasodilators in the therapy of shock, Surg Gynecol Obstet 132:51, 1971.

Shubin H, Weil MH: Practical considerations in the management of shock complicating acute myocardial infarction; a summary of current practice, Am J Cardiol **26**:603, 1970.

Sladen A, Laver MD, Pontoppidan H: Pulmonary complications and water retention in prolonged mechanical ventilation, N Engl J Med **279**:448, 1968.

Swan, HJC, Danzig R, et al: Current status of treatment of power failure of the heart in acute myocardial infarction with drugs and blood volume replacement, Circulation **39,40** (Suppl 4):277, 1969.

Swan HJC, et al: Hemodynamic spectrum of myocardial infarction and cardiogenic shock; a conceptual model, Circulation **45**:1097, 1972.

Tahir AH: Prevention of air embolism during subclavian venipuncture, Letter, JAMA **223**:79, 1973.

Thomas M, Malmcrona R, Shillingford, J: Haemodynamic effects of morphine in patients with acute myocardial infarction, Br Heart J **27**:863, 1965.

Thomas TV: Location of catheter tip and its impact on central venous pressure, Chest **61**:668, 1972.

Walters MB, et al: Complications with percutaneous central venous catheters, JAMA **220**:1455, 1972.

Weil MH, Shubin H: Symposium on shock and syncope, Am J Cardiol **26**:553, 1970.

Weil MH, Shubin H: Cardiogenic shock; medical management, Cardiovasc Rev, 1973, p 32.

Wilson JN, Grow JB, et al: Central venous pressure in optimal blood volume maintenance, Arch Surg **85**:563, 1962.

Wilson JN, Owens JC: Pitfalls in monitoring central venous pressure, Hosp Med, April 1970, p 86.

Wilson RF, Sarver E, Birks R: Clinical venous pressure and blood volume determinations in clinical shock, Surg Gynecol Obstet **132**:631, 1971.

Yang SS, Bentivoglio LG, Maranhao V, Goldberg H: From cardiac catheterization data to hemodynamic parameters, Philadelphia, 1972, FA Davis Co.

Zucker G, Eisinger RP, Floch MH, Singer MM: Treatment of shock and prevention of ischemic necrosis with levarterenol-phentolamine mixtures, Circulation **22**:935, 1960.

Zucker G, Levine J: Pressor and diminished local vasoconstrictor effects of levarterenol-phentolamine mixtures, Arch Intern Med **104**:607, 1959.

4 / The cardiac arrhythmias

The heart begins to beat automatically and rhythmically during early embryonic life and continues to beat until death occurs. (After cardiac arrest, the heart may continue to show signs of electrical activity even when clinical signs of death are present; see Chapter 2.) The cardiac stimuli arise in the neuromuscular tissues of the heart (the sinus node, the AV node, the bundle of His and its right and left branches, and the Purkinje fibers).

THE SINUS NODE

The sinus node (SA node) is a small, comma-shaped mass of neuromuscular tissue. It is about 15 mm long and about 5 mm wide and lies in a groove, the sulcus terminalis, between the opening of the superior vena cava and the right atrial appendage.

There are three neuromuscular bands between the sinus node and the AV node: the anterior, middle, and posterior internodal conduction pathways. When sinus rhythm is present, the most direct path from the sinus node to the AV node is through the posterior internodal tract.

The sinus node artery (ramus ostii cavae superioris), which arises from the right coronary artery in more than 50% of persons (and from the left coronary artery in the others) supplies the sinus node.

THE AV NODE AND THE AV JUNCTION

The AV node is a specialized neuromuscular bridge between the atria and ventricles. It is about 5 mm long and 2 to 3 mm wide. It lies in both the interatrial and interventricular septa, below and to the right of the opening of the coronary sinus.

The region traditionally known as the AV node is now divided into the following 3 regions.

1. The atrionodal (AN) region, located between the atrium and the anatomic AV node.
2. The nodal (N) region. This corresponds approximately to the AV node, which is seen on ordinary light microscopic slides.
3. The nodal-His (NH) region. This is situated between the N region and the bundle of His.

These three regions are now called collectively the *AV junction*.

These observations are important for the following reasons. It is now known that the N region of the AV junction does not have any true pacemaker cells and that so-called AV nodal rhythm does not arise in the N region. Instead, it actually arises in either the AN or NH regions of AV junction or in the bundles of His. This is the reason that the term *AV junctional rhythm* is better than the old term AV nodal rhythm.

The ramus septi fibrosi, which arises from the right coronary artery in approximately 90% of persons (and from the circumflex branch of the left coronary artery in the others) supplies the AV node.

THE BUNDLE OF HIS, ITS BRANCHES, AND THE PURKINJE FIBERS

The bundle of His is a direct continuation of the AV node. It is about 10 mm long and 3 mm wide. It runs along the top of the ventricular septum and then divides into a right bundle and a left bundle. The right bundle lies under the endocardium of the interventricular septum. It runs along the septum, and when it reaches the endocardium of the right ventricle, it divides into smaller branches and finally ends in a fine network of Purkinje fibers, which penetrate the right ventricular muscle.

The left bundle crosses over to the left side of the interventricular septum. We know now that it has a complicated structure, with an anterior (superior) and posterior (inferior) branch. The branches of the left bundle of His also terminate in Purkinje fibers that penetrate the left ventricle.

There are also additional neuromuscular connections between the atria and ventricles (accessory Kent's bundles and Mahaim's fibers). In the Wolff-Parkinson-White syndrome, a stimulus may pass from the atria to the ventricles by way of these connections in addition to passing through the AV node (Chapter 8).

CLASSIFICATION OF CARDIAC ARRHYTHMIAS

Normally, the sinus node forms stimuli at a faster rate than the other neuromuscular tissues of the heart. Therefore, the sinus node is the primary pacemaker of the heart and controls the rate at which the heart normally beats.

When stimulus formation in the sinus node is depressed or ceases, secondary pacemakers, such as the AV junction, the bundle of His or its branches, or the Purkinje fibers, can form stimuli and keep the heart beating. Stimulus formation in the AV junction is usually slower than in the sinus node. It is still slower in the branches of the bundle of His, and it is slowest in the Purkinje fibers. However, under abnormal conditions, stimuli can be formed in any of these secondary pacemakers at a very rapid rate.

Although stimulus formation is automatic, it can be modified by way of the sympathetic and vagal fibers that act on the sinus and the AV nodes. The sympathetic nervous system has a stimulating (positive chronotropic) action on the heart, and the parasympathetic nervous system has a depressing (negative chronotropic) effect. However, the sympathetic and vagus nerves influence different portions of the heart unequally. The sinus node and the AV node are predominantly under vagal influence, and an increased heart rate is often due to a decreased vagus tone rather than to increased sympathetic activity. There is some evidence that the right vagus nerve controls the sinus node and that the left vagus nerve controls the AV node. The ventricles are under sympathetic control only.

There are numerous ways of classifying cardiac arrhythmias. They can be classified on the basis of the site of origin of the arrhythmia (sinus node, AV junction, ventricle), on the basis of the ventricular rate of the arrhythmia (slow ventricular rate, or bradyarrhythmia; fast ventricular rate, or tachyarrhythmia), or on the basis of the clinical significance of the arrhythmia (minor arrhythmias, which usually do not need to be treated; major arrhythmias, which may need emergency treatment; life-threatening arrhythmias, which need emergency treatment) and on the basis of the presence or absence of conduction disturbances.

In this book, cardiac arrhythmias are classified as follows.

Bradyarrhythmias—arrhythmias due primarily to decreased stimulus formation

Sinus bradycardia—usually minor; may become major

Sinus arrhythmia—minor

SA block—minor; may become major

Wandering pacemaker—minor

AV junctional rhythm—minor; may become major

Escape beats (AV junctional or ventricular)—minor

Conduction disturbances

Intra-atrial block—minor

AV block

First-degree AV block—usually minor

Second-degree AV block

Wenckebach type (Mobitz type I)—usually minor

Conduction disturbances—cont'd

        Mobitz type II—major

        Complete AV block—major; may become life threatening

    AV dissociation—minor

    Fascicular (intraventricular) blocks

        Unifascicular blocks

           Right bundle branch block—usually minor; may become major

           Left anterior hemiblock—minor

           Left posterior hemiblock—minor

           Left bundle branch block—usually minor; may become major

        Bifascicular blocks—major

        Trifascicular blocks—major

Tachyarrhythmias—arrhythmias due primarily to increased stimulus formation

    Sinus tachycardia—minor

    Atrial premature contractions—usually minor; may become major

    AV junctional premature contractions—usually minor

    Supraventricular tachycardias—major

        Paroxysmal atrial tachycardia

        Multifocal atrial tachycardia

        AV junctional tachycardia (paroxysmal or nonparoxysmal)

        Atrial flutter and atrial fibrillation

        Paroxysmal atrial tachycardia with AV block

    Ventricular premature contractions—may be minor or major

    Ventricular tachycardia—major or life-threatening

    Bidirectional tachycardia—major or life-threatening

    Ventricular flutter—life-threatening

    Ventricular fibrillation—life-threatening

    Bradyarrhythmia-tachyarrhythmia syndromes—major; when severe bradycardia occurs or when a ventricular tachycardia occurs, the arrhythmia becomes life threatening

    Tachyarrhythmias associated with the Wolff-Parkinson-White syndrome—major

The major and life-threatening arrhythmias and the conduction disturbances are discussed, but the minor arrhythmias are only briefly mentioned.

REFERENCES

Bellet S: Clinical disorders of the heart beat, ed 3, Philadelphia, 1971, Lea & Febiger.

Bilitch M: A manual of cardiac arrhythmias, Boston, 1971, Little, Brown and Co.

Chung EK: Principles of cardiac arrhythmias, Baltimore, 1971, The Williams & Wilkins Co.

Cranefield PF, Wit AL, Hoffman BF: Genesis of cardiac arrhythmias, Circulation **47**:190, 1973.

Goldberger E: Unipolar lead electrocardiography and vectorcardiography, ed 3, Philadelphia, 1953, Lea & Febiger.

Hecht HH, et al: Atrioventricular and intraventricular conduction; revised nomenclature and concepts, Am J Cardiol **31**:232, 1973.

Hurst JW, Myerburg RJ: Cardiac arrhythmias; evolving concepts, Mod Concepts Cardiovasc Dis **37**:73, Jan 1968, part 1; **37**:79, Feb 1968, part 2.

James TN: The connecting pathways between the sinus node and the AV node, and between the right and left atrium in the human heart, Am Heart J **65**:498, 1963.

Scherlag BJ, Samet P, Helfant RH: His bundle electrogram; a critical appraisal of its uses and limitations, Circulation **46**:601, 1972.

5 / The bradyarrhythmias and conduction disturbances

Abnormal rhythms are described in terms of a reference rhythm, normal sinus rhythm, which consists of:

1. Regularly recurring sequences of P waves QRS complexes, and T waves.

2. P waves of sinus origin. The P wave is characteristically upward in lead II and in precordial leads V_3 to V_6 and downward in lead aV_R. The P wave is usually upward in lead I and may be flat, upward, or downward in leads aV_L, aV_F, and III.

3. Constant and normal P-R interval (from 0.12 to 0.2 sec). The P-R interval becomes shorter as the heart rate increases.

4. Heart rate between 60 and 100 beats per min.

SINUS BRADYCARDIA

A minor arrhythmia; may become major.

Sinus bradycardia is arbitrarily described as a sinus rhythm slower than 60 beats per min. The rate may even be 35 per min or slower.

Etiology. Sinus bradycardia is due to increased vagal tone. It occurs in normal persons, especially athletes. It often occurs during sleep. It can also occur in many abnormal conditions, such as intracranial lesions, jaundice, inanition, hypothyroidism, acute myocardial infarction, an infection such as typhoid fever, or acute rheumatic fever, or during convalescence from an infection. It can be produced by drugs such as digitalis, quinidine, procainamide, propranolol, reserpine, and guanethidine.

Clinical aspects. Symptoms are usually absent. Some patients may experience dizziness or lightheadedness. Sudden bradycardia may cause syncope.

Treatment. No specific treatment is ordinarily needed unless the bradycardia is associated with symptoms or with signs of a decreased cardiac output. In such patients atropine, ephedrine sulfate, or isoproterenol can be used. The treatment of sinus bradycardia associated with acute myocardial infarction is discussed in Chapter 10.

SA BLOCK

A minor arrhythmia; may become major.

When SA block occurs, the sinus node fails to initiate one or more stimuli, or there is a block or delay in the spread of the stimulus through the sinus node into the atria. Therefore, neither the atria nor the ventricles are stimulated, and the ECG shows a long pause (Figs. 5-1 and 5-2).

Electrocardiogram. SA block has been divided into several types.

1. First-degree SA block
2. Second-degree SA block
3. Third-degree SA block

First-degree SA block. The conventional ECG is not capable of recording the electrical activity in the sinus node, and this type of SA block cannot be recognized.

Second-degree SA block. Two types may occur.

1. Wenckebach type (Fig. 5-2). The P-P intervals become progressively shorter until a long pause occurs between two successive beats. For example, every third, fourth, or fifth beat may drop out, or the beats may

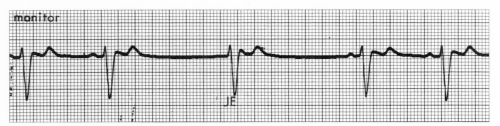

Fig. 5-1. SA block. An AV junctional escape beat *(JE)* is present.

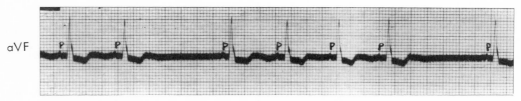

Fig. 5-2. SA block. A Wenckebach type of SA block is present. (Note the progressive shortening of the P-P intervals in the third to sixth beats.)

drop out in an irregular sequence. This type of SA block must be differentiated from sinus arrhythmia.

2. Mobitz type. The long pause that occurs is a multiple of the regular P-P cycle. Single beats may drop out regularly or irregularly. If alternate beats drop out, the heart rate will decrease to one half, and sinus bradycardia will occur. (This may explain the bradycardia of some long-distance runners.) Frequently, two or even three successive dropped beats may occur.

Third-degree SA block. This is characterized by standstill of the heart for a variable period of time. It has also been called sinus arrest, sinus standstill, sinoatrial arrest, sinoatrial standstill, and atrial standstill. It may be transient or permanent. When a long period of SA block or sinus arrest occurs, AV junctional or ventricular escape beats may occur (Fig. 5-1).

Etiology. Second-degree SA block due to excessive vagal stimulation can occur in normal persons. It can also occur in many abnormal conditions, such as acute myocarditis and acute myocardial infarction (particularly inferior myocardial infarction

with occlusion of the right coronary artery, which supplies the sinus node in about 60% of persons), and as a result of drugs, such as digitalis, quinidine, acetylcholine, and potassium salts.

Third-degree SA block (sinus arrest), which does not occur normally, can also be produced by the conditions listed above.

Clinical aspects. Physical examination will reveal pauses in the pulse due to "dropped beats." When the pauses are long, the patient may experience dizziness and faintness. Syncope can also occur.

SA block is often associated with other arrhythmias, such as various types of AV block.

The differentiation of sinus arrest from AV junctional rhythm is described on p. 56.

Treatment. No specific treatment is needed if the pauses are short and the patient does not have any symptoms. If the SA block is due to drugs, the dosage should be decreased or the drug stopped temporarily.

If the patient has symptoms associated with the slow heart rate or if the SA block has produced frequent long pauses (with more than two consecutive beats missed), atropine,* isoproterenol, or even transvenous cardiac pacing may be necessary.

AV JUNCTIONAL RHYTHM

A minor arrhythmia; may become major.

When AV junctional rhythm is present, the atria and ventricles are stimulated more or less simultaneously by a pacemaker in the AV junction (either in the AN or NH region; p. 50).

Electrocardiogram. The stimulus that starts in the AV junction spreads in a normal way to the ventricles. More or less simultaneously, the stimulus spreads in a retrograde way to the atria. As a result, the P waves may appear before or after the QRS complexes or may be hidden within the QRS complex (Figs. 5-3 and 5-4). In addition, the retrograde spread of the stim-

---

*This and other drugs are described in Part three.

ulus from the AV junction to the atria produces changes in the shapes of the P waves. The P waves in leads V_2, V_3, and aV_F become downward. The P waves in leads V_3 to V_6 are also downward. The P waves in lead aV_R become upward. The P waves in leads I and aV_L usually remain upward.

The position of the P wave in relation to the QRS complex may be fixed or may vary from beat to beat. When the P waves occur simultaneously with the QRS complex, they cannot be seen unless esophageal leads are taken. When the P waves appear before the QRS complex, the P-R interval is usually less than 0.1 sec.

In this condition the heart beats regularly at a rate between 30 and 60 beats per min.

Etiology. AV junctional rhythm is caused by depression of the sinus node as a result of vagal stimulation or by organic heart disease. It often occurs normally. It may also appear in acute infections and in acute

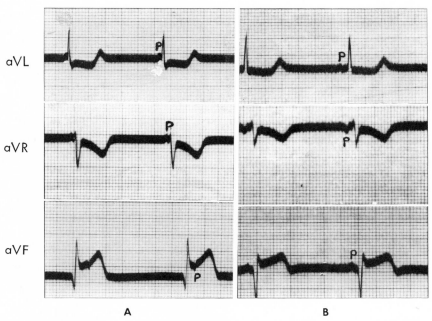

	A	B
aVL		
aVR		
aVF		

Fig. 5-3. Transient AV junctional (nodal) rhythm in a patient with an acute inferior wall myocardial infarction. Notice that the P waves appear either before or after the QRS complexes. **A,** Two days after the infarction occurred. **B,** Sinus bradycardia; ECG taken a week later.

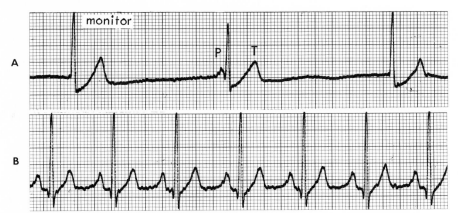

Fig. 5-4. Transient AV junctional rhythm in a patient with acute inferior wall myocardial infarction, monitor lead. **A,** AV junctional rhythm. Simultaneously, the patient's blood pressure fell, and he became diaphoretic. He was given 0.8 mg atropine IV. **B,** A few minutes later; sinus rhythm is present.

myocardial infarction (particularly inferior infarction or infarction of the atria), during inhalation anesthesia, and in association with acidosis (with or without hyperkalemia), hypoxia, or shock.

It can be produced by drugs such as digitalis, quinidine, procainamide, propranolol, and reserpine or by a vagotonic drug such as morphine sulfate. Atropine may even produce transient AV junctional rhythm in a normal person. This occurs if the atropine releases the vagal control of the AV node more quickly than it releases vagal control of the sinus node.

Clinical aspects. A regular slow radial pulse in association with large systolic pulsations in the neck veins is typical of AV junctional rhythm. The large neck vein pulsations occur because the atria may contract simultaneously with the ventricles. Therefore, the AV valves are closed, and blood is propelled from the right atrium into the superior vena cava and the neck veins during systole.

When AV junctional rhythm occurs and the P waves are hidden within the QRS complex, the ECG may simulate atrial fibrillation with fine fibrillatory (*f*) waves, but the diagnosis of AV junctional rhythm can be made from the following.

1. The base line between the complexes is completely flat. This indicates that there is no electrical activity present between the end of T wave and the beginning of the QRS complex.
2. Precordial leads V_1 and V_2 show no *f* waves.
3. If esophageal leads are taken at the atrial level, biphasic P waves can be seen within the QRS complex.

AV junctional rhythm can be differentiated from atrial standstill in the following ways.

1. In AV junctional rhythm, large systolic pulsations occur in the neck veins; whereas in atrial standstill, the neck veins show a normal systolic collapse.
2. Esophageal leads at the atrial level show P waves within the QRS complex in AV junctional rhythm, but not in atrial standstill.
3. In AV junctional rhythm, phonocardiograms show additional vibrations superimposed on the first portion of the first heart sound; but in atrial standstill, the initial vibrations of the first heart sound remain normal.

Treatment. AV junctional rhythm is usually transitory, and no treatment is needed. However, if the patient is receiving digitalis or a cardiac-depressant drug, the dosage should be reduced or the drug stopped temporarily.

If the patient shows symptoms due to the slow heart rate, atropine, ephedrine, or iso-

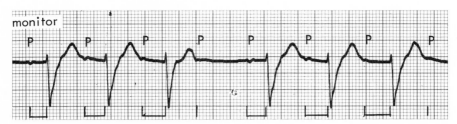

Fig. 5-5. Wenckebach type of AV block. A patient with acute myocardial infarction. Shortly after this ECG was taken, the patient developed cardiac arrest.

proterenol can be used. If the patient is hospitalized, the lower extremities can be temporarily raised approximately 45° to increase the venous return to the heart and to increase the heart rate in this way. Ace bandages can also be applied from the toes to the groins. Rarely, transvenous atrial or ventricular pacing is needed.

AV BLOCK

AV block, or heart block, exists when conduction of the stimulus from the atria to the ventricles through the AV node is slowed or blocked. The AV block may be transient, intermittent, or permanent. It may be incomplete or complete. A patient may show various types of AV block in one ECG.

Incomplete AV block occurs in two forms.

1. First-degree AV block (prolonged P-R interval)
2. Second-degree AV block

First-degree AV block

A minor arrhythmia.

Etiology. Digitalis may cause first-degree AV block, but this is not considered a sign of digitalis toxicity unless the P-R interval becomes longer than 0.26 sec.

Clinical aspects. First-degree AV block produces no symptoms. The intensity of the first heart sound tends to decrease as the P-R interval becomes longer.

Treatment. No treatment is needed for first-degree AV block.

Second-degree AV block
Wenckebach type (Mobitz type I)

A minor arrhythmia; may become major.

This is the common type of second-degree AV block.

Electrocardiogram. In the Wenckebach type of AV block each successive stimulus from the atria finds it more difficult to pass through the AV node. This produces progressive prolongation of the P-R interval with each beat. Finally, an atrial stimulus is not able to penetrate the AV node, and a P wave not followed by a QRS complex and T wave appears (Fig. 5-5). When the next atrial stimulus reaches the AV node, the node has recovered its ability to conduct, and a short P-R interval results. The next beat often shows a prolongation of the P-R interval, and the cycle may be repeated. (In association with the progressive lengthening of the P-R interval, there is progressive shortening of the R-R interval, until a P wave is not followed by a QRS complex.)

The ventricular rhythm depends on the frequency with which the AV node fails to respond to the atrial stimulus. For example, a condition in which every fourth P wave is blocked at the AV node can be called a 4:3 type of incomplete AV block, because there are 4 P waves to every 3 QRS complexes and T waves. However, it is common to see varying cycles of the Wenckebach phenomenon in the same ECG. Similarly, the prolongation of the

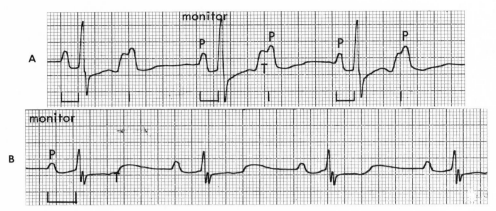

Fig. 5-6. A, Mobitz type II AV block. Notice that every alternate P wave is blocked. **B,** First-degree AV block. The P-R interval is 0.32 sec. **A** and **B** from the same patient, who had an acute myocardial infarction. **B** taken a day after **A.**

P-R interval in successive beats is not necessarily uniform.

Etiology. The etiology of the Wenckebach type of AV block is similar to that of first-degree AV block (see above). However, a Wenckebach type of AV block occurring in a patient receiving digitalis is a sign of digitalis toxicity.

Clinical aspects. The most obvious physical sign is an irregular heartbeat due to periodically occurring pauses (dropped beats). The patient may complain of palpitations, which are caused by this irregular heartbeat and by the fact that the beat after a pause may be forceful.

Treatment. Since the Wenckebach type of AV block is usually transient, no treatment is indicated. However, if the patient is taking digitalis or a cardiac-depressant drug, the dosage should be reduced or the drug temporarily stopped.

Mobitz type II

A major arrhythmia.

This occurs much less frequently than the Wenckebach type of second-degree AV block.

Electrocardiogram. In this type of incomplete AV block, the AV node fails to respond to sinus stimuli at regular intervals. The ventricular rate in these patients

is regular. The ventricular rate depends on the frequency with which the AV node responds to the atrial stimuli. For example, the AV node often responds to every alternate atrial stimulus, producing a 2:1 AV block (Fig. 5-6, *A*). In other patients, the AV node may respond only to every third atrial stimulus, producing a 3:1 AV block.

In the Mobitz type II AV block, the P waves that are followed by QRS complexes always show a constant P-R interval. (This pattern differentiates this type of incomplete AV block from complete AV block, in which the ventricular rate is also regular but there is no constant P-R interval; see below). In addition, the interval between any two successive P waves that are not separated by a QRS complex is often longer than the interval between two successive P waves that are separated by a QRS complex.

The QRS width may be normal or widened, depending on whether the block is in the AV node or in one or both branches of the bundle of His.

Etiology. The Mobitz type II AV block is associated with organic heart disease. It does not occur normally. It may be a precursor of complete AV block or of cardiac arrest.

Clinical aspects. The patient may be

aware of the slow forceful heart beats. On auscultation, atrial sounds may be heard over the heart during diastole, in addition to the regular heart sounds.

Treatment. This depends on the etiology of the Mobitz type II AV block. If it occurs in an asymptomatic patient with chronic organic heart disease, no treatment is indicated. If it occurs in acute myocardial infarction, active treatment may be indicated to prevent cardiac arrest (Chapter 10). If it is due to digitalis, the drug must be stopped immediately.

Complete AV block

A major arrhythmia.

Electrocardiogram. When complete AV block is present, all the atrial stimuli are blocked at the AV node. Therefore, stimuli must form in the heart in a distal normal portion of the AV node, in the bundle of His, in one of its right or left branches, or in the Purkinje fibers. This ventricular pacemaker is known as an idioventricular pacemaker, and the rhythm is known as idioventricular rhythm.

When the stimulus for the ventricles arises in the AV node, the shape of the QRS complex is more or less normal. When the ventricles are stimulated by a pacemaker below the AV node, the QRS complexes become wide and aberrant and may resemble the patterns of right or left bundle branch block.

The ventricles usually beat at a slow regular rate, between 30 and 60 per min, but the rate may be as low as 12 per min. Rarely, it is faster than 60 per min. When the stimulus arises in the AV node or in the bundle of His, the heart rate is usually faster than when the stimulus arises in the right or left bundle or in the Purkinje fibers.

Complete AV block is recognized by P waves that appear regularly and by QRS complexes that also appear regularly, but at a much slower rate. There is no constant P-R interval, and the presence of a P wave closely followed by a QRS complex is coincidental and is not due to the spread of the stimulus from the atria to the ventricles (Fig. 5-7).

The ventricular rate in complete AV block may be irregular for several reasons.

1. The location of the idioventricular pacemaker may shift. When this occurs, the shape of the QRS complex also changes in any one lead from beat to beat.
2. The ventricles may stop beating temporarily (ventricular standstill) (Fig. 5-8). During this period, AV junctional or ventricular escape beats may also occur.
3. Ventricular premature contractions, ventricular tachycardia, or transient ventricular fibrillation may occur (Figs. 5-9 and 5-10).
4. Even in a patient with apparently complete AV block, an occasional stimulus from the atria may penetrate the AV node and cause the ventricles to beat (Fig. 5-11).

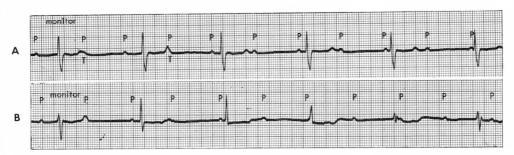

Fig. 5-7. Complete AV block. **A** and **B** taken several hours apart. **A,** Atrial rate of 75 per min. The ventricles are beating independently at a slow rate of approximately 40 beats per min. **B,** A few hours later, same patient; variations in the shape of the QRS from beat to beat.

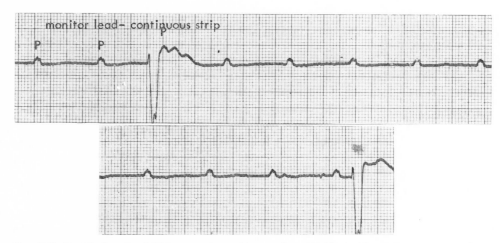

Fig. 5-8. Ventricular standstill in a patient with complete AV block. The atria continue to beat (P waves). A temporary transvenous pacemaker was immediately inserted.

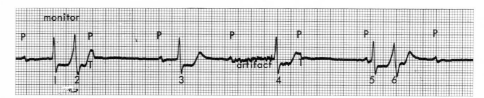

Fig. 5-9. Complete AV block with occasional ventricular premature contractions (beats 2 and 6). The atria are beating at a rate of approximately 60 per min. The ventricles are beating at a slow rate of approximately 40 per min.

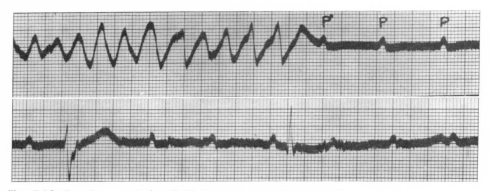

Fig. 5-10. Transient ventricular fibrillation and ventricular standstill in a patient with complete AV block. This ECG was taken before pacemakers were available. The patient had numerous similar attacks over a period of many years.

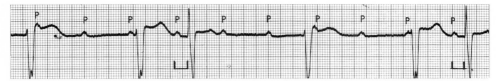

Fig. 5-11. Almost complete AV block. The atria are beating at a rate of approximately 75 per min. The ventricles are beating independently at a slow rate of approximately 33 per min. Occasional P waves reach the AV node and are able to penetrate it and stimulate the ventricles in a normal way (the third and sixth QRS complexes), causing the ventricular rhythm to become irregular.

Etiology. A common cause of complete AV block is coronary artery disease, acute or chronic. Other patients show fibrosis of the AV node without significant coronary artery disease. Other causes include calcific aortic stenosis; cardiac surgery; collagen vascular disease; myocarditis; infiltrative diseases such as amyloidosis, syphilitic gumma, or sarcoidosis; nonpenetrating cardiac trauma; digitalis; and cardiac-depressant drugs. Congenital complete AV block can also occur. (Complete AV block associated with acute myocardial infarction is discussed in Chapter 10.)

Clinical aspects. The slow ventricular rate causes the stroke volume to increase. As a result, the forceful ejection of blood from the left ventricle causes the systolic blood pressure to rise even above 150 mm Hg. The long diastolic period allows the diastolic blood pressure to fall even to 70 or 60 mm Hg.

The radial pulse rate is usually slow and regular, as mentioned above. Examination of the neck veins may show atrial pulsations in the intervals between heartbeats. Occasionally, when atrial and ventricular systole coincide, a large jugular vein pulsation (cannon wave) may be noted.

The patient usually does not have symptoms when the ventricular rate remains regular. However, there may be awareness of the slow forceful beating of the heart; and when the ventricular rate is very slow, dizziness may occur. In addition, attacks of syncope (Adams-Stokes syndrome) may occur.

Adams-Stokes syndrome. Syncope associated with complete AV block may occur in several ways. The ventricular rate may slow markedly or the ventricles may stop beating temporarily, but the atria continue to beat (Fig. 5-8). Both the ventricles and atria may stop beating. The syncope may be associated with attacks of ventricular tachycardia or transient ventricular fibrillation (Fig. 5-10). (Also see Chapter 1.)

Treatment of acute complete AV block. Symptomatic acute complete AV block can be treated in several ways.

Emergency treatment

1. Start the emergency treatment of syncope, described in Chapter 1. Treatment for cardiac arrest (Chapter 2) may also be necessary.

2. You can pound rhythmically with your closed fist over the patient's lower sternum at a rate of 60 per min until more definitive treatment is available (see below). The heart has been kept beating in this way for hours. However, chest thumping should be done only with electrocardiographic monitoring, because the thumps may produce cardiac standstill or ventricular fibrillation rather than heartbeats.

Definitive treatment

1. A temporary transvenous cardiac pacemaker can be inserted into the right ventricle until the factors that produced the complete AV block disappear. The rate of pacing is approximtaely 70 beats per min. This is the treatment of choice for acute complete AV block. (Also see p. 223.)

Fixed rate pacemakers have been used

in many patients. However, regular sinus rhythm often returns. When this happens, a fixed rate pacemaker will compete with the patient's spontaneous rhythm. If a stimulus from the pacemaker occurs in the vulnerable period of a spontaneous beat (at the apex, or nadir, of the T wave), it may produce ventricular fibrillation. This possibility can be avoided by using a demand pacemaker instead of a fixed rate pacemaker (p. 199).

If the patient has been receiving an infusion of isoproterenol, the infusion should be stopped just before the catheter electrode is inserted into the heart because the isoproterenol increases the irritability of the myocardium.

2. If a pacemaker cannot be inserted, the following drug therapy can be tried.

Isoproterenol is the drug of choice. In an emergency it can be given intracardiac, or it can be given IV, IM, subcutaneously, sublingually, or rectally. The usual method is to give an IV drip containing 1 mg isoproterenol dissolved in 500 ml 5% dextrose in water. (Each ml of this dilution therefore contains 2 μg isoproterenol.) The initial flow can be 2 μg per min, using a microdrip bulb. (If the microdrip bulb is calibrated to deliver 60 drops per ml, each 60 drops contains 4 μg isoproterenol.) Some patients may require doses as large as 40 μg isoproterenol per min to raise the heart rate to a satisfactory rate of 50 to 60 beats per min. However, if too much isoproterenol is given, a sinus tachycardia, ventricular premature contractions, or ventricular tachycardia may develop.

A trial dose of atropine, 0.4 to 0.8 mg, can be given IV. If sinus rhythm is restored or if the heart rate increases to 50 per min, one can continue to give atropine therapeutically, either IV, subcutaneously, or orally. However, it is usually not possible to continue therapeutic doses of atropine for more than 48 hours, because toxic reactions usually develop.

Corticosteroids can be given either orally or parenterally. Theoretically, corticosteroids may be beneficial by decreasing inflammation or edema in the region of the AV node. However, corticosteroids have been helpful even when the complete AV block is not associated with inflammation or edema in the region of the node.

Prednisone, given orally in a daily dose of 60 mg, methylprednisolone (Solu-Medrol), given IM in a dose of 20 mg twice a day, or other similar corticosteroids can be used. If improvement does not occur within 48 hours, the corticosteroid should be stopped.

If the complete AV block is associated with acidosis, alkalinizing therapy with sodium bicarbonate may make the heart responsive to catecholamines, such as isoproterenol or epinephrine. Alkalinizing therapy should not be used if an acidosis is not present, because this therapy may precipitate ventricular tachycardia or ventricular fibrillation.

Epinephrine is very effective when cardiac standstill (asystole) develops (Chapter 2).

Chlorothiazide or similar thiazide diuretics have been used particularly in patients with intermittent complete AV block. The mechanism of action is the lowering of the serum potassium concentration (to below 4 mEq/L) produced by the thiazide. When this occurs, the resting membrane potential of cardiac muscle fibers and cardiac pacemaker cells is increased. This results in increased cardiac conduction.

The dosage of chlorothiazide is 0.5 to 2.0 gm a day for at least 8 weeks. A therapeutic effect may be noted before the serum potassium concentration decreases.

3. If congestive heart failure is present, diuretics such as the thiazides, furosemide (Lasix) or ethacrynic acid (Edecrin), which cause a loss of potassium ions from the urine, can be used (see above). A diuretic such as spironolactone (Aldactone A) or triamterine (Dyrenium), which raises the

serum potassium concentration, should not be used.

Digitalis has been used to treat congestive heart failure in patients with complete AV block. However, there is always the possibility that it may produce cardiac arrest. Therefore, it should be used only after a transvenous cardiac pacemaker has been inserted.

4. If second-degree or complete AV block is due to digitalis toxicity, the digitalis should be stopped immediately. It may take several days for the toxicity to disappear if the patient has been taking a short-acting digitalis preparation, or it may take a week or more if a long-acting digitalis drug has been given. In addition, if renal insufficiency is present, the digitalis toxicity may last longer because digitalis drugs (except digitoxin) are excreted primarily by the kidneys.

Potassium salts must not be used if second-degree or complete AV block occurs as a result of digitalis toxicity, because they can increase the degree of AV block and may cause cardiac arrest. However, potassium salts can be used in patients with paroxysmal atrial tachycardia with AV block due to digitalis toxicity (Chapter 8).

5. If ventricular premature contractions are present or if ventricular tachycardia or ventricular fibrillation occur, quinidine, procainamide, propranolol, lidocaine, diphenylhydantoin, or any other cardiac-depressant drug should not be used unless a transvenous cardiac pacemaker has been inserted.

6. Every patient with complete AV block who requires surgery with general anesthesia should have a transvenous demand pacemaker inserted for possible use during the surgery and in the immediate postoperative period.

7. The treatment of complete AV block complicating acute myocardial infarction is described in Chapter 10.

Treatment of chronic complete AV block. If the patient does not have symptoms, treatment is not needed.

Treatment is indicated if the patient has symptoms of the Adams-Stokes syndrome, such as syncope; congestive heart failure that does not respond to diuretics; angina that does not respond to nitrites; signs of cerebral anoxia, such as excessive weakness, mental irritability, or depression; mental deterioration (organic brain syndrome); or signs of increasing azotemia. The goal of the treatment, which can be accomplished in several ways, is to restore normal AV conduction, if possible, or to increase the ventricular rate to approximately 60 beats per min and to make the ventricular rhythm more stable.

A long-term transvenous cardiac pacemaker can be implanted (Chapter 17). If the relation of the patient's symptoms and signs to the complete AV block is not obvious, a temporary transvenous cardiac pacemaker can be inserted, and the patient can be observed for signs of improvement. I believe that a cardiac pacemaker should be implanted after the first episode of syncope in a patient with complete AV block. Some cardiologists prefer to use a trial of drug therapy first.

The following drugs can be used.

Isoproterenol is the drug of choice. It can be given sublingually, orally, or rectally to a patient with symptomatic complete AV block. To prevent hypertension or coronary insufficiency, the total daily dose of sublingually administered isoproterenol should not exceed 50 mg. An extended-release oral preparation of isoproterenol (Proternol) is also available. This can be used in a dose of 15 to 30 mg every 3 to 4 hours, for a total daily dose of 30 to 180 mg.

Ephedrine sulfate given orally in a dose of 25 to 50 mg daily every 4 to 6 hours can be used as a substitute for isoproterenol. However, it is less effective than isoproterenol.

Atropine should not be given for long-term use, because toxic reactions quickly develop.

Chlorothiazide has already been mentioned on p. 62.

AV DISSOCIATION

AV dissociation is a minor arrhythmia. However, since it is often mistaken for complete AV block, its salient characteristics are described here.

AV dissociation exists when the atria and ventricles beat independently, the ventricular rate being the same or slightly faster than the atrial rate. It represents an attempt of the ventricles to escape from the depressive effect of vagal stimulation on the sinus node. AV dissociation may be complete or incomplete.

Some cardiologists describe complete AV block as a form of AV dissociation because in both conditions the atria and ventricles are beating independently. Other cardiologists include ventricular and AV junctional tachycardia as forms of AV dissociation because the atria and ventricles also beat independently in these tachyarrhythmias. However, this classification obscures the characteristics of AV dissociation.

Electrocardiogram. In the bradyarrhythmias that have been previously described, either the sinus node or some other neuro-

muscular tissue is the pacemaker of the heart. In AV dissociation there are two pacemakers competing with each other for dominance. The sinus node stimulates the atria, and the AV node stimulates the ventricles more or less simultaneously so that when the stimulus from the sinus node reaches the AV node, the AV node is still refractory as a result of its own previous stimulus. Therefore, the stimulus from the sinus node is not able to penetrate the AV node and spread through the ventricles. This is known as *complete AV dissociation* (Figs. 5-12 to 5-15). In some ways it is similar to what happens in complete AV block. However, there is an important difference between these two conditions. In AV dissociation, a stimulus that reaches the AV node when it is not refractory will penetrate the AV node and cause the ventricles to beat prematurely. (This is known as *incomplete AV dissociation* or *AV dissociation with interference* [Fig. 5-15]). However, when complete AV block is present, no stimulus is able to penetrate the AV node to cause the ventricles to beat prematurely.

AV dissociation can also occur in association with first-degree AV block (Fig. 5-15).

Etiology. Both complete and incomplete

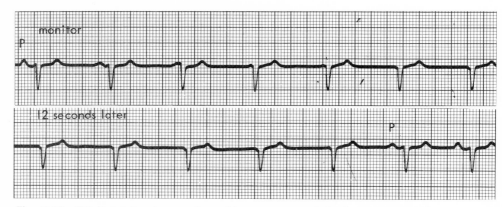

Fig. 5-12. AV dissociation in a patient with acute myocardial infarction. In the first strip, the P waves move into the QRS complexes. In the second strip, taken 12 sec later, the P waves emerge again.

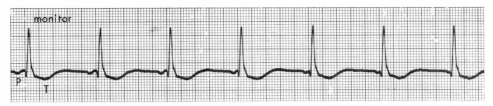

Fig. 5-13. AV dissociation, possibly due to procainamide. The downward P waves do not indicate AV junctional rhythm. This monitor lead was taken with reversed polarity.

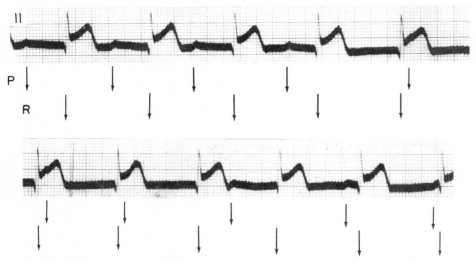

Fig. 5-14. AV dissociation in a patient with acute inferior wall myocardial infarction. The upper and lower rows form a continuous strip.

AV dissociation can occur normally and abnormally; for example, during acute infections, acute myocardial infarction, acute rheumatic fever, increased intracranial pressure, vagal stimulation produced by ocular pressure or carotid sinus massage, or forced inspiration. Drugs such as digitalis, quinidine, procainamide, propranolol, and other cardiac-depressant drugs can also produce it.

Treatment. No treatment is usually needed. However, if the AV dissociation is due to digitalis toxicity, the dosage should be decreased or the digitalis stopped temporarily. If it is due to quinidine or any other drug, the drug should be stopped temporarily.

FASCICULAR (INTRAVENTRICULAR) BLOCKS

The ventricular conduction system is composed of three major divisions (fascicles): (1) the right bundle of His, (2) the left anterior division, and (3) the left posterior division of the (left) main bundle of His. Unifascicular, bifascicular, or trifascicular block can occur, depending on which of the fascicles of the conduction system is involved.

Unifascicular heart block

There are four types of unifascicular heart block.

1. Right bundle branch block occurs when the right bundle of His is blocked.

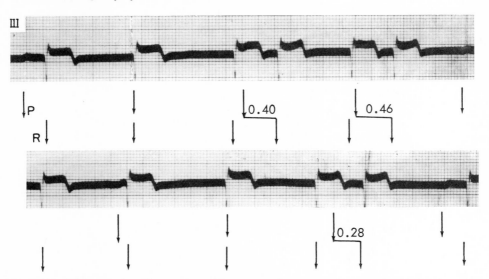

Fig. 5-15. AV dissociation. The upper and lower rows form a continuous strip. Notice that some of the atrial stimuli penetrate the AV node. When this happens, the cardiac rhythm becomes irregular. This tracing is unusual because the conducted beats show prolonged P-R intervals.

2. Left anterior hemiblock occurs when the anterior division of the left bundle of His is blocked.
3. Left posterior hemiblock occurs when the posterior division of the left bundle of His is blocked.
4. Left bundle branch block occurs when the left main branch of the bundle of His or both its anterior and posterior branches are blocked.

The diagnosis of these fascicular blocks is made by the ECG.

Right bundle branch block

Usually a minor conduction disturbance; may become major.

Clinical aspects. Right bundle branch block often occurs in normal persons. It may be transient or permanent. Transient right bundle branch block also may occur normally. It frequently occurs after massive pulmonary embolism (see Fig. 11-1) or acute myocardial infarction. Permanent right bundle branch block is often found in association with rheumatic heart disease, hypertensive heart disease, and coronary artery disease.

When acute myocardial infarction, pulmonary embolism, or left anterior hemiblock (see below) is absent, the prognosis of right bundle branch block is excellent.

Electrocardiogram. The QRS width is 0.12 sec or more. Precordial leads near the sternum, such as lead V_1, usually show an rsR', with a slurred R'. Precordial leads on the left side of the chest, such as leads V_5 and V_6, show a qRS with a wide final S. When incomplete right bundle branch block is present, the pattern is similar, but the QRS width is less than 0.12 sec.

Treatment. The patient should be treated for the underlying condition, not for the right bundle branch block.

Left anterior hemiblock

A minor conduction disturbance. However, if it is associated with right bundle branch block, it becomes a major conduction disturbance.

Electrocardiogram. Marked left axis deviation (superior axis deviation) is present. The mean electrical axis of the QRS complex in the frontal plane is approximately −60° or more.* When this occurs, the depth of S_3 is 2⅓ or more greater than the height of R_1. The QRS width is normal or may be prolonged to 0.10 sec.

Etiology. Left anterior hemiblock may be caused by numerous conditions, including acute myocardial infarction, diffuse arteriosclerotic fibrosis, myocarditis following cardiac catheterization or cardiac surgery, or massive pulmonary embolism.

Clinical aspects. Left anterior hemiblock and left axis deviation are not synonymous. A frontal plane axis of −30° may be completely normal ("horizontal" electrical position of the heart). Left axis deviation is also commonly associated with left ventricular hypertrophy. Furthermore, marked left axis deviation (approximately −90°) may occur in emphysema, probably related to the position of the heart.

Treatment. The patient should be treated for the underlying condition, not specifically for the left anterior hemiblock. (Also see Bifascicular Blocks, below.)

Left posterior hemiblock

A minor conduction disturbance. When it is associated with right bundle branch block, it becomes major.

Electrocardiogram. Right axis deviation is present, with a mean electrical axis of the QRS +120° or greater. When this occurs, the height of R_3 is 2⅓ greater than the depth of S_1. In addition, lead II shows an S, and lead aV_R shows a QR type of pattern.

The QRS width may be normal or 0.10 sec.

Clinical aspects. Left posterior hemiblock can occur as an isolated conduction disturbance or can be due to ischemic heart disease, myocarditis, and so on. It can also be associated with right bundle

branch block as a form of bilateral bundle branch block.

A diagnosis of left posterior hemiblock is difficult because the pattern can occur normally in persons with a "vertical heart" and in patients with emphysema or chronic pulmonary or rheumatic heart disease, when the heart is electrically vertical.

Treatment. The patient's underlying condition should be treated.

Left bundle branch block

Usually a minor conduction disturbance; may become major.

Electrocardiogram. The QRS width is 0.12 sec or more.

Precordial leads on the left side of the chest, such as V_5 and V_6, show wide, notched, or slurred R waves, depressed RS-T segments, downward T waves, and absent q waves.

Precordial leads near the sternum, such as V_1 and V_2, show wide QS or rS patterns with elevated RS-T segments and upward T waves.

When incomplete left bundle branch block is present, the pattern is similar, but the QRS width is less than 0.12 sec.

Clinical aspects. Left bundle branch block may be transient or permanent. Transient left bundle branch block may rarely occur normally or may occur after acute myocardial infarction, congestive heart failure, acute infections, or as a result of quinidine or procainamide toxicity. Permanent left bundle branch block is almost always due to organic heart disease, either hypertensive, coronary, rheumatic, or syphilitic. It is associated with a decreased life expectancy.

Treatment. The patient should be treated for the underlying heart condition, not for the left bundle branch block.

Bifascicular blocks

A major conduction disturbance.

Bifascicular block occurs when right bundle branch block occurs simultaneously

---

*Different authors use varying criteria for the electrical axis in left anterior hemiblock, ranging from −30° to −60°. The lower the cutoff criterion, the more false positive diagnoses will be reported. Therefore, I prefer to use −60°.

with left anterior hemiblock or simultaneously with left posterior hemiblock.

Lasser and others have shown that about 10% of patients who have right bundle branch block associated with marked left axis deviation (left anterior hemiblock) develop complete AV block and syncope. However, I believe that an asymptomatic patient with bifascicular heart block should merely be followed with periodic ECGs. If such a patient needs a surgical operation, it should be done with constant electrocardiographic monitoring, and facilities should be available for the immediate insertion of a temporary transvenous ventricular demand pacemaker if complete AV block develops during surgery.

Trifascicular blocks

A major conduction disturbance.

Trifascicular block occurs when all three fascicles of the conduction system are blocked, either temporarily or permanently. The following types of trifascicular block can occur.

1. Complete AV block
2. Right bundle branch block with alternating left anterior hemiblock and with left posterior hemiblock
3. Right bundle branch block with left anterior (or posterior) hemiblock and with first- or second-degree AV block

The treatment of these patients is the same as for bifascicular block.

Fascicular block complicating acute myocardial infarction

This is discussed in Chapter 10.

REFERENCES

Aronow WS: Jugular venous pulse in 2:1 atrioventricular block, Ann Intern Med **73:**277, 1972.

Aronson R, Kaplinsky E, Neufeld HN: Isorhythmic dissociation; a physiologic arrhythmia, Chest **64:** 387, 1973.

Beregovich J, et al: Management of acute myocardial infarction complicated by advanced atrioventricular block; role of artificial pacing, Am J Cardiol **23:**54, 1969.

Burchell HB: Modes of therapy of bradycardia, Bull N Y Acad Med **47:**1011, 1971.

Criscitiello MG: Therapy of atrioventricular block, N Engl J Med **279:**808, 1968.

Donoso E, et al: Unusual forms of second-degree atrioventricular block, including Mobitz type II block, associated with Morgagni-Adams-Stokes syndrome, Am Heart J **67:**150, 1964.

Dreifus LS, Watanabe Y, et al: Atrioventricular block, Am J Cardiol **28:**371, 1971.

Fisch C, Martz BL, Priebe FH: Enhancement of potassium-induced atrioventricular block by toxic doses of digitalis drugs, J Clin Invest **39:**1885, 1960.

Goldberger E: Unipolar lead electrocardiography and vectorcardiography, ed 3, Philadelphia, 1953, Lea & Febiger.

Greenwood RJ, Finkelstein D: Sinoatrial heart block, Springfield, Ill, 1964, Charles C Thomas, Publisher.

Lasser RP, Haft JI, Friedberg CK: Relationship of right bundle branch block and marked left axis deviation to complete heart block and syncope, Circulation **37:**429, 1968.

Marriott HJL, Menendez MM: A-V dissociation revisited, Prog Cardiovasc Dis **8:**522, 1966.

Pick A, Langendorf R: Recent advances in the differential diagnosis of A-V junctional arrhythmias, Am Heart J **76:**553, 1968.

Waldo AL, James TN: A retrospective look at A-V nodal rhythms, Circulation **47:**222, 1973.

6 / Supraventricular tachyarrhythmias

The term supraventricular tachyarrhythmia includes the following types of tachyarrhythmias: paroxysmal atrial and AV junctional tachycardia, atrial flutter, atrial fibrillation, paroxysmal atrial tachycardia with AV block (PAT with block), and tachyarrhythmias associated with the Wolff-Parkinson-White syndrome. Sinus tachycardia is not a supraventricular tachycardia. However, it is discussed in this chapter because it can be confused with PAT.

SINUS TACHYCARDIA

A minor arrhythmia.

Sinus tachycardia is arbitrarily described as a sinus rhythm faster than 100 beats per min. The rate may become as rapid as 180 or more per min, particularly in young persons during exercise. Usually the rate is between 100 and 160 per min.

Electrocardiogram. P waves with a normal axis (upward in lead II, downward in lead aV_R) are present, indicating their origin from the sinus node. When the heart rate becomes rapid, the P waves tend to merge with the preceding T waves. The P-R and Q-T intervals shorten as the rate increases. The differentiation of sinus tachycardia from PAT is described on p. 73.

Clinical aspects. Sinus tachycardia commonly occurs in normal persons during exercise, with anxiety, after drinking coffee, tea, or alcoholic beverages, or after smoking. It can be produced by nitrites, by sympathomimetic drugs such as ephedrine, epinephrine, or isoproterenol, or by anticholinergic drugs such as atropine and the phenothiazines.

Sinus tachycardia can also occur in abnormal conditions, such as hyperthyroidism, congestive heart failure, rheumatic fever and most febrile illnesses, shock, and acute myocardial infarction. Persistent sinus tachycardia occurring in acute myocardial infarction is usually associated with complications such as congestive heart failure, cardiogenic shock, pulmonary embolism, or extension of the infarct.

The patient may complain of palpitations during sinus tachycardia.

Treatment. The underlying condition should be treated. It is important to differentiate sinus tachycardia, which does not need emergency treatment, from PAT, which may require emergency treatment.

ATRIAL PREMATURE CONTRACTIONS

A minor arrhythmia; may become major.

The term premature contraction, premature systole, or extrasystole indicates that the atria or ventricles are stimulated prematurely—that is, before the next regular beat is due—from an ectopic focus or foci. The premature contractions are called atrial premature contractions when they arise in some portion of the atria. AV junctional premature contractions arise in the AV junction. Ventricular premature contractions arise in one of the branches of the bundle of His or in the Purkinje fibers.

Premature contractions may also arise in the sinus node. However, the conventional ECG provides no way of differentiating a sinus premature contraction from an atrial premature contraction.

Electrocardiogram. An atrial premature

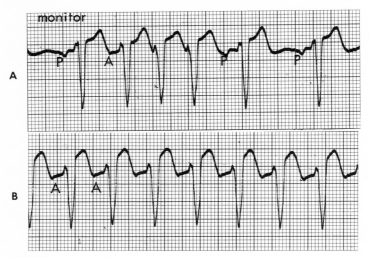

Fig. 6-1. Atrial premature contractions and paroxysmal atrial tachycardia. **A** and **B** taken a few seconds apart. **A,** Sinus beat *(P)* followed by three atrial premature contractions *(A)*. **B,** Atrial tachycardia has developed.

contraction has the following characteristics.

1. A premature P wave is present. It may be superimposed on the preceding T wave because it is premature. The premature P wave is usually followed by a QRS complex and a T wave. Occasionally, it is not followed by a QRS and T *(blocked atrial premature contraction)*.

2. The atrial premature contraction may or may not show an aberrant shape; that is, it may or may not resemble the other P waves in the lead in which it appears. When multiple atrial premature contractions arise from a single focus, they show a similar shape in any one lead (Fig. 6-1). When they arise from varying foci, their shape in any one lead varies (Fig. 6-4).

3. The P-R interval of the atrial premature contraction is usually longer than the normal P-R intervals in the ECG. However, it may be the same or shorter.

4. The QRS and T waves that follow the premature P waves usually resemble the other QRS and T waves in the lead, but aberrations of QRS and T waves may occur (p. 72).

Clinical aspects. Atrial premature con-

tractions occur spontaneously in normal persons and may also occur in many abnormal conditions, such as congestive heart failure, acute and chronic pulmonary disease, and acute myocardial infarction. They are often a precursor of PAT, atrial fibrillation, or atrial flutter. When frequent atrial premature contractions are present, the pulse becomes very irregular and may simulate atrial fibrillation.

Treatment. Generally, no treatment is needed. However, if the patient complains of palpitations, the atrial premature contractions can be abolished by sedatives, digitalis, quinidine, procainamide, or propranolol.* The patient should avoid drinking coffee, tea, and other caffeine-containing beverages.

The treatment of atrial premature contractions associated with acute myocardial infarction is discussed in Chapter 10.

AV JUNCTIONAL PREMATURE CONTRACTIONS

A minor arrhythmia; may become major. The anatomy and physiology of the AV

---

*These and other drugs are described in Part three.

node and AV junction have already been described in Chapter 4.

Electrocardiogram. Two types of AV junctional premature contractions may appear.

1. A premature AV junctional P wave (p. 55) is followed by a QRS and T wave (Fig. 6-6).

2. A premature normal-appearing QRS complex without a P wave appears. The AV junctional P wave is hidden within the QRS complex in such a patient. Occasionally, an AV junctional P wave occurs after the QRS complex and is superimposed on the T wave.

Clinical aspects. AV junctional premature contractions are common in coronary artery disease, especially in acute inferior myocardial infarction. They are also common in rheumatic heart disease and congenital heart disease.

Treatment. AV junctional premature contractions are treated like atrial premature contractions.

SUPRAVENTRICULAR TACHYCARDIAS

The term supraventricular tachycardia includes PAT, AV junctional tachycardia, and atrial flutter or atrial fibrillation with a rapid ventricular rate, because it may be impossible to determine the exact atrial rhythm when the heart is beating rapidly (even if esophageal or intracavity leads are used).

Clinically, it is important to determine whether a tachyarrhythmia is supraventricular or ventricular because the etiology, prognosis, and treatment of these two types of tachyarrhythmias are different. However, distinction between the two may be difficult or impossible at times (see below).

Paroxysmal atrial tachycardia

A major arrhythmia.

Electrocardiogram. PAT is a succession of three or more atrial premature contractions that may arise from a single focus or from varying foci in the atria. It shows the following characteristics.

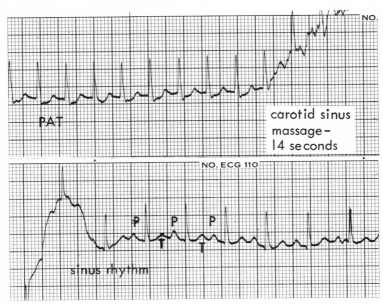

Fig. 6-2. Effect of carotid sinus massage on paroxysmal atrial tachycardia. The upper and lower rows are part of a continuous strip. In the upper row no definite P waves are visible. The diagnosis of this ECG is therefore merely "supraventricular tachyarrhythmia." The ventricular rate is approximately 185 per min. In the lower strip, taken at the end of the carotid sinus massage, sinus rhythm has appeared. However, the heart rate is still rapid (approximately 135 per min).

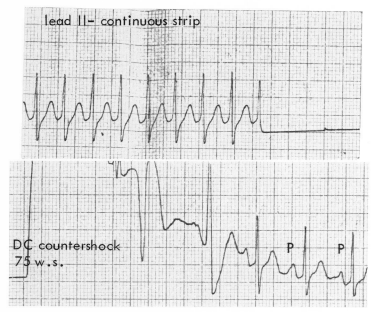

Fig. 6-3. Effect of synchronized DC shock on paroxysmal atrial tachycardia. Notice that no definite P waves are visible during the tachycardia. This ECG can be described simply as "supraventricular tachyarrhythmia." The ventricular rate is approximately 185 per min. Immediately after the DC shock, sinus rhythm appeared at a rate of approximately 90 per min.

1. The heart rate is rapid, usually between 160 and 250 per min (Figs. 6-2 and 6-3). However, the rate may be 140 per min or less, particularly if the patient is receiving quinidine, procainamide, or digitalis.

2. P waves are present. They usually show an abnormal shape but resemble sinus P waves rather than AV junctional P waves. In some patients the P waves may be superimposed on the T waves and may not be obvious.

3. The heart rate is often very regular. However, an irregular heart rate may occur in several ways: the PAT may be the result of atrial premature contractions that occur at irregular intervals; some of the atrial premature contractions may be blocked; or AV junctional or ventricular premature contractions may also occur, producing an irregular ventricular rate.

4. The QRS and T may be normal or aberrant.

Supraventricular tachyarrhythmias with aberration of the QRS complex and T wave. The term aberrant ventricular complex describes a widened and altered QRS complex, usually associated with some change in the shape of the T wave, following a premature supraventricular beat. The supraventricular beat may be an atrial premature contraction or an AV junctional premature contraction, or atrial fibrillation or atrial flutter may be present.

Aberration of the QRS and T can occur in the following ways.

The refractory period of the right branch of the bundle of His is longer than the refractory period of the AV node. Therefore, in certain instances, a premature beat that arises in the atria (or in the AV junction) can penetrate the AV node normally but may reach the right bundle of His when it is still partially refractory from the previous beat. Therefore, this premature beat will show a QRS pattern similar to right bundle branch block. Rarely, the left bundle shows a longer refractory period than the AV node. In such a case, an atrial or AV junctional premature contraction will be followed by an aberrant QRS complex of the left bundle branch block type.

When a paroxysmal supraventricular tachyarrhythmia is present with a rapid ventricular rate, the atrial stimuli may reach the ventricles when one of the bundles is still refractory from the previous beat. The exact ventricular rate at which this occurs varies with patients and also depends on whether one of the bundles of His is diseased.

When aberration of QRS and T occurs, the differentiation of a supraventricular tachyarrhythmia from a ventricular tachyarrhythmia may be difficult or impossible, particularly if a supraventricular tachyarrhythmia occurs in a patient with the Wolff-Parkinson-White syndrome. (Also see p. 102.)

The following criteria suggest that an aberrant QRS and T are due to a *supraventricular premature contraction*.

1. A premature P precedes the aberrant QRS and T. If P waves are not apparent, they may become obvious in bipolar lead S5. Lead S5 is taken as follows. The electrocardiograph is set to take standard lead I. A suction cup electrode is placed over the manubrium, and the RA cable of the electrocardiograph is connected to this electrode. Another suction cup electrode is placed over the fifth intercostal space at the right sternal border. The LA cable is connected to this electrode. Lead I is taken (Lian).

Esophageal or intracardiac leads have also been used to differentiate supraventricular from ventricular tachyarrhythmias. However, even with these leads, a differential diagnosis may be impossible because ventricular tachycardia can occur with retrograde 1:1 conduction from the ventricles through the AV node to the atria.

These observations also show that one of the main characteristics of ventricular tachycardia—namely, that the atrial rate and the ventricular rate are dissociated and different—is not always valid. (See also p. 97.)

2. The aberrant QRS shows a right bundle branch pattern (a triphasic QRS—rsR', rSR', or rsr'—in lead V1, with the initial deflection of the aberrant QRS identical to the initial normal QRS deflection).

3. A varying coupling interval is present between the premature aberrant QRS and the preceding normal QRS.

4. There is no compensatory pause after the premature aberrant QRS.

5. If atrial fibrillation is present, the aberrant QRS and T tend to occur when there has been a long pause between the preceding previous beat and the beat before this (long cycle–short cycle phenomenon) (Fig. 6-10). Criteria 2, 3, and 4 above are also present.

6. A similar aberrant QRS appears in previous ECGs of the patient when sinus rhythm is present.

The following criteria suggest that an aberrant QRS and T are due to a *ventricular premature contraction*.

1. When atrial fibrillation is present, the ventricular premature contraction also tends to occur when there has been a long cycle–short cycle phenomenon. However, the ventricular premature contraction usually shows fixed coupling and is usually followed by a compensatory pause (rule of bigeminy).

2. The QRS complex in lead V1 is monophasic or diphasic, consisting of a qR, Rs, R, or qr.

One must also realize that when atrial premature contractions or a supraventricular tachyarrhythmia occurs in a patient with bundle branch block, the QRS and T will be aberrant and the ECG may resemble a ventricular tachycardia (Fig. 6-12).

Differentiation of PAT from sinus tachycardia. It may be difficult to differentiate a PAT from a sinus tachycardia, especially when P waves appear normal. However, the following criteria can be used.

1. In sinus tachycardia the ventricular rate is usually less than 140 per min. In PAT the rate is usually 160 per min or faster. However, in both conditions the rate can be slower or faster than 140 per min.

2. In sinus tachycardia, deep inspiration or vagal stimulation by means of carotid sinus pressure often causes the heart rate to slow momentarily. Exercise increases the heart rate. Most cases of PAT do not respond to deep inspiration or to exercise; and when vagal stimulation is effective, the tachycardia abruptly stops and a slow, regular sinus rhythm begins again.

3. Sinus tachycardia usually has a gradual onset and gradually disappears, whereas PAT usually begins and ends abruptly. However, these patterns do not always occur.

4. The best way of differentiating these two conditions is to compare the P waves before and after the tachycardia. In sinus tachycardia, the P waves remain unchanged. In PAT, aberration of the P and aberration of the P-R interval usually occur.

5. Abnormal T waves may occur after an attack of any type of tachyarrhythmia (posttachycardia T wave inversion) but rarely occur after a sinus tachycardia. These abnormal T waves may persist for days or weeks.

Clinical aspects. PAT occurs in persons with normal hearts in approximately one third of cases. It can also occur in abnormal conditions, such as hyperthyroidism; acute or chronic pulmonary disease; congenital heart disease, especially atrial septal defects and Eisenmenger's complex; in association with the Wolff-Parkinson-White syndrome; in coronary artery disease and acute myocardial infarction (Chapter 10); and in rheumatic heart disease. It can also be produced by digitalis toxicity.

PAT is usually not serious. However, when the ventricular rate exceeds 180 per

min, the cardiac output decreases so that signs of congestive heart failure may appear. In addition, if the patient has a cardiac prosthesis with a ball valve, a rapid ventricular rate may prevent the ball valve from functioning adequately, and congestive heart failure can quickly develop. If coronary artery disease is present, angina may develop when the heart rate is only 150 or 160 per min. If acute myocardial infarction is present, the rapid ventricular rate is also detrimental.

PAT is often transient and disappears spontaneously. However, attacks can last hours and in some patients may last days, weeks, or longer. The frequency of attacks may vary from several times a day to one a year or less.

Treatment. The urgency of treatment of a PAT depends on the frequency of attacks, duration of previous attacks, duration of present attack, presence of circulatory collapse, congestive heart failure, angina, or previous effective medication.

The treatment of PAT associated with acute myocardial infarction is described in Chapter 10.

Emergency treatment. If the patient shows signs of cardiogenic shock, severe angina, or congestive heart failure, it is important to stop the tachycardia as quickly as possible. This can be done by means of vagal stimulation, by drugs that have a vagal or parasympathetic effect, or by drugs that have a hypertensive effect.

1. Carotid sinus massage is the most effective form of vagal stimulation. Carotid sinus massage for the *treatment* of a paroxysmal tachyarrhythmia is different from carotid sinus pressure for the *diagnosis* of carotid sinus sensitivity. *Therapeutic carotid sinus massage* is done as follows.

The carotid sinus is located anterior to the sternomastoid muscle at the upper level of the thyroid cartilage (Adam's apple) and sometimes 1/2 inch above it. The examiner should stand behind the patient, who should be lying with the neck extended and the head turned slightly to the opposite side of the examiner. With two fingers, the examiner presses the artery against the transverse process of the sixth cervical vertebra. The pulsating artery should be felt under the fingertips, and pressure should be maintained up to 15 to 20 sec if necessary. Simultaneously, the area should be massaged by the pressing fingers. The right carotid sinus should be compressed first. If the tachycardia persists, the left carotid sinus should be massaged after the examiner waits 2 to 3 min. Simultaneous bilateral massage of the carotid sinuses should never be done. The patient should be monitored with an ECG, and the carotid sinus massage should be stopped as soon as the heart rate slows.

Vagal stimulation by means of eyeball pressure should *not* be done, because it may cause injury to the cornea, or detachment of the retina in patients with myopia.

2. IV digitalization is the drug treatment of choice if carotid sinus massage is not successful. Deslanoside (Cedilanid-D) can be given IV in a dose of 0.4 to 0.8 mg (2 to 4 ml), or an IV injection of 0.75 to 1 mg (3 to 4 ml) digoxin (Lanoxin) can be given.

After ½ to 1 hour, carotid sinus massage should be tried again. If it is still not successful, another 0.4 mg (2 ml) deslanoside or 0.25 to 0.5 mg (1 to 2 ml) digoxin should be given IV. Carotid sinus massage should be repeated again in ½ to 1 hour.

3. Quinidine can be given orally if digitalis and carotid sinus massage are not effective. An oral test dose of 200 mg quinidine sulfate is given to rule out idiosyncracy. This is followed by 200 to 300 mg (0.2 to 0.3 gm) quinidine sulfate orally every 3 to 4 hours for 24 hours. If sinus rhythm does not reappear, synchronized DC shock can then be used (see below).

4. Parasympathomimetic drugs can be given instead of quinidine if digitalis and carotid sinus massage are not effective. The following parasympathomimetic drugs can be used.

Edrophonium hydrochloride (Tensilon) can be given as an IV bolus in a dose of 5 mg over a period of 30 to 60 sec, with constant monitoring of the ECG and blood pressure. If sinus rhythm does not reappear in 5 min, another 5 mg can be given. If the tachycardia continues, carotid sinus massage should be repeated.

Neostigmine can be given subcutaneously or IM in a dose of 0.5 to 2.0 mg (1 to 4 ml of a 1:2,000 solution). Carotid sinus massage should be tried in ½ to 1 hour if the tachycardia persists. The neostigmine can be repeated in 3 to 4 hours.

Neostigmine should *not* be given IV, because fatal cardiac arrest can occur.

5. Propranolol (Inderal) can be given instead of edrophonium hydrochloride, or it can be used if digitalis or edrophonium or both are not effective. Propanolol is given IV in a dose of 1 to 3 mg at a rate of 1 mg or less per min, with electrocardiographic and blood pressure monitoring. The injection should be stopped as soon as the heart rate slows or if the blood pressure falls significantly. If excessive bradycardia occurs, 0.5 to 1 mg atropine can be given IV. If the tachycardia continues, a second dose of propranolol may be repeated after 2 or more min. If this is not effective, no further propranolol should be given within 4 hours.

6. Methoxamine (Vasoxyl), metaraminol (Aramine), phenylephrine (Neo-Synephrine), levarterenol (Levophed), and other vasopressor drugs have also been used to treat PAT. They produce a sudden increase in blood pressure to 160 mm Hg or higher, which stimulates the vagal fibers in the carotid sinus and aortic arch, thus stopping the tachycardia. They should not be used in patients with hypertension, severe organic heart disease, or hyperthyroidism, or when a rise in blood pressure may be dangerous.

Phenylephrine hydrochloride in a dose of 0.5 to 1 mg (0.25 to 0.5 ml of a 0.2% solution) or metaraminol in a dose of 0.5

to 2.0 mg (0.05 to 0.2 ml) can be injected IV over a period of 2 to 3 min. These drugs should be diluted with 10 ml of 5% dextrose in water to prevent an excessive rate of administration. The blood pressure should be monitored and the injection stopped if the blood pressure rises above 160 mm Hg.

7. Synchronized precordial DC shock can be given if drug therapy is not effective (Chapter 18). However, if the patient has been taking digitalis or has received digoxin or deslanoside to stop the tachycardia, the DC shock should be withheld at least 24 hours.

8. Transvenous cardiac pacing can also be done to control a paroxysmal atrial tachyarrhythmia (Chapter 16).

Nonemergency treatment. If the patient's clinical condition is stable or if there is a history of repeated attacks of paroxysmal tachycardia, the emergency treatment described above can be done. However, the following simple treatment is often also successful.

The patient can often stop the paroxysmal tachycardia by using one of the following maneuvers, which increases vagal tone.

1. Arching the head backward as far as possible.

2. Blowing into a toy balloon, particularly one that is difficult to expand.

3. Performing Valsalva's maneuver (attempted forced inspiration with the glottis closed) or Müller's maneuver (attempted forced expiration with the glottis closed), or changing the posture by stooping or by bending the trunk.

4. Attempting to vomit by putting a finger deep in the throat or by inducing vomiting by taking Ipecac Syrup. The initial dose is 4 to 8 ml orally, repeated every hour until vomiting occurs. In some patients, the tachycardia may stop even before the vomiting occurs. Side effects such as weakness, sweating, decreased blood pressure, pallor, or diarrhea may occur but are not significant.

A sedative, such as diazepam (Valium), 5 to 10 mg orally, or phenobarbital, 60 to 100 mg orally, is also often effective.

Morphine sulfate, 15 mg given IM, may also stop the attack.

Prophylaxis. Every patient with repeated attacks of PAT or paroxysmal supraventricular tachyarrhythmia should receive thyroid function tests to determine if hyperthyroidism is present In addition, coffee, tea, and other caffeine-containing beverages should be stopped. The patient may require sedatives, maintenance doses of digitalis, with or without a cardiac-depressant drug such as quinidine or procainamide, or propranolol. Some patients may require a combination of digitalis, quinidine (or procainamide), and propranolol. When propranolol is used simultaneously with quinidine or with procainamide, smaller doses of each drug are required.

Multifocal atrial tachycardia

A major arrhythmia.

This type of supraventricular tachyarrhythmia has also been called repetitive multifocal paroxysmal atrial tachycardia or chaotic atrial tachycardia. In 1945 Dr. S. P. Schwartz and I described it as extrasystolic auricular tachycardia.

Electrocardiogram. The following signs are present (Fig. 6-4).

1. Two or more premature P waves with varying shapes and varying P-R intervals and with two or more different P-P cycles.

2. An atrial rate between 100 and 250 beats per min. However, the atrial rate is usually slower than in PAT.

3. An isoelectric line between the T-P intervals.

4. An irregular ventricular response because some of the premature P waves are blocked and are not followed by a QRS complex and T wave.

Clinical aspects. Multifocal atrial tachycardia does not occur normally. The most common underlying condition is hypoxia and chronic pulmonary disease, or conges-

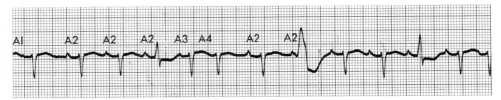

Fig. 6-4. Multifocal atrial tachycardia. *A1, A2, A3,* and *A4* show premature atrial contractions from varying foci. Notice that the fourth, eighth, and eleventh QRS complexes are aberrant.

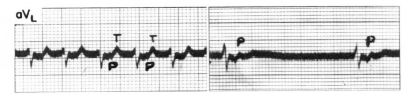

Fig. 6-5. Paroxysmal AV junctional tachycardia. **B,** Taken several hours after **A.** During the tachycardia it is difficult to see the AV junctional P waves.

tive heart failure. It may also occur as a result of digitalis toxicity or hypokelemia. Many of the patients are diabetic. It is often a precursor of atrial fibrillation or atrial flutter.

Treatment. No satisfactory treatment is available. Digitalis is usually not effective and may increase the atrial premature contractions. If the tachycardia is due to digitalis, potassium salts can be used. The cardiac-depressant drugs are also not effective. A patient with pulmonary disease should receive adequate oxygenation.

AV junctional tachycardia

A major arrhythmia.

AV junctional tachycardia consists of a succession of AV junctional premature contractions. Two types of AV junctional tachycardia have been described: paroxysmal and nonparoxysmal.

Paroxysmal AV junctional tachycardia

The etiology, clinical aspects, and treatment of paroxysmal AV junctional tachycardia are the same as in PAT. It is often very difficult to differentiate these two conditions unless atrial or AV junctional P waves are clearly visible (Fig. 6-5). When

P waves are not obvious, the term supraventricular tachycardia can be used to describe the ECG.

Nonparoxysmal AV junctional tachycardia

The heart rate is only moderately accelerated to approximately 70 to 130 beats per min (Figs. 6-6 and 6-7). The tachycardia does not show the abrupt onset and termination that is characteristic of paroxysmal AV junctional or atrial tachycardia.

Common causes of nonparoxysmal AV junctional tachycardia are digitalis toxicity, myocarditis due to acute rheumatic fever or other causes, and acute inferior myocardial infarction. Less common causes are open heart surgery, hypertensive heart disease, and congenital heart disease, especially Ebstein's disease.

When nonparoxysmal AV junctional tachycardia occurs as a result of digitalis toxicity, the underlying atrial rhythm is almost always atrial fibrillation (Fig. 6-7).

Emergency treatment. If the patient with nonparoxysmal AV junctional tachycardia is taking digitalis, it should be stopped immediately. If the tachycardia

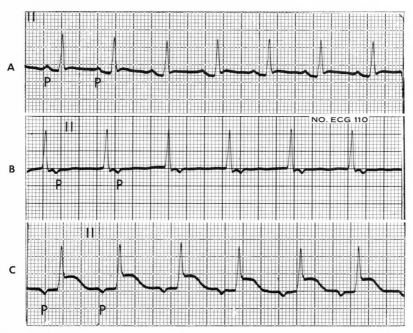

Fig. 6-6. Nonparoxysmal AV junctional tachycardia in a patient with acute inferior wall myo-cardial infarction and cardiogenic shock. **A, B,** and **C,** Taken a few minutes apart. **A,** Sinus rhythm with a rate of approximately 95 per min. **B,** Nonparoxysmal AV junctional tachycardia has developed. The heart rate has slowed slightly to 88 per min. Notice the AV junctional P waves after the QRS complexes. **C,** Heart rate is unchanged. However, the AV junctional P waves are now in front of the QRS complexes (with a prolonged P-R interval of 0.2 sec). Notice the marked RS-T elevations, due to the acute myocardial infarction, that have developed.

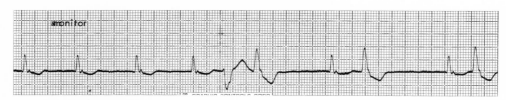

Fig. 6-7. Nonparoxysmal AV junctional tachycardia due to digitalis toxicity. The ventricular rate is 75 per min. The basic rhythm is atrial fibrillation. Ventricular premature contractions, pro-ducing a bigeminal rhythm, and bidirectional ventricular premature contractions, due to digitalis toxicity, are also present.

continues and the patient's clinical condi-tion worsens (from congestive heart fail-ure, for example) diphenylhydantoin can be used to slow the ventricular rate.

No treatment is usually indicated for nonparoxysmal AV junctional tachycardia due to other causes. However, quinidine,

procainamide, or propranolol can be used, if necessary, to slow the heart rate.

Atrial flutter and atrial fibrillation

Atrial flutter and atrial fibrillation can be considered variants of the same phe-nomenon; namely, an atrial tachyarrhy-

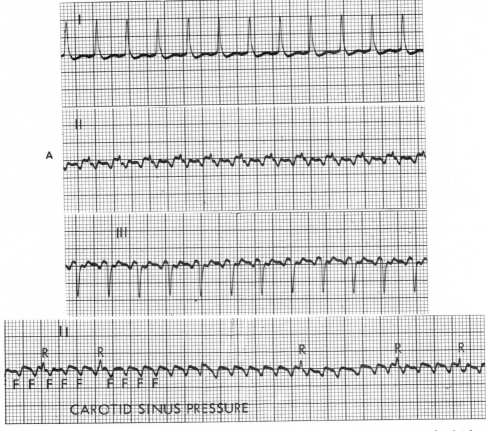

Fig. 6-8. Atrial flutter. **A,** Leads I, II, and III. The flutter waves are not apparent in lead I but are obvious in leads II and III. **B,** Carotid sinus pressure slowed the ventricular rate but did not change the atrial flutter rate.

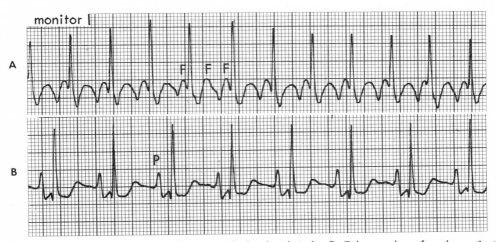

Fig. 6-9. Atrial flutter converted to sinus rhythm by digitalis. **B,** Taken a day after the patient had been fully digitalized orally.

thmia. The major difference between the two conditions is that in atrial flutter the stimulus spreads through the atria at a slower rate and through a more regular path than in atrial fibrillation. When atrial flutter is present, the atrial rate is usually between 200 and 300 per min. When the atrial rate exceeds 380 to 400 per min, the stimulus spreads irregularly through the atria, and atrial fibrillation results.

Atrial flutter or atrial fibrillation can be described as paroxysmal or chronic, depending on whether it has been present for less or more than 2 weeks.

Atrial flutter

A major arrhythmia.

Electrocardiogram. The atrial flutter (F) waves show the following characteristics.

1. One complete flutter cycle consists of an upward wave followed by a downward wave or vice versa (Figs. 6-8 and 6-9). The peak and nadir of the F wave may be sharp, rounded, or notched. In precordial leads V_1 and V_2 and in the esophageal leads the F waves may resemble large biphasic P waves. Some leads show the F waves better than others, depending on the direction in which the stimulus spreads through the atria. The downward deflections of the F waves are often marked in leads II, III, and aV_F (suggesting that atrial flutter may be a variant of an AV junctional tachycardia). Lead I usually does not show the F waves clearly.

2. A continuous sequence of F waves occurs, often producing a sawtooth effect. The F waves become distorted where they are superimposed on the QRS, RS-T, and T.

There is no isoelectric period between the F waves. This differentiates atrial flutter from PAT with block (p. 89).

3. The rate at which the atria flutter varies from approximately 200 to 380 or 400 per min, with an average rate of 300 per min. Quinidine or procainamide may slow the atrial flutter rate to below 200 per

min, and in addition, may make the F waves slower and blunter.

The atrial flutter rate in any one patient is very constant even over a long period of time. (The flutter rate is measured from the interval between the peaks of any two successive F waves; p. 230.)

4. Although the AV node can occasionally respond to stimuli as rapid as 300 per min, producing a 1:1 atrial flutter, some degree of AV block is usually present. Thus, if the atria are fluttering at a rate of 300 per min and every other stimulus that reaches the AV node is blocked, the ventricules beat at a regular rate of 150 per min (2:1 atrial flutter).

5. Although it is not possible to describe a P-R interval in a case of atrial flutter, the QRS complexes usually have a fixed relation to the peaks of the F waves throughout the ECG, in association with a regular ventricular rate Occasionally, the ventricles do not respond regularly to the F waves, and slight irregularity of the ventricular rhythm occurs. When the ventricular rate is rapid, it may be impossible to recognize the F waves, and the ECG must be described merely as supraventricular tachyarrhythmia.

6. Vagal stimulation by means of carotid sinus pressure and so on tends to aggravate the degree of AV block so that transient slowing of the ventricles occurs, but the atrial flutter rate remains unchanged (Fig. 6-8). Rarely, carotid sinus pressure increases the atrial rate so that transient atrial fibrillation occurs. (One must remember that carotid sinus pressure may be dangerous in a patient with coronary artery disease or in a fully digitalized patient; p. 8).

7. The ventricular rate may be used as a means of differential diagnosis. Since the atrial rate in most cases of atrial flutter is approximately 200 to 360 per minute and since there is usually some degree of AV block present, the ventricular rate is usually 160 per min or less. Therefore, a ven-

tricular rate of 200 indicates that the atria are fluttering at a rate of 200 and that a 1:1 atrial flutter is present. Such a slow atrial flutter rate is very rare unless quinidine or procainamide has been given. Therefore, a ventricular rate of approximately 200 per min itself suggests that atrial flutter is not present.

Similarly, if a patient with atrial flutter is given light exercise, such as bending forward and backward or bending the knees, the ventricular rate may suddenly double rather than increase slightly. For example, if a 4:1 atrial flutter is present and the atrial rate is 300, the ventricular rate is 75 per min. Exercise may convert the rhythm to a 2:1 atrial flutter. Therefore, the ventricular rate will suddenly increase to 150 per min.

8. When paroxysmal atrial flutter with a 1:1 conduction occurs, the shape of the QRS complexes may become aberrant and may resemble the pattern of a ventricular tachycardia. It may be difficult and at times impossible to make a differential diagnosis when this occurs. However, the ventricular rate in a 1:1 atrial flutter is faster than 250 beats per min, whereas the ventricular rate in a ventricular tachycardia is seldom faster than 200 per min and does not exceed 250 per min.

Carotid sinus pressure can be used if a 1:1 atrial flutter is suspected. This will slow the ventricular rate of atrial flutter and will allow the F waves to become obvious. It will not slow the ventricular rate of a ventricular tachycardia.

Etiology. Atrial flutter rarely occurs normally. It usually occurs in abnormal conditions, such as acute or chronic pulmonary disease, acute myocardial infarction, pericarditis, myocarditis, trauma to the heart, hyperthyroidism, and rheumatic heart disease, particularly mitral stenosis. Drugs such as quinidine or procainamide may produce atrial flutter when given to a patient with atrial fibrillation (see below). Digitalis rarely causes atrial flutter.

Clinical aspects. The symptoms of atrial flutter depend on the ventricular rate. When a 1:1 atrial flutter occurs, the ventricular rate may be almost 300 per min. When a 2:1 atrial flutter is present, the ventricular rate may be 150 per min or faster. Under these circumstances, the clinical picture is that of a supraventricular tachyarrhythmia. When the ventricular rate is slow, the patient may not even be aware of the arrhythmia. Usually some degree of AV block is present, and the ventricular rate is usually between 70 and 80 per min. The flutter waves may sometimes be visible in the neck veins. In addition, auscultation of the heart may reveal faint extra sounds due to the atrial flutter.

Treatment. The treatment of atrial flutter depends on the duration of the flutter, the underlying heart condition, and cardiovascular signs, such as rapid ventricular rate, hypotension, or congestive heart failure. The treatment of atrial flutter associated with acute myocardial infarction is described in Chapter 10.

Emergency treatment. Emergency treatment should be used when a rapid ventricular rate (150 per min or faster) is associated with decreased cardiac function, such as increasing congestive heart failure or decreasing blood pressure in a patient with severe organic heart disease.

1. Synchronized DC shock is the emergency treatment of choice. Practically all patients with atrial flutter respond to DC shock (Chapter 18). Usually a very low energy charge is needed (even 25 ws or less). If the patient reverts to atrial flutter after the DC shock, one can attempt to convert the rhythm to atrial fibrillation by giving a very low energy charge of 5 to 10 ws.

If one is planning to convert the atrial flutter with DC shock, one should not digitalize the patient. In addition, if the patient has been taking digitalis, it should be withheld, if possible, for at least 24 hours. (Also see Chapter 18.)

2. Digitalis is the second choice for the emergency treatment of atrial flutter. Digitalis increases the rate at which the atria flutter and therefore converts atrial flutter into atrial fibrillation. When this occurs, the digitalis should be stopped. The atrial fibrillation usually spontaneously disappears, and sinus rhythm reappears. This may take 1 to 2 days or even 1 week or longer. However, if atrial fibrillation is still present a week after the digitalis is stopped, a spontaneous change to sinus rhythm will probably not occur. In some patients, the atrial fibrillation reverts to atrial flutter when the digitalis is stopped. In other patients, the atrial fibrillation may revert to sinus rhythm even when a maintenance dose of digitalis is continued after the initial digitalization.

When digitalis is used for the emergency treatment of atrial flutter, a rapid-acting preparation such as deslanoside or digoxin should be given IV or IM. Enough digitalis should be given to convert the atrial flutter to atrial fibrillation and to slow the ventricular rate to approximately 70 per min. This often requires even 2 or more times the usual digitalizing doses, even when the patient has been taking digitalis. However, if the patient has severe organic heart disease or has hypokalemia, hyponatremia, or hypercalcemia, such large digitalis doses may be dangerous.

The digitalis is then stopped for 48 hours. If sinus rhythm has not yet appeared, the patient should be placed on an oral maintenance dose of digitalis, and nonemergency treatment should be continued with quinidine, procainamide, or a combination of quinidine and propranolol (see below).

3. Right atrial pacing with a transvenous cardiac pacemaker has also been used to convert atrial flutter to sinus rhythm (p. 224).

Nonemergency treatment. Atrial flutter in all patients should be converted to sinus rhythm, if possible (unless the atrial flutter has been present for years), because the ventricular rate tends to be unstable and tends to increase abruptly with exercise, as was mentioned above.

If the ventricular rate is below 100 per min and the patient does not show signs of acute congestive heart failure or hypotension, the following nonemergency treatment can be given.

1. Digitalis can be given orally, rather than parenterally, to convert the rhythm to atrial fibrillation and to slow the ventricular rate to approximately 70 per min.

2. If sinus rhythm has not reappeared 48 hours after the digitalis has been stopped, the patient should be given a maintenance dose of oral digitalis, and quinidine should also be given orally. Quinidine acts by slowing the rate at which the atria flutter. It therefore restores sinus rhythm. Occasionally, it merely produces a slow atrial flutter and a slow ventricular rate without restoring sinus rhythm. This is the reason that quinidine therapy of atrial flutter should be monitored electrocardiographically.

Quinidine often transiently increases the ventricular rate when given to a patient with either atrial flutter or atrial fibrillation. This can occur in two ways. First, quinidine has a vagolytic effect on the AV node and in this way allows more stimuli to penetrate the AV node and to reach the ventricles. Second, quinidine slows the atrial flutter rate. For example, if the patient has a 4:1 atrial flutter with a flutter rate of 360 per min, the ventricular rate is 90 per min. If quinidine reduces the atrial rate to 300 per min and decreases the AV block so that a 2:1 atrial flutter results, the ventricular rate may transiently increase to 150 per min. Therefore, quinidine must always be given in combination with digitalis (or propranolol) when used to treat atrial flutter. The digitalis (or the propranolol) acts to maintain a high degree of AV block.

3. Procainamide can be used instead

of quinidine if the patient is sensitive to quinidine. However, it is much less effective than quinidine in converting atrial flutter to sinus rhythm.

4. Propranolol can be used to increase the degree of AV block and slow the ventricular rate when atrial flutter is present. By itself, it rarely is successful in restoring sinus rhythm. However, it can be given instead of quinidine after the patient has been digitalized, or it can be given in combination with quinidine after the patient has been digitalized. When this is done, smaller doses of both propranolol and quinidine are needed. (Since propranolol can precipitate or aggravate congestive heart failure, the patient should be digitalized before it is used to treat atrial flutter.)

Prophylaxis. If sinus rhythm has been restored by digitalis, the patient should be given digitalis orally. If digitalis and quinidine have been required to restore sinus rhythm, a maintenance dose of both drugs should be used to prevent further attacks of paroxysmal atrial flutter. Some patients may require a combination of digitalis, quinidine, and propranolol. If synchronized DC shock or right atrial pacing has been used, maintenance doses of digitalis or quinidine or both may also be necessary.

The duration of maintenance therapy depends on the condition that precipitated the atrial flutter and the severity of the cardiovascular signs that occurred with the atrial flutter. I believe that maintenance therapy should be continued for a minimum of 3 months after sinus rhythm is restored. When atrial flutter is associated with an acute condition, such as acute pulmonary disease or acute myocardial infarction, prophylactic treatment may not be needed after sinus rhythm has been restored

Atrial fibrillation

A major arrhythmia.

When atrial fibrillation is present, the normal atrial contractions are replaced by a continuous series of rapid, irregular, fibrillatory *(f)* waves at a rate of 380 to 600 or more per min. These waves are ineffective in emptying the atria so that functionally the atria remain in diastole.

Electrocardiogram. The *f* waves show the following characteristics.

1. They appear as fine, irregular undulations on the tracing (Figs. 6-10 and 6-11). In precordial leads near the sternum, in esophageal leads, and in lead S_5 (p. 73) large biphasic *f* waves may appear.

2. The *f* waves are continuous, and when they are superimposed on the RS-T and T, they can distort the shape of the RS-T and T.

3. The rate of the *f* waves varies from 380 to 600 or more per min. The average rate is approximately 450 per min. (The fibrillation rate is measured from the interval between the peaks of two successive *f* waves; p. 230.)

4. Marked irregularity in the size and

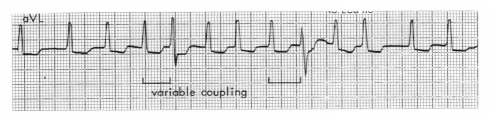

Fig. 6-10. Atrial fibrillation with aberration of QRS complexes. The fifth and ninth QRS complexes are aberrant. Notice the variable coupling between these QRS complexes and the preceding QRS.

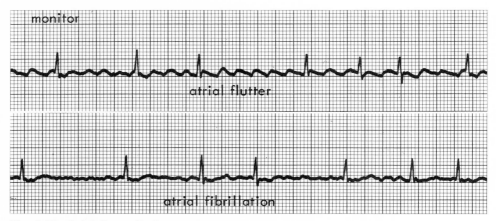

Fig. 6-11. Atrial flutter–fibrillation. The upper and lower rows are part of a continuous strip. The interval between them is approximately 5 sec.

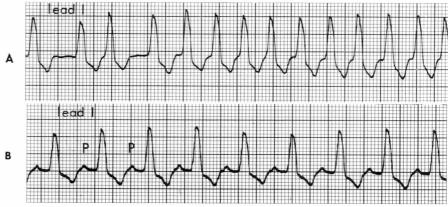

Fig. 6-12. Paroxysmal atrial fibrillation in a patient with left bundle branch block. **A,** Atrial fibrillation at a rate of approximately 160 per min. It is difficult to see the f waves. The widened QRS complexes (due to the left bundle branch block) make the tracing resemble a ventricular tachycardia. **B,** Taken 2 hours after the patient received 0.5 mg digoxin orally. Sinus rhythm has now appeared. The QRS complexes are typical of left bundle branch block.

shape of the f waves occurs from moment to moment.

The fibrillatory waves have been divided into coarse f waves (amplitude greater than 0.5 mm in lead V_1) or fine f waves (amplitude less than 0.5 mm in lead V_1). It has been stated that coarse f waves occur characteristically in rheumatic heart disease but that fine f waves occur characteristically in coronary artery disease. However, this is not an absolute differentiation.

In addition, digitalis increases the rate at which the atria fibrillate and in this way produces very fine f waves that sometimes are difficult to see.

When the atria are fibrillating at a relatively slow rate, the f waves tend to resemble the F waves of atrial flutter. When this happens, the tracing can be called coarse atrial fibrillation, impure atrial fibrillation, or flutter-fibrillation (Fig. 6-11).

5. Aberration of the QRS complexes

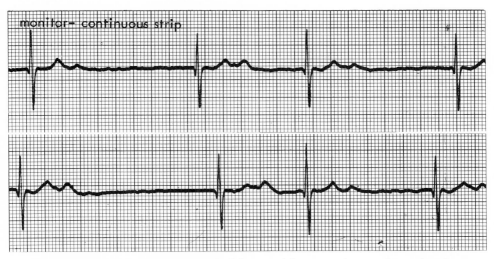

Fig. 6-13. Atrial fibrillation with marked slowing of the ventricular rate due to digitalis.

may occur when the ventricular rate is rapid, especially when it reaches and exceeds 200 per min and when a long R-R interval occurs before a short R-R interval (long cycle–short cycle phenomenon) (Fig. 6-10). (Also see p. 95.) The aberrant QRS complexes usually show a right bundle branch block type of pattern (Gouaux-Ashman phenomenon).

6. The ventricular rate in paroxysmal atrial fibrillation is often faster than 150 per min. When this occurs, it may be difficult to recognize the *f* waves, (Fig. 6-12). Such a tracing can therefore be described merely as a supraventricular tachyarrhythmia.

When chronic atrial fibrillation is present, the ventricular rate is often slower than 100 per min, even without medication.

7. The ventricular rate is also usually totally irregular because many of the atrial stimuli are blocked at the AV node or are too weak to penetrate it. In addition, ventricular premature contractions may be present. When the patient is digitalized, the ventricular rate becomes slower and more regular. (A regular ventricular rate between 70 and 100 per min or faster in a patient with atrial fibrillation who is receiving digitalis may indicate a nonparoxysmal AV junctional tachycardia due to digitalis toxicity; see p. 77.)

8. Digitalis can also cause marked slowing of the ventricular rate in a patient with atrial fibrillation (Fig. 6-13) and can produce a bradyarrhythmia similar to complete AV block (Fig. 6-14).

Etiology. Atrial fibrillation is one of the most common cardiac arrhythmias. It may occur in otherwise normal persons. However, it is also common in hypertensive or coronary artery disease, acute myocardial infarction; rheumatic heart disease, particularly mitral insufficiency or mitral stenosis; hyperthyroidism; and constrictive pericarditis. It can occur after cardiac surgery, especially after mitral valve surgery, or after trauma to the heart or to the head, and it may be precipitated by severe physical exertion or emotional excitement. It is rarely due to digitalis toxicity. However, sympathomimetic drugs can precipitate it.

Paroxysmal atrial fibrillation (less than 2 weeks' duration) is common in hyperthyroidism, the Wolff-Parkinson-White syndrome, and acute myocardial infarction.

Chronic atrial fibrillation (more than 2

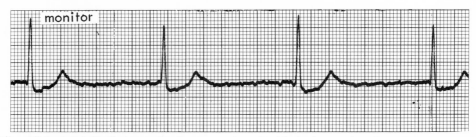

Fig. 6-14. Atrial fibrillation with almost complete AV block due to digitalis. (There are slight variations in the ventricular rate.)

weeks' duration) is common in rheumatic heart disease or in hypertensive heart disease (particularly in elderly patients). Hyperthyroidism may also produce chronic atrial fibrillation.

Atrial fibrillation may be precipitated by atrial premature contractions. A prolonged P-R interval also predisposes to it.

Clinical aspects. The patient's symptoms depend on the ventricular rate. When paroxysmal atrial fibrillation occurs with a ventricular rate above 150 per min, a patient may develop congestive heart failure or angina. Atrial fibrillation often produces congestive heart failure even in a normal person. The reason for this is that the loss of atrial systole decreases the cardiac output 25% to 33% or more. When the ventricular rate is slow, the patient may be unaware of the arrhythmia.

There is usually complete irregularity of the rate, rhythm and force of the heartbeat, which is easily determined by palpation of the radial artery. When the ventricular rate is rapid, many of the ventricular beats may be too weak to open the aortic valve so that the radial artery pulse may be much slower than the apical heart rate (pulse deficit). This is the reason that the ventricular rate of a patient with atrial fibrillation must always be determined by auscultation of the cardiac apex.

Patients with atrial fibrillation may be very sensitive to carotid sinus pressure, which may produce syncope.

Thrombosis in the right or left atrial appendage often occurs in patients with chronic atrial fibrillation due to stasis of blood caused by the lack of atrial contractions or due to actual myocarditis of the atria in rheumatic heart disease. Small fragments of such thrombi may break off and embolize from the left atrium to the systemic circulation or from the right atrium to the lungs and can produce serious and even lethal embolization. These emboli may first appear shortly after the atrial fibrillation has been converted to sinus rhythm (due to the forceful atrial contractions that occur). This is one of the reasons that patients with chronic atrial fibrillation must receive anticoagulation therapy before conversion to sinus rhythm is attempted either with quinidine or with synchronized DC shock (Chapter 18). However, emboli from thrombi in the atrial appendages often occur while atrial fibrillation is present. Such patients may be benefited by restoration of sinus rhythm.

Treatment. The treatment of atrial fibrillation depends on the duration of the atrial fibrillation, the ventricular rate, the etiology, and cardiovascular signs such as congestive heart failure, angina, and hypotension.

Emergency treatment. The goal of emergency treatment is to slow a rapid ventricular rate and to treat congestive heart failure, if present.

The treatment of paroxysmal atrial fibrillation associated with acute myocardial infarction is described in Chapter 10.

1. Digitalis is the drug of choice for the emergency treatment of atrial fibrillation. It slows the ventricular rate by increasing the degree of AV block. (It can also produce complete AV block as a toxic sign.) It also slows the ventricular rate indirectly by its positive inotropic effect on the heart muscle. The goal of digitalis treatment of atrial fibrillation is to slow the ventricular rate to approximately 60 to 80 per min. If the ventricular rate is slowed to below 60 per min, a decrease in cardiac output may develop. One should remember that if the atrial fibrillation is due to hyperthyroidism, digitalis may not be able to slow the ventricular rate below 100 per min until the hyperthyroidism is treated.

Digitalization should be done with a rapid-acting digitalis preparation such as deslanoside or digoxin given IV or IM. If the clinical condition is not too serious, the patient can be digitalized orally.

Some patients with paroxysmal atrial fibrillation will respond to digitalization with the reappearance of sinus rhythm. Most patients will respond with the persistence of the atrial fibrillation but with a slower ventricular rate.

2. DC shock can be used if digitalization is contraindicated (Chapter 18).

Nonemergency treatment. It is not always necessary to treat atrial fibrillation. For example, treatment is unnecessary if the ventricular rate is between 60 and 80 per min and does not increase above 90 per min with exercise.

1. If the patient does not show signs of acute severe congestive heart failure or if the ventricular rate is approximately 100 per min, the patient can be digitalized over a period of several days with oral doses of digitalis.

2. Combined quinidine and digitalis therapy can be given. When digitalization slows the ventricular rate but the atrial fibrillation persists, it may be desirable to try to convert the atrial fibrillation to sinus rhythm. This can be done with administra-

tion of either quinidine or DC shock (Chapter 18). Either of these procedures may be successful. However, it is important to decide whether the patient will benefit from restoration of sinus rhythm. The indications and contraindications for conversion of atrial fibrillation to sinus rhythm are discussed in Chapter 18.

If quinidine is used to convert the atrial fibrillation to sinus rhythm, it must be used in combination with digitalis for reasons already discussed (p. 82).

In addition, if atrial fibrillation has been present for more than 1 month, the patient must receive anticoagulation therapy before quinidine or DC shock is used (p. 250).

3. If signs of digitalis toxicity appear before the ventricular rate slows, propranolol can be given orally in combination with the digitalis to increase the AV block and to further slow the ventricular rate. Propranolol can also be used in combination with quinidine to try to restore sinus rhythm after the ventricular rate has been slowed by digitalis and while the patient is maintained on digitalis.

4. Procainamide can be given to treat atrial fibrillation. (See the treatment of atrial flutter above.)

Prophylaxis. When atrial fibrillation has been converted to sinus rhythm, the patient should be given quinidine, or quinidine plus propranolol, indefinitely, to maintain the sinus rhythm (unless toxicity to the drug [or drugs] occurs). Propranolol alone should not be used. If the patient has congestive heart failure, digitalis should also be given.

Paroxysmal atrial tachycardia with AV block (PAT with block)

A major arrhythmia.

The relationship between PAT with block and organic heart disease has been known for some time. More recently, Barker, Lown and Levine, and others have stressed its relation to digitalis toxicity.

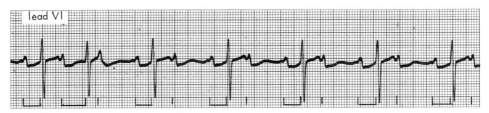

Fig. 6-15. PAT with block, due to digitalis. Lead VI was taken at two times normal standardization to accentuate the P waves. The first part of the strip shows a Wenckebach type of AV block. This changes to a 2:1 AV block. The diagrams below the ECG indicate the P waves and the P-R intervals.

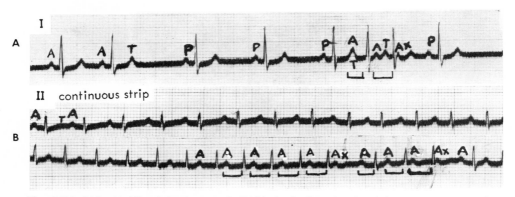

Fig. 6-16. PAT with Wenckebach type of AV block. **A,** Occasional atrial premature contractions *(A)*. At the end of the strip, three atrial premature contractions occur with progressive prolongation of the P-R interval, until the third atrial premature contraction is blocked *(Ax)*. **B,** An attack of PAT in the same patient. In the lower row, the P-R intervals progressively prolong until an atrial premature contraction is blocked *(Ax)*, producing an irregular ventricular rate. The patient had not received digitalis. The diagrams indicate the P-R intervals.

However, only about 10% of digitalis-induced arrhythmias show PAT with block.

Electrocardiogram

1. The atrial rate is usually between 150 and 200 per min. Rarely, it is faster or slower.

2. AV block is present (Fig. 6-15). It may be the Wenckebach type of AV block (Figs. 6-16 to 6-17), or it may be the Mobitz type II AV block. A 2:1 type of AV block is usually present (Fig. 6-15). In other patients complete AV block may occur transiently or chronically.

3. The baseline between the P waves is isoelectric.

4. Vagal stimulation will aggravate the degree of AV block.

5. The interval between successive P waves is often not constant and may vary by as much as 0.12 sec.

6. Occasionally, a double atrial tachycardia is present rather than the usual type of PAT with block described above. In these patients one pacemaker in the atria stimulates the atria. The other pacemaker in the AV junction stimulates the ventricles.

7. The P waves are usually upward in leads II, III, and aV_F (rarely downward in these leads). They are often very small and may not be visible in the limb leads. However, they can be seen in lead V_1, lead V_2, the esophageal leads, or lead S_5 (p. 73).

Etiology. PAT with a Wenckebach type

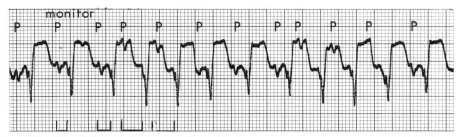

Fig. 6-17. PAT with Wenckebach type of AV block in a patient with acute myocardial infarction. The diagrams below the ECG show the progressive prolongation of the P-R interval. The ventricular rate is irregular and varies from 135 to 160 per min.

Table 1. Differentiation between PAT with block and atrial flutter*

Clinical aspects	PAT with block	Atrial flutter
Atrial rate	Usually 150 to 200 per min.	Usually faster than 200 per min
P wave shape (leads II, III, aV$_F$)	Usually upward	Downward
P-P baseline	Isoelectric	Undulating
P-P interval	Regular or irregular	Regular
A-V relationship	Variable	Regular (2:1, 3:1, 4:1, and so on) AV conduction
Carotid sinus pressure	AV block more severe	AV block more severe
Onset and offset	Gradual	Abrupt
Potassium chloride administration	Restores sinus rhythm	Has no effect

*Adapted from Lown B, Levine HD: Atrial arrhythmias, digitalis, and potassium, New York, 1958, Landberger Medical Books, Inc, and from Rosner, SW: Circulation **29:**614, 1964.

of AV block can occur in normal persons. However, PAT with a Mobitz type II AV block rarely if ever occurs normally. Either type can be produced by digitalis, particularly if there is associated potassium depletion (due to diuretics, vomiting, diarrhea, and so on) even when the serum potassium concentration is normal. Quinidine, atropine, or isoproterenol can also cause it. It also occurs in association with acute myocardial infarction, acute or chronic pulmonary disease, rheumatic heart disease, and hypertensive heart disease, and particularly if there is potassium depletion.

Clinical aspects. PAT with block is often serious, regardless of whether or not is it due to digitalis toxicity, because many of the patients have severe organic heart disease. It may occur transiently, or it may be present for months or years. Digitalis

may cause PAT with either the Wenckebach or the Mobitz type II AV block. When PAT with block is produced by digitalis toxicity, other signs of the digitalis toxicity, such as ventricular premature contractions, may also be present.

The differential diagnosis between patients with PAT with block, and those with atrial flutter is sometimes difficult. Table 1 shows some of the differences between the two conditions. PAT with block can also be confused with sinus tachycardia because the small P waves may be overlooked (Fig. 6-18).

Treatment

Emergency treatment. Since the ventricular rate in PAT with block is usually relatively slow because of the AV block, this arrhythmia usually does not cause severe

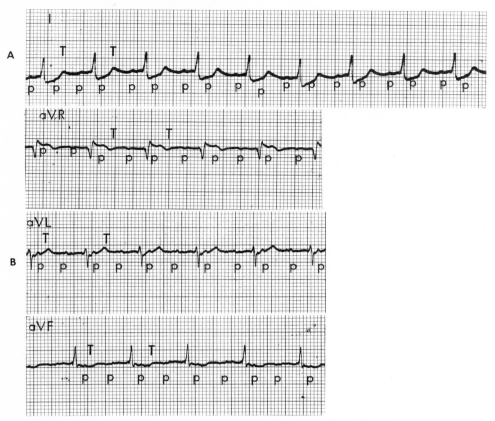

Fig. 6-18. PAT with block, not related to digitalis. **A** and **B** taken a week apart on the same patient. Both show PAT with block with a 2:1 AV block. **A,** Atrial rate is approximately 215 per min. **B,** Atrial rate has slowed to 185 per min.

disturbances in cardiovascular function. Therefore, emergency treatment is not generally indicated. However, if the tachycardia is due to digitalis toxicity, if the ventricular rate is rapid (140 per min or faster), or if the patient shows signs of severe congestive heart failure or shock (regardless of whether digitalis toxicity is the cause of the tachycardia), emergency treatment should be given.

PAT with block is most effectively and safely treated if the arrhythmia is divided into two groups: (1) digitalis-induced and (2) non–digitalis-induced. When there is doubt about the cause of PAT with block, always assume that digitalis toxicity is present, and treat accordingly.

Digitalis-induced PAT with block should be treated as follows.

1. Digitalis must be stopped immediately.

2. Potassium chloride is the drug of choice for the emergency treatment of PAT with block due to digitalis toxicity. (It is not effective in PAT with block due to other conditions.) Potassium chloride should preferably be given orally. A dose of 5 gm (67 mEq) potassium chloride, mixed with orange juice, can be given over a 30-min period. If sinus rhythm does not reappear in 2 hours, another 2.5 gm (33.5 mEq) can be given.

When the potassium chloride is effective, a 1:1 atrial tachycardia may develop before sinus rhythm reappears. The rapid ventricular rate associated with this 1:1 atrial tachycardia may aggravate congestive heart failure. However, this rapid heart rate is transient and will disappear when the patient is given more potassium chloride.

If the patient appears to be critically ill and if potassium is not contraindicated (see below), potassium chloride should be given IV rather than orally. Three gm (40 mEq) potassium chloride are dissolved in 500 ml 5% dextrose in water and infused in approximately 2 hours. The patient must be monitored with ECGs, and the infusion should be stopped if signs of potassium toxicity, such as peaking or tenting of the T waves, occur. If sinus rhythm does not reappear when the infusion is completed, another 3 gm (40 mEq) potassium should be infused.

Potassium toxicity can be treated by an IV infusion of 50 ml 50% dextrose with 5 units of regular insulin or by IV administration of sodium bicarbonate. This must be done with electrocardiographic monitoring.

3. Procainamide (Pronestyl) can be used if potassium chloride is contraindicated; for example, if uremia is present, if the ECG shows signs of hyperkalemia, or if hyperkalemia is present. Procainamide can also be used when a large amount of potassium chloride has been given without results. Procainamide can also be used in combination with potassium chloride if hyperkalemia is not present.

4. Diphenylhydantoin (Dilantin) can also be used. IV doses of 50 mg per min are given until a total dose of 100 to 250 mg is reached.

5. Propranolol (Inderal) can also be used. It can be given orally or IV. However, one should remember that propranolol has a negative inotropic effect and can aggravate congestive heart failure.

6. Quinidine can also be given orally.

Non–digitalis-induced PAT with block should be treated as follows.

1. Rapid digitalization (orally or parenterally) is the treatment of choice if the PAT with block is *not* due to digitalis toxicity. However, one should remember that if renal insufficiency is present, the digitalis may not be eliminated for 7 or more days, even when a rapid-acting digitalis preparation has been used.

2. Procainamide, propranolol, or quinidine may be tried if digitalis fails to convert the PAT with block to sinus rhythm.

Prophylaxis. If the patient has been taking a diuretic such as the mercurials, the thiazides, furosemide (Lasix), or ethacrynic acid (Edecrin), which depletes the body of potassium ions, the diuretic should be changed to a potassium-sparing diuretic, such as spironolactone (Aldactone) or triamterene (Dyrenium). However, if this is done, supplemental potassium chloride cannot be given.

If digitalis is needed for congestive heart failure, the smallest possible effective doses should be used after the PAT with block disappears.

REFERENCES
Paroxysmal atrial and AV junctional tachycardia

Barrow JG: Treatment of paroxysmal supraventricular tachycardia with lanatoside C, Ann Intern Med **32**:116, 1950.

Berger AJ, Rackliffe RL: Treatment of paroxysmal supraventricular tachycardia with methoxamine, JAMA **152**:1132, 1953.

Bernstein H: Treatment of paroxysmal supraventricular tachycardia with Neo-Synephrine, N Y State J Med **56**:2570, 1956.

Boyd LJ, Scherf D: Magnesium sulfate in paroxysmal tachycardia, Am J Med Sci **206**:43, 1943.

Cantwell JD, Dawson JE, Fletcher GF: Supraventricular tachyarrhythmias; treatment with edrophonium Arch Intern Med **130**:221, 1972.

Chung EK: Appraisal of multifocal atrial tachycardia, Br Heart J **33**:500, 1971.

Conkle DM, Hannah HH, Reis RL: Effects of tachycardia on the function of the Starr-Edwards mitral ball valve prosthesis, Am J Cardiol **31**:105, 1973.

Dolara A, Possi L: Persistent supraventricular tachycardia, Am J Cardiol **16**:449, 1965.

Dreifus LS, Rabbino MD, Watanabe Y: Newer agents in the treatment of cardiac arrhythmias, Med Clin North Am **48**:371, 1964.

Durham JR: Severe reaction to methoxamine hydrochloride; report of a case occurring during treatment of paroxysmal supraventricular tachycardia, JAMA 167:1835, 1958.

El Etr AA: Pharyngeal stimulation in treatment of arrhythmias, Letter, JAMA 204:740, 1968.

Furman RH, Geiger AJ: Use of cholinergic drugs in paroxysmal supraventricular tachycardia; serious untoward reactions and fatality from treatment with methacholine and neostigmine, JAMA 149:269, 1952.

Gold H, Corday E: Vasopressor therapy in the cardiac arrhythmias, N Engl J Med 260:1151, 1959.

Goldberger E, Schwartz SP: Extrasystolic auricular tachycardia, N Y State J Med 45:1229, 1945.

Gould L, Zahir M, Shariff M, Giulani MG: Treatment of cardiac arrhythmias with phentolamine, Am Heart J 78:189, 1969.

Han J: The mechanism of paroxysmal atrial tachycardia, Am J. Cardiol 26:329, 1970.

Heyl AF: Auricular paroxysmal tachycardia caused by digitalis; report of case, Ann Intern Med 5:858, 1932.

Kistin AD: Problems in the differentiation of ventricular arrhythmias from supraventricular arrhythmias with abnormal QRS, Prog Cardiovasc Dis 9:1, 1966.

Klein H: Nonparoxysmal junctional tachycardia complicating acute myocardial infarction, Letter, Circulation 46:831, 1972.

Konecke LL, Knoebel SB: Nonparoxysmal junctional tachycardia complicating acute myocardial infarction, Circulation 45:367, 1972.

Langendorf R, Pick A, Winternitz M: Mechanisms of intermittent ventricular bigeminy; appearance of ectopic beats dependent upon length of ventricular cycle, "rule of bigeminy," Circulation 11:422, 1955.

Lian, et al: Intérêt de la dérivation précordiale auriculaire S5 dans le diagnostic des troubles du rhythm auriculaire, Arch Mal Coeur 45:481, 1952.

Lipson MJ, Naimi S: Multifocal atrial tachycardia (chaotic atrial tachycardia), Circulation 42:397, 1970.

Luria MH, et al: Paroxysmal tachycardia with polyuria, Ann Intern Med 65:461, 1966.

Marriott HJL: Differential diagnosis of supraventricular and ventricular tachycardia, Geriatrics 25:91, 1970.

Marriott HJL, Sandler IA: Criteria, old and new, for differentiating between ectopic ventricular beats and aberrant ventricular conduction in the presence of atrial fibrillation, Prog Cardiovasc Dis 9:18, 1966.

Massumi RA, Tawakkol AA, Kistin AD: Reevaluation of electrocardiographic and bedside criteria for diagnosis of ventricular tachycardia, Circulation 36:628, 1967.

Miller R, et al: Paroxysmal auricular tachycardia at a rate of 80 per minute, Am Heart J 35:134, 1948.

Rosen KM: Junctional tachycardia, Circulation 47:654, 1973.

Shine KI, Kastor JA, Yurchak PM: Multifocal atrial tachycardia; clinical and electrocardiographic features in 32 patients, N Engl J Med 279:344, 1968.

Ticzon AR, Whalen RW: Refractory supraventricular tachycardias, Circulation 47:642, 1973.

Waldman S, Pelner L: Action of neostigmine in supraventricular tachycardias, Am J Med 5:164, 1948.

Weiss S, Sprague HB: Vagal reflex irritability and treatment of paroxysmal auricular tachycardia with ipecac, Am J Med Sci 194:53, 1937.

Wolff L: Clinical manifestation of paroxysmal tachycardia; anginal pain, N Engl J Med 232:491, 1945.

Youmans WB, et al: Neo-Synephrine in treatment of paroxysmal supraventricular tachycardia, Am Heart J 37:359, 1949.

Zipes DP, Fisch C: Supraventricular arrhythmia with abnormal QRS complex, Arch Intern Med 130:129, 1972.

Atrial flutter and atrial fibrillation

Aberg H: Atrial fibrillation, Acta Med Scand 184:425, 1968.

Brest AN, Durge NG, Goldberg H: Conversion of atrial fibrillation to atrial flutter as a manifestation of digitalis toxicity, Am J Cardiol 6:682, 1960.

Cohen SI, et al: Concealed conduction during atrial fibrillation, Am J Cardiol 25:416, 1970.

Delman AJ, Stein E; Atrial flutter secondary to digitalis toxicity, Circulation 29:593, 1964.

Edmands RE, Greenspan K: Hemodynamic consequences of atrial fibrillation, Geriatrics 26:99, 1971.

Finkelstein F, and Gold H, Bellet S: Atrial flutter with 1:1 conduction, Am J Med 20:65, 1956.

Friedberg HD: Atrial fibrillation and digitalis toxicity, Am Heart J 77:429, 1969.

Goldberger E, Baer A: Observations on etiology and treatment of auricular flutter, Am Practit 2:124, 1951.

Gouaux JL, Ashman R: Auricular fibrillation with aberration simulating ventricular paroxysmal tachycardia, Am Heart J 34:366, 1947.

Haft JI, et al: Termination of atrial flutter by rapid electrical pacing of the atrium, Am J Cardiol 20:239, 1967.

James TN: Myocardial infarction and atrial arrhythmias, Circulation 24:761, 1961.

Jensen JB, et al: Electroshock for atrial flutter and atrial fibrillation, JAMA 194:1181, 1965.

Killip T, Gault JH: Mode of onset of atrial fibrillation, Am Heart J 70:172, 1965.

Lamb LE, Pollard LW: Atrial fibrillation in flying personnel, Circulation 29:694, 1964.

Peter RH, et al: A clinical profile of idiopathic atrial fibrillation, Ann Intern Med 68:1288, 1968.

Rabbino MD, Dreifus LS, Likoff W: Cardiac arrhythmias following intracardiac surgery, Am J Cardiol 7:681, 1961.

Soloff LA, Zatuchni J: The hyperactive carotid sinus reflex of the cardioinhibitory type in individuals with auricular fibrillation, Am J Med Sci 226:281, 1954.

Stern S: Conversion of chronic atrial fibrillation to sinus rhythm with combined propranolol and quinidine treatment, Am Heart J 74:170, 1967.

Thurmann M, Janney JG Jr: The diagnostic importance of fibrillatory wave size, Circulation 25:991, 1962.

Wessler S, Avioli LV: Propranolol therapy in patients with cardiac disease, JAMA 206:357, 1968.

Wilkand B, et al: Atrial fibrillation and flutter treated with synchronized DC shock; a study on immediate and long-term results, Acta Med Scand 182:665, 1967.

Zeft HJ, et al: Right atrial stimulation in the treatment of atrial flutter, Ann Intern Med 70:447, 1969.

Paroxysmal atrial tachycardia with AV block

Barker PS, Wilson FN, Johnson FD, Wishart SW: Auricular paroxysmal tachycardia with auriculoventricular block, Am Heart J 25:765, 1943.

Claiborne TS: Auricular tachycardia with auriculoventricular block of 12 years duration in a 16-year-old girl, Am Heart J 39:444, 1950.

Conn RD: Diphenylhydantoin sodium in cardiac arrhythmias, N Engl J Med 272:277, 1965.

Corwin ND, Klein MJ, Friedberg CK: Countershock conversion of digitalis-associated paroxysmal atrial tachycardia with block, Am Heart J 66:804, 1963.

Decherd GM Jr, Herrmann GR, Schwab EH: Paroxysmal supraventricular tachycardia with A-V block, Am Heart J 26:446, 1943.

El-Sharif N: Supraventricular tachycardia with A-V block, Brit Heart J 32:46, 1970.

Enselberg CC, Simmons HB, Mintz AA: The effects of potassium upon the heart, with special reference to the possibility of treatment of toxic arrhythmias due to digitalis, Am Heart J 39:713, 1950.

Freiermuth LJ, Jick S: Paroxysmal atrial tachycardia with atrioventricular block, Am J Cardiol 1:584, 1958.

Goldberg LM, et al: Paroxysmal atrial tachycardia with atrioventricular block, Circulation 21:449, 1960.

Lown B, Levine HD: Atrial arrhythmias, digitalis, and potassium, New York, 1958, Landberger Medical Books, Inc.

Lown B, Wyatt NF, Levine HD: Paroxysmal atrial tachycardia with block, Circulation 21:129, 1960.

Mark H, Shaw R: Non–digitalis-induced paroxysmal atrial tachycardia with block; management with cardioversion, J Electrocardiol 2:171, 1960.

Morgan W, Breneman G: Atrial tachycardia with block treated with digitalis, Circulation 25:787, 1962.

Rosner SW: Atrial tachysystole with block, Circulation 29:614, 1964.

Shmagranoff GL, Jick S: Simultaneous atrial and nodal tachycardia, Ann Heart J 54:417, 1957.

Spritz N, Frimpter GW, Braverman WS, Rubin AL: Persistent atrial tachycardia with atrioventricular block, Am J Med 24:442, 1958.

7 / Ventricular tachyarrhythmias

Ventricular tachyarrhythmias include ventricular premature contractions, ventricular tachycardia, ventricular flutter, and ventricular fibrillation.

VENTRICULAR PREMATURE CONTRACTIONS

A minor arrhythmia; may become major.

Ventricular premature contractions may arise in one of the branches of the bundle of His or in the Purkinje fibers of the ventricles.

Electrocardiogram. A ventricular premature contraction has the following characteristics.

1. The QRS complex is premature, is 0.12 sec or more wide, and is aberrant, notched, or slurred. It is associated with a T wave that usually points in a direction opposite to the main deflection of the QRS (Fig. 7-1).

2. The premature QRS is not preceded by a P wave.

3. Multiple ventricular premature contractions that arise from a single focus show a similar shape and coupling interval (distance from the preceding normal QRS) in any one lead (Fig. 7-1). (Also see parasystole, below.)

4. Occasionally, a ventricular premature contraction will occur simultaneously with the apex (or nadir) of the preceding T wave (R on T phenomenon) (Figs. 7-2 and 7-3). When this occurs, it may be a precursor of a ventricular tachycardia, particularly if the patient has an acute myo-

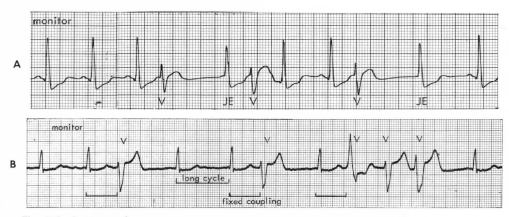

Fig. 7-1. A, Ventricular premature contractions *(V)* in a patient with acute myocardial infarction. The first ventricular premature contraction is followed by a very long pause and an AV junctional escape beat *(JE)*. The second ventricular premature contraction is followed by a very short pause. **B,** Ventricular premature contractions *(V)* in a patient with atrial fibrillation. The multiple premature ventricular contractions occur at the same time after a normal beat (fixed coupling).

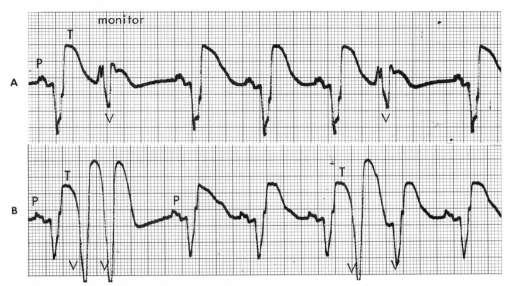

Fig. 7-2. Ventricular premature contractions in a patient with acute myocardial infarction. **A** and **B** taken a few seconds apart. **A,** Isolated ventricular premature contractions (V). **B,** Multiple ventricular premature contractions are present. The first ventricular premature contraction of each series occurs simultaneous with the apex of the preceding T wave (R on T phenomenon).

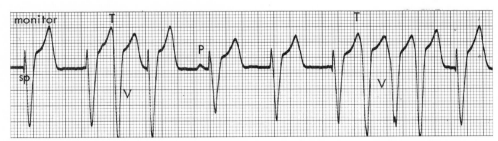

Fig. 7-3. Ventricular premature contractions (V) in a patient with a ventricular demand pacemaker. The first ventricular premature contraction occurs simultaneously with the apex of the preceding T wave (R on T phenomenon) but is merely followed by another pacemaker contraction. However, at the end of the strip the second ventricular premature contraction, which also occurs simultaneously with the apex of the preceding T wave, is followed by two more ventricular premature contractions. These ventricular premature contractions were suppressed with IV doses of lidocaine. In this ECG the pacemaker spikes (sp) are not visible in every pacemaker contraction. This often occurs in monitor leads.

cardial infarction. However, ventricular premature contractions may show an R on T pattern and may not be followed by a ventricular tachycardia. Conversely, ventricular tachycardia often starts with a ventricular premature contraction that does not show an R on T pattern.

A ventricular premature contraction is often followed by a fully compensatory pause (the sum of the R-R intervals immediately before and after the ventricular premature contraction equals the sum of two regular R-R intervals). However, this does not always occur and has no diagnostic significance.

5. The long cycle–short cycle phenome-

non may be present. When atrial fibrillation is present and the ventricular rate is irregular, a bigeminal rhythm may occasionally occur. This may be due to ventricular premature contractions or to normal beats with wide aberrant QRS complexes. The differentiation of these two conditions is described on p. 97.

6. A sinus or AV junctional P wave may or may not be present within the premature QRS complex.

Clinical aspects. Ventricular premature contractions are the most common cardiac arrhythmia. They frequently occur in normal persons. They can be produced by tea, coffee, alcohol, or emotional excitement. Digitalis toxicity often produces coupled ventricular premature contractions that occur every second beat (particularly if atrial fibrillation is present). However, such coupled ventricular premature contractions can occur in the absence of digitalis toxicity. Digitalis can also cause ventricular premature contractions from varying foci and may produce a ventricular tachycardia or a bidirectional tachycardia (Chapter 8). Ventricular premature contractions from varying foci do not occur in normal persons. When ventricular premature contractions occur in patients with myocardial infarction, they may show abnormal Q waves and abnormal RS-T segments, indicative of the myocardial infarction.

Treatment. The treatment of ventricular premature contractions depends on their etiology and characteristics.

When ventricular premature contractions occur simultaneously with the apex (or nadir) of the preceding T wave, when they are multifocal, or when they occur in a succession of three or more, they should be immediately treated with a cardiac-depressant drug such as lidocaine, procainamide, or quinidine.* (If acute myocardial

---

*These and other drugs are described in Part three.

infarction is present, lidocaine is the drug of first choice; see Chapter 10.)

Ventricular premature contractions may also occur in congestive heart failure. When the patient is treated for the congestive heart failure, including digitalization, the ventricular premature beats often disappear.

Isolated ventricular premature contractions ordinarily do not need to be treated. If they produce annoying palpitations, they can often be eliminated by the patient's receiving mild sedatives, not drinking coffee or tea, or by receiving oral doses of potassium salts, quinidine, or procainamide.

VENTRICULAR TACHYCARDIA

A major or life-threatening arrhythmia.

Ventricular tachycardia is a succession of three or more ventricular premature contractions that may arise from a single focus or from varying foci in the ventricles.

Electrocardiogram. A ventricular tachycardia shows the following characteristics.

1. The QRS complexes are 0.12 sec or more wide, are aberrant, and are followed by aberrant RS-T segments and T waves. The QRS complexes resemble isolated ventricular premature contractions recorded before the start of the tachycardia.

2. Occasionally, it is difficult to separate the QRS from the RS-T and T. If this occurs, the tachycardia is called ventricular flutter (see below).

3. The ventricular rhythm may be regular or slightly irregular. Cycle lengths may vary by 0.02 to 0.03 sec.

4. The atria beat independently of the ventricles, usually but not necessarily at a slower rate; and when P waves are seen in the ECG, they have no constant relation to the QRS complexes. The atrial rhythm can consist of a sinus tachycardia, atrial tachycardia, AV junctional tachycardia, atrial flutter, or atrial fibrillation. Rarely, some or all of the stimuli from the ventricles may penetrate the AV node and

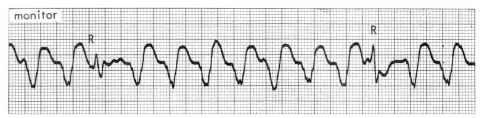

Fig. 7-4. Ventricular tachycardia in a patient with acute myocardial infarction. Occasional capture beats *(R)* are present. The patient was treated with IV doses of lidocaine.

Table 2. Differential diagnosis of ventricular tachycardia and supraventricular tachycardia with aberrant QRS complexes*

	Ventricular tachycardia	Supraventricular tachycardia
Rate	120 to 200 per min; occasionally as fast as 250 per min	150 to 240 per min; occasionally as fast as 290 per min
Rhythm	Regular or irregular	Regular or irregular
Right bundle branch block type QRS complex	Rare	Common
Relation of P waves (if visible) to QRS complex	AV dissociation or AV junctional P waves	Usually a 1:1 P-QRS relationship; occasionally, a Wenckebach or Mobitz type II AV block
Relationship of QRS shape to premature contractions prior to the tachycardia	Similar	Usually different; it may be similar if bundle branch block is present or if supraventricular premature contractions show aberrant QRS complexes
Capture and/or fusion beats	Diagnostic	Do not occur
Vagal stimulation	Almost always not effective	Often effective

*Adapted from Willerson JT, Yurchak PM, DeSanctis RW: Cardiovasc Clin **2**:69, 1970.

stimulate the atria in a retrograde fashion. When this occurs, AV junctional P waves will appear, following the QRS complexes. It may be impossible to determine the nature of the P waves unless esophageal or intra-atrial leads are taken.

5. Fusion or capture beats or both may appear. Occasionally, atrial stimuli may reach the AV node when it is not refractory to forward conduction to the ventricles. When this occurs, the stimulus will penetrate the AV node and spread through the ventricles in a normal way. This is known as a *capture beat* (Fig. 7-4). On other occasions, as a normal atrial stimulus is spreading through the AV node to the ventricles, the stimulus from the ectopic

ventricular focus is also spreading through the ventricles. The result is a *fusion beat,* which partially resembles a normal QRS complex and T wave and partially resembles a ventricular premature contraction (Fig. 7-7). A capture beat or a fusion beat is preceded by a P wave. Although capture and fusion beats have been considered diagnostic of ventricular tachycardia, they are usually not found during an attack of ventricular tachycardia.

6. An atrial premature contraction may be associated with a wide, aberrant QRS complex, as was pointed out in Chapter 6. This may also occur with a supraventricular tachycardia. When this happens, it may be difficult to distinguish the supra-

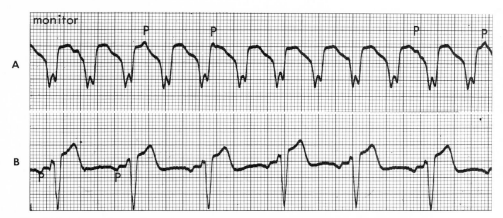

Fig. 7-5. Ventricular tachycardia in a patient with arteriosclerotic heart disease. **A,** Occasional P waves can be seen. The atrial rate is approximately 75 per min; the ventricular rate is approximately 140 per min. **B,** A few seconds after the patient received a bolus of lidocaine IV; sinus rhythm is present.

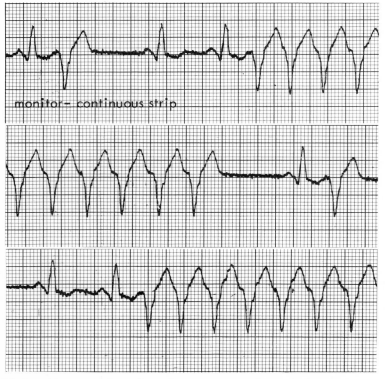

Fig. 7-6. Repetitive ventricular tachycardia in a patient with arteriosclerotic heart disease.

ventricular tachyarrhythmia with aberrant QRS complexes from a ventricular tachycardia. Table 2 shows some of the differences between the two conditions. (Also see p. 73.)

7. Posttachyarrhythmia T wave inversion may occur. After an attack of paroxysmal supraventricular or ventricular tachyarrhythmia, downward T waves may appear in the precordial and limb leads (upward in lead aV_R) and may last for several days to several weeks. The mechanism for these T wave changes is not known. However, they should not be diagnosed as a sign of myocardial infarction.

8. There are three general types of ventricular tachycardia. The first type is *extrasystolic ventricular tachycardia* (Figs. 7-4 and 7-5). The tachycardia consists of a succession of at least three ventricular contractions. If multiple attacks of ventricular tachycardia occur in any one person, each paroxysm usually starts with a ventricular premature contraction that occurs after the normal QRS by an interval that is relatively constant (although it may vary by as much as 0.08 sec). The tachycardia is usually followed by a long pause, similar to the compensatory pause of an ordinary ventricular contraction, before sinus rhythm returns.

Repetitive ventricular tachycardia is a relatively rare type of extrasystolic ventricular tachycardia. The successive ventricular premature contractions occur in short cycles of three to twelve beats, alternating with sinus rhythm or single ventricular premature contractions (Fig. 7-6). Repetitive ventricular tachycardia may occur in otherwise normal persons. However, symptoms, such as palpitations, breathlessness, precordial pain, or syncope can occur.

The second general type of ventricular tachycardia is *accelerated idioventricular tachycardia* (accelerated idioventricular rhythm) (Fig. 7-7). When the heart rate slows, pacemakers in the AV junction, the bundle of His, or in the Purkinje fibers may become active and begin to beat slowly, producing either an idioventricular AV junctional rhythm or an idioventricular ventricular rhythm with a rate less than 60 per min (p. 55). Occasionally, these idioventricular pacemakers may become accelerated. This sometimes occurs in acute inferior myocardial infarction, digitalis toxicity, and hyperkalemia. The ventricular rate increases to 60 to 110 beats per min.

The accelerated idioventricular tachycardia usually lasts for not more than 30 successive beats. Then sinus rhythm re-

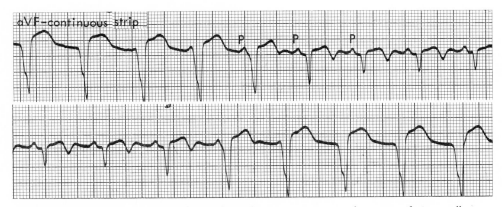

Fig. 7-7. Accelerated idioventricular tachycardia in a patient with acute inferior wall myocardial infarction. The first four beats show the idioventricular tachycardia. The fifth and sixth beats are fusion beats. Then sinus rhythm reappears, but is followed again in the lower strip by the idioventricular tachycardia. No treatment was needed.

appears. Isolated ventricular premature contractions may also occur in addition to the accelerated idioventricular tachycardia.

The third type of ventricular tachycardia is *parasystolic ventricular tachycardia*. Parasystole describes a syndrome in which premature ventricular contractions occur at a fixed rate from an ectopic focus in either the atria or ventricles. It shows the following characteristics.

a. The premature contractions are formed at a regular rate. The intervals between every two premature contractions are the same or are simple multiples that have a common denominator.

b. Since the parasystolic focus forms stimuli independently of the regular rhythm of the heart, the premature contractions that occur in the ECG have no constant relation to the regular heartbeats. In other words, the coupling interval varies. The situation is similar to the lack of relation between the P waves and the QRS complexes that occurs in complete AV block or in complete AV dissociation.

c. Occasionally, a regular sinus stimulus and a parasystolic stimulus reach the ventricles almost simultaneously. When this occurs, a fusion beat is formed.

d. The regular sinus stimulus that spreads through the heart does not penetrate the parasystolic focus because of *entrance block*.

e. Premature contractions may not appear at their regular time because of an *exit block* that prevents the premature stimulus from passing out of the ectopic focus.

The clinical aspects of parasystole are the same as for regular ventricular premature contractions.

Bidirectional tachycardia is a tachyarrhythmia in which alternate wide QRS complexes in any one lead point in opposite directions (see Fig. 8-11). It is almost always due to digitalis toxicity. In spite of the widened QRS complexes, it is now believed that bidirectional tachycardia is a form of supraventricular tachycardia (Chapter 8).

Clinical aspects. Ventricular tachycardia can occur in normal persons. Most commonly it occurs in association with serious heart disease, particularly coronary artery disease and acute myocardial infarction. It can also occur in myocarditis and in the cardiomyopathies. Mechanical irritation to the heart during cardiac catheterization or during the placement of a transvenous catheter electrode can also produce it.

It can be initiated by a fixed rate pacemaker when the pacemaker spike occurs when the ventricles are most vulnerable, namely at the apex (or nadir) of the T wave (R on T phenomenon) (also see p. 199). Ventricular tachycardia can also be produced by a "runaway" pacemaker. This has occurred with both fixed rate and demand pacemakers.

Drugs such as digitalis, quinidine, procainamide, papaverine, thioridazine tranquilizers, sympathomimetic drugs such as epinephrine or isoproterenol, or IV doses of mercurial diuretics can also cause a ventricular tachycardia.

Occasionally, a ventricular tachycardia occurs because of a reentrant mechanism. This can be precipitated when the heart slows for any reason (p. 110).

Various clinical signs of ventricular tachycardia, such as slight irregularities of the ventricular rate, splitting of the first and second heart sound, cannon waves in the neck veins, or variations in systolic blood pressure from beat to beat, have been used to differentiate ventricular tachycardia from paroxysmal atrial tachycardia with QRS aberration. Table 2 shows some of the differences between the two conditions.

Ventricular tachycardia must also be differentiated from the supraventricular tachyarrhythmias that occur with the Wolff-Parkinson-White syndrome because the wide QRS complexes that occur may simulate a ventricular tachycardia (Chapter 8).

A similar situation occurs in paroxysmal atrial flutter with a 1:1 AV conduction. The wide, aberrant QRS complexes that occur because of the rapid ventricular rate (above 250 per min) also simulate ventricular tachycardia. Atrial flutter can be suspected in such patients because a ventricular rate faster than 250 per min is rare in ventricular tachycardia. If carotid sinus pressure is used, the ventricular rate will often momentarily slow, and the atrial flutter waves will become apparent.

When a supraventricular tachyarrhythmia occurs in a patient with bundle branch block or with the Wolff-Parkinson-White syndrome, the ECG can also simulate ventricular tachycardia (see Fig. 6-12).

Emergency treatment. Treatment depends on the etiology of the ventricular tachycardia and on the presence of signs such as increasing congestive heart failure, shock, and intractable angina. If any of these signs are present or if the patient has an acute myocardial infarct, the following emergency treatment should be given.

1. A sharp thump with the closed fist over the lower sternum may restore sinus rhythm (see Fig. 2-2).

2. Lidocaine (Xylocaine), given IV, is the drug of first choice. Give an IV bolus immediately, and follow it with an IV drip.

3. If acute myocardial infarction is present or if the patient appears critically ill, administer synchronized DC shock immediately after the lidocaine bolus if the ventricular tachycardia persists. DC shock is effective in 95% of patients with ventricular tachycardia. The initial shock should be 50 ws. If this is not effective, increase each additional charge by 50 ws until a maximum of 400 ws have been given. If the ventricular tachycardia persists or reappears after this last charge, administer other treatment.

DC shock usually causes prompt return of sinus rhythm. Occasionally, the ventricular tachycardia may persist for a few seconds until sinus rhythm reappears. DC shock is, of course, contraindicated if the ventricular tachycardia is due to digtalis toxicity.

4. Procainamide can also be used par-enterally if lidocaine is not effective and if DC shock apparatus is not available. Procainamide may be more effective than quinidine in the treatment of ventricular tachycardia.

5. Bretylium tosylate is also excellent. However, it is not yet commercially available.

6. Diphenylhydantoin, given IV, is the drug of choice if the ventricular tachycardia is due to digitalis toxicity.

7. Propranolol has only a fair effect on ventricular tachycardia.

8. Electrical pacing can also be used if DC shock or drug therapy is not effective. (Chapter 16).

9. The following general therapy should also be given.

   a. If the ventricular tachycardia is due to a drug such as digitalis or quinidine, stop the drug immediately.

   b. If arterial hypoxemia is present, correct it at once by making certain that the patient has an adequate airway and by giving oxygen, if necessary.

   c. If the ventricular tachycardia is due to mechanical irritation, such as a transvenous catheter electrode in the right heart chamber, withdraw or reposition the catheter electrode.

   d. If hyperkalemia or hypokalemia is present, correct it as soon as possible.

   e. Accelerated idioventricular tachycardia does not ordinarily require treatment, because it represents an escape mechanism to overcome a bradyarrhythmia. However, it may be associated with ventricular premature contractions from the same idioventricular focus. When this occurs, the ventricular rate may become faster than 110 per min, and a typical ventricular tachycardia may occur. Such ventricular premature contractions can be suppressed by increasing the basic heart rate with atropine given IV or with isoproterenol. Cardiacdepressant drugs such as lidocaine, procainamide, or quinidine have also been used for this type of ventricular tachycardia, but there is a danger that they may cause cardiac arrest.

f. Repetitive ventricular tachycardia responds to synchronized DC shock. However, the ventricular tachycardia usually reappears. Quinidine or procainamide can also be used. If congestive heart failure occurs, the patient can be treated in the usual way with digitalis and diuretics.

g. Parasystolic ventricular tachycardia is treated the same as extrasystolic ventricular tachycardia.

Prophylaxis. An IV drip of lidocaine should be continued when the ventricular tachycardia has been stopped either with lidocaine or with synchronized DC shock. The lidocaine should be continued for at least 48 to 72 hours after sinus rhythm returns.

Before the lidocaine infusion is stopped, the patient should be given oral doses of procainamide or quinidine (or diphenylhydantoin if the ventricular tachycardia was due to digitalis toxicity). If the ventricular

tachycardia has occurred during an acute myocardial infarction, procainamide or quinidine should be continued for at least 3 months. If the patient has a recurrent attack of ventricular tachycardia during the acute infarction, prophylactic therapy with oral doses of procainamide or quinidine should be continued indefinitely.

VENTRICULAR FLUTTER

A life-threatening arrhythmia.

Ventricular flutter is similar to ventricular tachycardia. However it is not possible to separate the QRS complexes from the RS-T segments and the T waves. Instead, regular large or small undulations appear (Figs. 7-8 and 7-9). The small ventricular flutter waves may become irregular so that the ECG resembles both ventricular flutter and ventricular fibrillation (ventricular flutter–fibrillation).

The ventricular rate in ventricular flutter usually varies from 180 to 250 beats per min, as in a patient with the usual type of ventricular tachycardia. However, the ventricular rate of ventricular flutter may become faster. When this occurs and when the ventricular flutter waves are large, the ECG may be very similar to atrial flutter with 1:1 conduction (p. 81) or to a supraventricular tachyarrhythmia in a patient with the Wolff-Parkinson-White syndrome (p. 113).

Ventricular flutter is a very serious tachyarrhythmia and is often a precursor

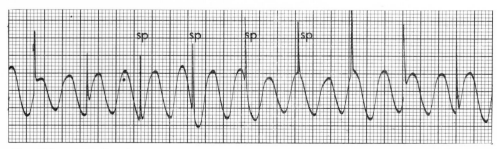

Fig. 7-8. Ventricular flutter. The ventricular rate is approximately 185 per min. Pacemaker spikes *(sp)* are also present, but the pacemaker is not functioning. The patient developed ventricular fibrillation shortly after this ECG was taken, and died.

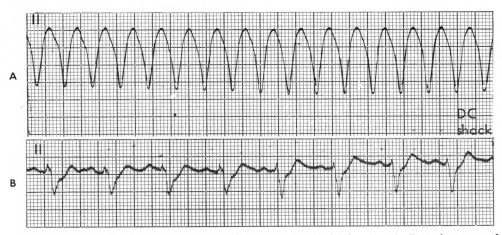

Fig. 7-9. Ventricular flutter in a patient with acute myocardial infarction. **A,** Typical pattern of ventricular flutter. The ventricular rate is approximately 185 per min. Since the patient had become unconscious and had no palpable pulse or measurable blood pressure, *unsynchronized* precordial DC shock (400 ws) was given. **B,** Return of regular sinus rhythm a few seconds later.

of either ventricular fibrillation or cardiac standstill.

Emergency treatment. A sharp blow with the closed fist to the lower sternum may restore sinus rhythm (also see p. 15). If this is not effective, the emergency treatment for ventricular tachycardia (see above) or for cardiac arrest (Chapter 2) should be given.

VENTRICULAR FIBRILLATION

A life-threatening arrhythmia.

When ventricular fibrillation occurs, the heart stops contracting effectively because an ineffective stimulus spreads rapidly through the ventricles in an irregular path.

Electrocardiogram. The ECG shows small (fine) or large (coarse) waves that are irregular in size, shape, width, and rate (see Fig. 2-8). The rate can vary from 150 to 300 per min.

Clinical aspects. Ventricular fibrillation can occur in the dying heart. It often occurs in acute myocardial infarction; during hypoxia from any cause, including surgical anesthesia; and after electrocution. It can also be precipitated by drugs such as digitalis, quinidine, and procainamide. It can

occur with hyperkalemia, hypokalemia, and hypercalcemia. Transient ventricular fibrillation can occur in patients with complete AV block (see Fig. 5-10).

Because effective cardiac contractions stop when ventricular fibrillation occurs, the patient becomes unconscious in a few seconds.

Emergency treatment. A sharp blow with the closed fist to the lower sternum may restore sinus rhythm (see Fig. 2-2 and p. 15). If this is not effective, the emergency treatment of cardiac arrest should be started immediately (Chapter 2).

REFERENCES

Ayres SM, Grace WJ: Inappropriate ventilation and hypoxemia as causes of cardiac arrhythmias, Am J Med **46:**495, 1969.

Cass RN: Repetitive tachycardia; a review of 40 cases with no demonstrable heart disease, Am J Cardiol **19:**597, 1967.

Cohen HC, et al: Ventricular tachycardia with narrow QRS complexes (left posterior fascicular tachycardia), Circulation **45:**1035, 1972.

Cohen LS, et al: Recurrent ventricular tachycardia and fibrillation treated with a combination of beta-adrenergic blockade and electrical pacing, Ann Intern Med **66:**945, 1967.

Cohn LJ, Donoso E, Friedberg CK: Ventricular tachycardia, Prog Cardiovasc Dis **9:**29, 1966.

DeSanctis RW, Kastor JA: Rapid intracardiac pacing for treatment of recurrent ventricular tachyarrhythmias in the absence of heart block, Am Heart J 76:168, 1968.

Devorss J, Winters WG: Repetitive ventricular tachyarrhythmia; result of pacemaker failure, Letter, JAMA 220:1494, 1972.

Dhurandhar RW, et al: Primary ventricular fibrillation complicating acute myocardial infarction, Am J Cardiol 27:347, 1971.

Easley RM Jr, Goldstein S: Differentiation of ventricular tachycardia from junctional tachycardia with aberrant conduction; the use of competitive atrial pacing, Circulation 37:1015, 1968.

Feldman AE, Hellerstein HK, et al: Repetitive ventricular fibrillation in myocardial infarction refractory to bretylium tosylate subsequently controlled by ventricular pacing, Am J Cardiol 27:227, 1971.

Giles TD, Modlin RK: Death associated with ventricular arrhythmia and thioridazine hydrochloride, JAMA 205:98, 1968.

Greenwood RJ, Finkelstein D: Ventricular tachycardia responding solely to digitalis therapy, Am J Cardiol 7:441, 1961.

Harden K, Mackenzie IL, Ledingham I McA: Spontaneous reversion of ventricular fibrillation, Lancet 2:1140, 1963.

Langendorf R, Pick A, Winternitz M: Mechanisms of intermittent ventricular bigeminy; appearance of ectopic beats dependent upon length of ventricular cycle, "rule of bigeminy," Circulation 11:422, 1955.

Ledwich JR, Fay JE: Idiopathic recurrent ventricular fibrillation, Am J Cardiol 24:255, 1969.

Lesch M, Lewis E, et al: Paroxysmal ventricular tachycardia in the absence of organic heart disease, Ann Intern Med 66:950, 1967.

Lown B, Temte JV, Arter WJ: Ventricular tachyarrhythmias; clinical aspects, Circulation 47:1364, 1973.

Massumi RA, Tawakkol AA, Kistin AD: Reevaluation of electrocardiographic and bedside criteria for diagnosis of ventricular tachycardia, Circulation 36:628, 1967.

McCallister BD, McGoon DC, Connolly DC: Paroxysmal ventricular tachycardia and fibrillation without complete heart block, Am J Cardiol 18:898, 1966.

Papadopoulos C, Blazek CJ: Ventricular tachycardia of 70 days' duration with survival, Am J Cardiol 11:107, 1963.

Pennington JE, Taylor J, Lown B: Chest thump for reverting ventricular tachycardia, N Engl J Med 283:1192, 1970.

Pick A, Langendorf R: Differentiation of supraventricular and ventricular tachycardia, Prog Cardiovasc Dis 2:391, 1960.

Ring A, Blankfein J: Paroxysmal ventricular tachycardia in an apparently normal heart, Ann Intern Med 42:680, 1955.

Rubeiz GA, el-Hajj M, Toumà A: Successful use of external electrical cardioversion in the treatment of ventricular fibrillation caused by quinidine, Am J Cardiol 16:118, 1965.

Smirk FH, Palmer DG: A myocardial syndrome with particular reference to the occurrence of sudden death and of premature systoles interrupting antecedent T waves, Am J Cardiol 6:620, 1960.

Stern TN: Paroxysmal ventricular fibrillation in the absence of other disease, Ann Intern Med 47:552, 1957.

Thind GS: Intractable ventricular tachycardia, Letter, Ann Intern Med 72:603, 1970.

Verska JJ: Potassium parenterally in treatment of uncontrolled ventricular arrhythmia, Letter, JAMA 219:220, 1972.

Vogel JHK, Tabari K, et al: A simple technique for identifying P waves in complex arrhythmias, Am Heart J 67:158, 1964.

Wallace WA, Ableman WH, Norman JC: Runaway demand pacemaker, Ann Thorac Surg 9:209, 1970.

Willerson JT, Yurchak PM, DeSanctis RW: Ventricular tachycardia, Cardiovasc Clin 2:69, 1970.

Zipes DP, Fisch C: Ventricular tachycardia, Arch Intern Med 128:815, 1971.

Zipes DP, Fisch C: Initiation of ventricular tachycardia, Arch Intern Med 128:988, 1972.

Zipes DP, Fisch C: Accelerated ventricular rhythm, Arch Intern Med 129:650, 1972.

8 / Other emergency arrhythmias

In this chapter arrhythmias associated with periods of both bradycardia and tachycardia (bradyarrhythmia-tachyarrhythmia syndromes), tachyarrhythmias associated with the Wolff-Parkinson-White syndrome, and bradyarrhythmias and tachyarrhythmias associated with digitalis toxicity are discussed.

BRADYARRHYTHMIA-TACHYARRHYTHMIA SYNDROMES

Major arrhythmias. When severe bradycardia occurs or when a ventricular tachycardia occurs, the arrhythmia becomes life threatening.

Isolated case reports of transient atrial fibrillation or paroxysmal atrial tachycardia (PAT) complicating SA block appeared prior to Short's report in 1954, when he described "the syndrome of alternating bradycardia and tachycardia." However, he pointed out that in these previous cases the attacks of tachyarrhythmias were brief and relatively symptomless and were associated with SA block. His patients showed sinus bradycardia alternating with PAT or atrial flutter.

Actually, at least three types of bradycardia-tachycardia syndromes occur.

1. Short's classical syndrome of *alternating* bradycardia and tachycardia (Figs. 8-1 and 8-2)
2. Bradycardia induced by drugs used in the treatment of paroxysmal tachyarrhythmias (Figs. 8-3 and 8-4)
3. Primary bradyarrhythmias complicated by ventricular tachyarrhythmias (Fig. 8-5)

The term sick sinus syndrome has been used to describe bradyarrhythmia-tachyarrhythmia syndromes, as well as bradyarrhythmias produced by synchronized DC shock (p. 250).

Syndrome of alternating bradycardia and tachycardia

Clinical aspects. During the periods of sinus bradycardia, the heart rate is between 30 and 50 per min and may be slower. Sinus arrhythmia, wandering pacemaker, and SA block with nodal or ventricular escape beats may occur. Dizziness or syncope may occur when the heart rate slows. The bradycardia may last from minutes to months or longer. If the patient exercises during the period of bradycardia, the heart rate increases.

During the periods of supraventricular tachyarrhythmias, the ventricular rate may be as fast as 200 per min. However, if AV block is present with the atrial tachyarrhythmia, the ventricular rate may be slow. When the ventricular rate is fast, the patient may complain of palpitations or of any of the symptoms of a PAT (Chapter 6). The duration of the tachycardia can vary from minutes to months or longer. Two of Short's patients had atrial tachycardia that lasted a whole year.

In the intervals between the bradyarrhythmias and the tachyarrhythmias, the patient may show normal sinus rhythm.

The exact cause of this syndrome is not known.

Emergency treatment

1. Digitalis is the drug of choice for the treatment of the tachyarrhythmias asso-

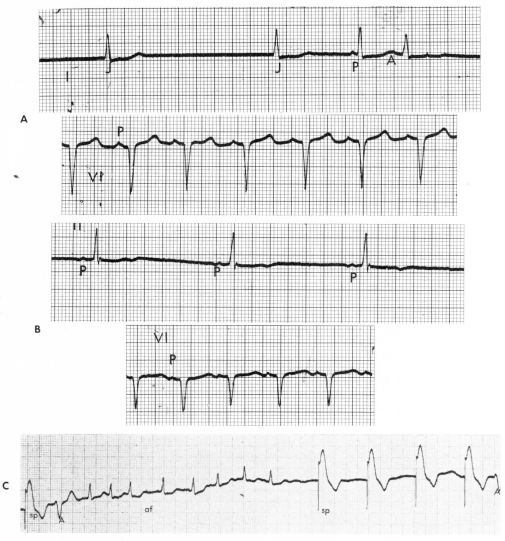

Fig. 8-1. Bradycardia-tachycardia syndrome in an 83-year-old patient. **A,** A period of SA block, AV junctional escape beats *(J),* and one atrial premature contraction *(A)* in lead I. A few moments later, when lead VI was taken, the rhythm had changed to a regular sinus rhythm at a rate of 90 per min. The patient was not receiving any medication. **B,** Next day; an AV junctional rhythm with a ventricular rate of approximately 40 per min in lead II. When lead VI was taken, the rhythm spontaneously changed to a sinus tachycardia at a rate of approximately 115 per min. **C,** A transvenous demand pacemaker has been inserted. The patient was complaining of palpitations when this ECG was taken. It shows a pacemaker spike *(sp)* and contraction, followed by an atrial premature contraction *(A)* and a short period of paroxysmal atrial fibrillation *(af),* followed by pacemaker contractions at a rate of 72 per min. The patient was then given oral procainamide therapy, and the premature contractions and the tachyarrhythmias stopped.

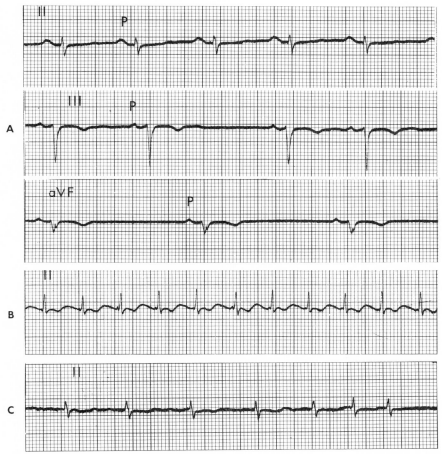

Fig. 8-2. Bradycardia-tachycardia syndrome in a 76-year-old patient. **A,** Regular sinus rhythm in lead II, transient SA block in lead III, and marked sinus bradycardia (rate approximately 35 per min) in lead aV$_F$. (These leads are part of one ECG.) **B,** Two months later; paroxysmal atrial flutter. **C,** Four months after **B**; paroxysmal atrial fibrillation. The patient was then digitalized and maintained on oral digitalis therapy, which prevented further attacks of either bradyarrhythmias or tachyarrhythmias.

ciated with the syndrome of alternating bradycardia and tachycardia. Digitalis will slow the ventricular rate and may maintain sinus rhythm. It may also convert a PAT or an atrial flutter to atrial fibrillation and maintain the atrial fibrillation with a slow ventricular rate.

2. Transvenous cardiac pacing with a ventricular demand pacemaker is the treatment of choice when severe symptomatic bradyarrhythmias occur. Cardiac pacing

will not prevent the attacks of tachyarrhythmias that are part of the syndrome (Fig. 8-1, C). However, when a transvenous pacemaker has been inserted, the tachyarrhythmia can then be treated with procainamide, quinidine, propranolol, or other cardiac-depressant drugs.*

3. Quinidine, procainamide, propranolol, or any other cardiac-depressant drug

---

*These and other drugs are described in Part three.

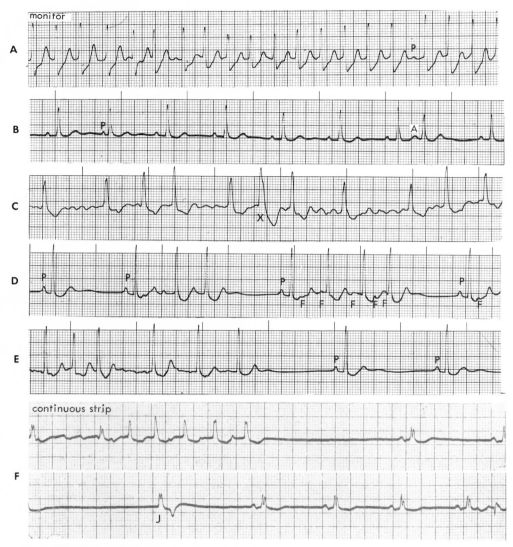

Fig. 8-3. Tachyarrhythmias complicated by bradyarrhythmias, secondary to drug therapy. **A** through **E**, Monitor leads, taken on separate days, of a patient who was having attacks of paroxysmal supraventricular tachyarrhythmias. **A**, Supraventricular tachyarrhythmia. It is difficult to determine if P waves are present. At the end of the strip the rate slowed, and sinus P waves became visible. **B**, Sinus rhythm. One atrial premature contraction (A) is present. **C**, Paroxysmal atrial fibrillation. X is an aberrant QRS complex (p. 73). **D**, Sinus rhythm associated with short periods of paroxysmal atrial flutter (F). **E**, End of an attack of paroxysmal atrial fibrillation and appearance of a slow sinus rhythm at a rate of approximately 36 per min. **F**, End of an attack of paroxysmal supraventricular tachyarrhythmia, followed by SA block, an AV junctional escape beat (J), sinus rhythm, and the recurrence of the tachyarrhythmia at the end of the lower strip. The patient had been receiving digitalis, quinidine, and propranolol because of the persistent and disturbing tachyarrhythmias. All drugs were stopped, and regular sinus rhythm reappeared.

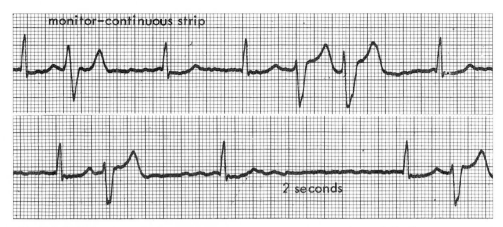

Fig. 8-4. Multiple ventricular premature contractions in a patient with atrial fibrillation associated with bradycardia, possibly due to procainamide.

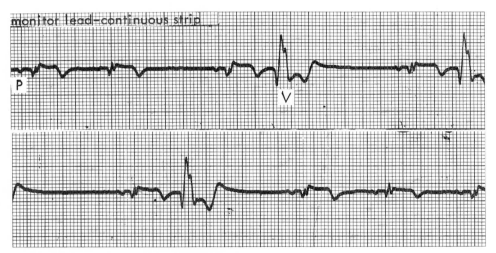

Fig. 8-5. Ventricular premature contractions associated with slowing of the heart rate in a patient with acute myocardial infarction. The first two heartbeats show a ventricular rate of approximately 70 per min. When the heart rate slowed to approximately 45 per min (third complex), each regular sinus beat was followed by a ventricular premature contraction (V). These disappeared when the heart rate became faster again.

must *never* be used to treat a patient with the bradycardia-tachycardia syndrome unless a pacemaker has been inserted, because the drugs can cause lethal cardiac arrest.

4. Short found that atropine administered IV could transiently increase the ventricular rate when given to a patient during a period of bradycardia. Orally administered atropine was not effective and merely produced side effects. Subcutaneously administered epinephrine also can increase the heart rate but also produces side effects such as ventricular premature contractions. Short also found that ephedrine and benzedrine (levo-amphetamine) gave only temporary improvement.

Tachyarrhythmias complicated by bradyarrhythmias secondary to drug treatment

Numerous potent cardiac-depressant drugs, such as quinidine, procainamide, lidocaine, edrophonium chloride, propranolol, and diphenylhydantoin, are now available for the treatment of tachyarrhythmias, and these drugs are often used in combination or successively. When this is done, there is a danger that when the tachyarrhythmia stops, a severe bradyarrhythmia even with cardiac standstill may develop, rather than regular sinus rhythm. Fig. 8-3, *F*, illustrates this.

The best treatment for this condition is prevention. If a severe bradyarrhythmia develops, all cardiac-depressant drugs should be stopped temporarily, until the cardiac rhythm becomes stable. Atropine or isoproterenol may be needed if long periods of SA block occur. One should also remember that the patient may be sensitive to a drug, such as quinidine, which can produce syncope due to transient ventricular fibrillation.

Primary bradyarrhythmias complicated by ventricular tachyarrhythmias

Normally, a stimulus spreads radially through the heart muscle cells. However, when the heart rate is slow, the stimulated heart muscle and the Purkinje fibers tend to return to the resting state in a nonuniform way, which may predispose the patient to reentrant tachyarrhythmias for the following reason. Some cardiac cells may still be refractory when the next stimulus reaches them. As a result, the radial spread of the stimulus is blocked in one direction but proceeds normally in another direction. The stimulus finally reaches cells on the far side of the cells that were refractory when the stimulus first started. However, these cells are no longer refractory. As a result, they are now stimulated in a retrograde way and in turn carry the stimulus to adjacent cells, causing a continuous re-entrant type of ventricular tachycardia. (Also see p. 266.)

Ventricular tachyarrhythmias can occur whenever the heart rate becomes slow (Fig. 8-5). The classical example of this phenomenon is the association of complete AV block with episodes of transient ventricular tachycardia or transient ventricular fibrillation (see Fig. 5-10).

The treatment of bradyarrhythmias associated with transient tachyarrhythmias depends on the etiology of the bradyarrhythmia, the drugs used, and the presence of complete AV block. The presence of complete AV block is an immediate indication for a transvenous ventricular demand pacemaker. If complete AV block is not present, the condition may disappear if all cardiac-depressant drugs are withdrawn. Because of the danger of producing cardiac standstill, one should not treat the premature contractions or tachyarrhythmia with cardiac-depressant drugs unless a temporary ventricular demand pacemaker has been inserted.

ARRHYTHMIAS ASSOCIATED WITH THE WOLFF-PARKINSON-WHITE SYNDROME

The Wolff-Parkinson-White pattern is a minor conduction disturbance. When a tachycardia is present, the condition becomes major.

Preexcitation (accelerated AV conduction) occurs when a stimulus spreads either partially or completely from the atria to the ventricles by ways of accessory conduction fibers before the stimulus can reach the ventricles by way of the AV node. These accessory conduction fibers include Kent's bundle, James' fibers, and Mahaim's fibers. Kent's bundle passes from the atria to the ventricles. James' fibers pass from the sinus node to the lowermost portion of the AV node near the origin of the bundle of His, by way of the posterior internodal pathway (p. 50). Stimuli spreading from the sinus node to the AV node in this way show a short P-R interval because they are **not** delayed in the AV node. Mahaim's fibers connect the lower AV node and the bundle of His or one of its branches with the ventricular septum, bypassing most of the His-Purkinje system.

Several types of preexcitation have been described.

1. The classical Wolff-Parkinson-White syndrome and its variants
2. The Lown-Ganong-Levine syndrome

The Wolff-Parkinson-White syndrome

Electrocardiogram. The classical ECG shows the following characteristics.

1. A short P-R interval of 0.11 sec or less.

2. Widening of the QRS complex to 0.11 sec or more.

3. A normal P-J interval, which does not exceed 0.26 sec. (J is the junction between the end of the QRS complex and the beginning of the RS-T segment.) The normal P-J interval indicates that the widening of the QRS complex is more apparent than

real and is due to the accelerated spread of the stimulus from the atria to the ventricles.

4. Slurring or notching of the first portion of the QRS complex. This is known as a delta wave (Figs. 8-6 and 8-7). Not all leads show the delta wave.

5. Aberration of the RS-T segment and T wave may occur in association with the widened and slurred QRS complex.

6. Two QRS patterns have been described. Type A shows large, slurred R waves over the precordium and resembles right bundle branch block (Fig. 8-6). This pattern may be due to premature excitation of the left ventricle. Type B shows deep S waves in precordial leads near the sternum and resembles the pattern of left bundle branch block (Fig. 8-7). This pattern may be due to premature excitation of the right ventricle. Either type may show an abnormal QS in leads II, III, and aV_F, which simulates inferior myocardial infarction (Fig. 8-6). Rarely, a patient will show

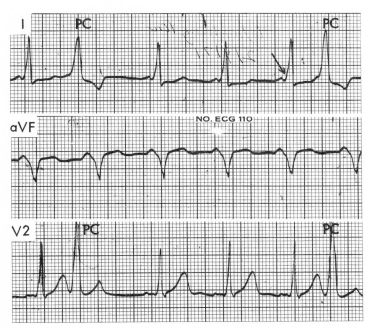

Fig. 8-6. Wolff-Parkinson-White syndrome, type A. Arrow points to the delta wave. Occasional premature contractions are present (PC).

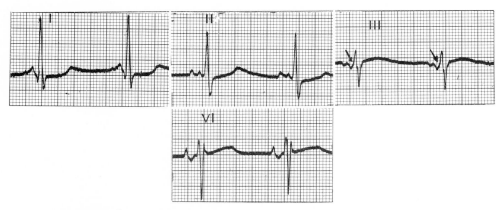

Fig. 8-7. Wolff-Parkinson-White syndrome, type B. Arrow points to the delta wave.

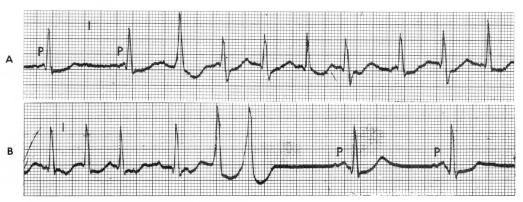

Fig. 8-8. Wolff-Parkinson-White syndrome. **A,** Beginning of an attack of paroxysmal atrial fibrillation. **B,** End of the attack a few minutes later. Same patient as in Fig. 8-7.

type A QRS complexes at one time and type B at another time, or vice versa.

Variations of the classical Wolff-Parkinson-White pattern may occur; for example, the P-R interval can be longer than 0.12 sec.

Clinical aspects. The Wolff-Parkinson-White syndrome can occur normally. However, about one third of patients with this syndrome have associated heart disease, chiefly hypertensive or coronary artery disease. Many of the patients with the syndrome who also have congenital heart disease show the Ebstein malformation. There is also an association between hyperthyroidism and the Wolff-Parkinson-White syndrome. In both normal persons and in patients with heart disease, the Wolff-Parkinson-White syndrome can occur transiently.

From 40% to 80% of patients have attacks of paroxysmal tachyarrhythmias. The usual type of tachyarrhythmia is a PAT, usually with QRS complexes of normal width. This type of supraventricular tachycardia is probably due to a reentrant type of mechanism. The stimulus passes down the AV node to the ventricles in a normal way and then travels retrograde (upward) through an accessory conduction pathway from the AV node into the atria. This circus movement cycle may repeat itself, causing a reentrant tachyarrhythmia.

Paroxysmal atrial fibrillation (Fig. 8-8) occurs less commonly and is usually associated with wide, aberrant QRS complexes, so that the ECG may resemble a ventricular tachycardia (pseudoventricular tachycardia) (Fig. 8-9). When this occurs, it may be difficult to differentiate it from a true ventricular tachycardia, unless the ventricular rate exceeds 250 per min, which rarely occurs in a true ventricular tachycardia.

Paroxysmal atrial flutter is still less common. It is also usually associated with wide, aberrant QRS complexes.

True ventricular tachycardia is not a part of the Wolff-Parkinson-White syn-

drome, although it may occur in a patient with underlying organic heart disease.

When sinus rhythm is present, atropine or epinephrine may increase conduction through the AV node and may restore a normal QRS width. Quinidine or procainamide also tends to restore the normal QRS width by blocking conduction through the accessory pathways from the atria to the ventricles.

Although patients with the Wolff-Parkinson-White syndrome may have attacks of paroxysmal tachyarrhythmias for many years, the condition is not always benign. A long attack of tachyarrhythmia may pre-

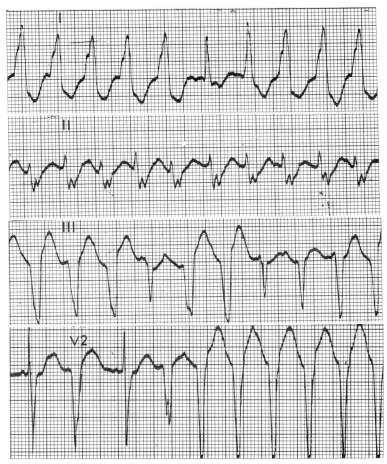

Fig. 8-9. Wolff-Parkinson-White syndrome, with pseudoventricular tachycardia. Occasional QRS complexes with a normal width are present. Same patient as in Fig. 8-7.

cipitate congestive heart failure. Also, death from ventricular fibrillation can occur.

Emergency treatment

1. If the patient shows signs of severe congestive heart failure, shock, or intractable angina, synchronized DC shock should be used. However, many patients have innumerable attacks of paroxysmal tachyarrhythmias over a period of many years. (One of my patients has had recurrent attacks for more than 30 years.) Therefore, synchronized DC shock should be used only in an emergency or when drug therapy is ineffective.

2. Quinidine or procainamide is the drug of choice when paroxysmal atrial fibrillation occurs because either drug depresses conduction through the anomalous pathways. In some patients, a combination of quinidine and procainamide may be more successful than either drug alone, or a combination of quinidine, procainamide, and digitalis may be needed.

3. Digitalis is the drug of choice for the treatment of PAT with a regular ventricular rate. Large doses of digitalis are sometimes needed to restore sinus rhythm. The situation is similar to the action of digitalis in atrial flutter. Therefore, one must be careful to avoid digitalis toxicity.

Digitalis tends to increase conduction through the accessory conduction pathways. Therefore, if it is given to a patient with both the Wolff-Parkinson-White syndrome and paroxysmal atrial fibrillation, it may aggravate the tachyarrhythmia by increasing the ventricular rate still further.

4. Propranolol is the next drug of choice for treatment of the tachyarrhythmias. However, it may be necessary to use it with digitalis because it has a negative inotropic effect and can precipitate or aggravate congestive heart failure. Here again, propranolol, quinidine, procainamide, and digitalis may be needed in a refractory tachyarrhythmia.

5. Carotid sinus pressure (p. 74) may occasionally stop the tachyarrhythmia.

6. Potassium chloride (given orally or parenterally) may also be helpful in stopping the tachyarrhythmia.

7. Recently, surgical operations on the conduction system have been tried in several patients. The AV node has been interrupted surgically in a few patients, and attempts have been made to cut the accessory conduction pathways in other patients.

8. Transvenous pacing (p. 223) can also be used to stop an attack of tachyarrhythmia associated with the Wolff-Parkinson-White syndrome.

Prophylaxis. Regardless of the treatment used, the attacks of paroxysmal tachyarrhythmias tend to recur. Digitalis quinidine, procainamide, and propranolol, either alone or in combination, may be helpful.

The Lown-Ganong-Levine syndrome

The Lown-Ganong-Levine syndrome is characterized by a short P-R interval (less than 0.12 sec) and a QRS of normal duration. There is no delta wave and no slurring of the QRS.

Paroxysmal supraventricular tachyarrhythmias are also common in these patients.

Treatment is the same as for the classical Wolff-Parkinson-White syndrome.

ARRHYTHMIAS ASSOCIATED WITH DIGITALIS TOXICITY

Although gastrointestinal symptoms such as anorexia, nausea, or vomiting are usually considered to be the most common early signs of digitalis toxicity, digitalis can induce cardiac arrhythmias without gastrointestinal symptoms. This is particularly common because purified digitalis preparations are available.

The development of signs of digitalis toxicity depends on many factors.

1. The type of digitalis preparation used and the method of administration. Digitalis toxicity occurs more frequently when it is given parenterally and also when a long-

acting preparation, such as digitoxin or gitalin (Gitaligin), is given orally.

2. The age of the patient. Elderly patients are more sensitive to digitalis than are younger patients. Digitalis toxicity may last a week or more in an elderly patient, even when a rapidly excreted preparation, such as digoxin, is used. (A similar situation occurs in uremia.)

3. Hypoxia aggravates digitalis toxicity. Therefore, digitalis toxicity may occur after the usual therapeutic doses in acute myocardial infarction or in acute or chronic pulmonary disease.

4. Electrolyte disturbances, particularly hypokalemia, will also aggravate digitalis toxicity. The potassium loss may be due to diuretics, corticosteroids, vomiting, diarrhea, or any other mechanism. In these patients, the serum potassium concentration may be within normal in spite of the loss of total exchangeable body potassium content.

Hypomagnesemia (which is often associated with hypokalemia), hypercalcemia, or hyponatremia can also precipitate or aggravate digitalis toxicity.

Digitalis can produce every known type of cardiac arrhythmia, due to either a disturbance of conduction or a disturbance of impulse formation or to both factors. The type of arrhythmia may change rapidly, even in one ECG.

Common arrhythmias due to digitalis toxicity include ventricular premature contractions with or without a bigeminal rhythm, sinus bradycardia, wandering pacemaker, SA block, AV junctional rhythm, nonparoxysmal AV junctional tachycardia, all degrees of AV block, PAT with block, bidirectional tachycardia (see below), ventricular tachycardia, and ventricular fibrillation.

Uncommon arrhythmias include atrial flutter and atrial fibrillation.

It is sometimes very difficult to determine if an arrhythmia is due to digitalis toxicity or is a sign of the underlying heart disease. The ECG may or may not show signs of digitalis effects, such as a shortened Q-T interval, reversal of the direction of the T wave, and depression of the RS-T segment with a scooped-out appearance (see Fig. 9-2).

A tachyarrhythmia, such as a bidirectional tachycardia or ventricular premature

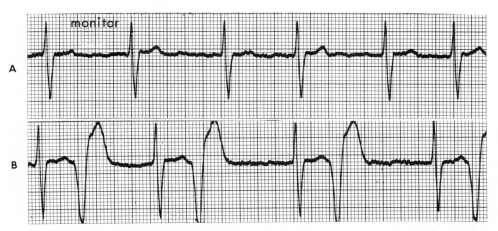

Fig. 8-10. Bigeminal rhythm with ventricular premature contractions, due to digitalis. The basic rhythm is atrial fibrillation. **A,** Patient had been digitalized, and the ventricular rate had slowed. **B,** A week later; ventricular premature contractions with a bigeminal rhythm are now present. The digitalis was stopped for several days, and the premature contractions disappeared.

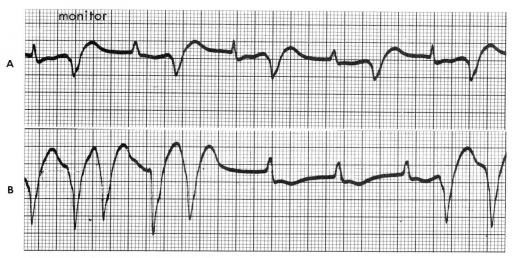

Fig. 8-11. Bidirectional tachycardia due to digitalis toxicity. **A,** Bidirectional tachycardia. **B,** A few hours later; ventricular tachycardia.

contractions with a bigeminal rhythm, occurring in a patient with atrial fibrillation, is very suggestive of digitalis toxicity (Figs. 8-10 and 8-11).

It is now possible to measure the concentration of digoxin or digitoxin in the blood by means of radioimmunoassay or nonradioactive methods. It has been found that when digitalis toxicity occurs, the plasma digitalis concentration is higher than when toxicity is not present. Unfortunately, toxicity can occur even when the plasma concentration of digoxin or digitoxin is within a therapeutic range.

Emergency treatment

1. Stop administering the digitalis immediately. The duration of toxicity will depend on the type of digitalis preparation that the patient has been taking, the route by which it has been given, the age of the patient, and whether the toxicity is associated with electrolyte or metabolic disturbances. Therefore, toxicity may last a few hours or a day or two if the patient has been receiving ouabain, digoxin, or deslanoside, or a week or more if the patient has been receiving digitoxin, gitalin, acetyldigitoxin, or digitalis leaf. In addition, elderly patients or patients with azotemia may continue to show digitalis toxicity 7 days or more even when a rapid-acting digitalis preparation has been used.

2. Stop administering diuretics, such as the mercurials, thiazides, furosemide, and ethacrynic acid, which can cause a loss of potassium ions in the urine. If diuretics are needed, use a potassium-sparing drug, such as triamterene (Dyrenium) or spironolactone (Aldactone).

3. Correct other electrolyte disturbances, particularly hypokalemia, hypercalcemia, and hypomagnesemia.

Prophylaxis

1. The patient should be digitalized slowly, and orally, if possible.

2. If digitalis is given orally, a quickly acting and quickly eliminated preparation should be used.

3. Rapid digitalization should be avoided if the patient's previous digitalis intake is not known. In addition, patients with hypokalemia, hypomagnesemia, hyponatremia, hypercalcemia, hypothyroidism, with acute myocardial infarction in the first 24 hours after the attack, or with acute or chronic pulmonary disease or azotemia

may require less than the usual digitalizing doses.

4. If the patient has atrial fibrillation and digitalis is not able to slow the ventricular rate below 100 per min without causing side-effects, propranolol can be used in addition to the digitalis. When this is done, smaller doses of both drugs will be effective.

5. If a patient has atrial fibrillation with a rapid ventricular rate that does not respond to digitalis, one should suspect that an underlying condition such as hyperthyroidism, acute pulmonary embolism, or the Wolff-Parkinson-White syndrome may be present.

Bradyarrhythmias associated with digitalis toxicity

Major arrhythmias.

A sudden sinus bradycardia below 50 per min or the development of an almost regular ventricular rate from 30 to 50 per min in a patient who has atrial fibrillation and who is taking digitalis is suggestive of digitalis toxicity. Sinus arrhythmia, wandering pacemaker, SA block, AV junctional rhythm, AV dissociation, and all degrees of AV block can also occur with digitalis toxicity.

Emergency treatment

1. A first-degree AV block needs no treatment if the P-R interval does not exceed 0.24 sec. However, if it measures 0.26 sec or more, reduce the digitalis dosage, or temporarily stop administering the drug.

2. If a Wenckebach type of AV block is present, decrease the digitalis dosage, or temporarily stop administering the drug.

3. If the Mobitz type II SA block occurs or if complete AV block occurs, immediately stop administering the digitalis. It may also be necessary to increase the ventricular rate if the patient has syncopal symptoms from the slow rate or if signs of increasing congestive heart failure or shock develop. This can be done with atropine given orally or IV. Isoproterenol

will also increase the heart rate, but it may increase ventricular irritability. Therefore, it should be used only when atropine is not effective. In such patients a temporary transvenous cardiac pacemaker may be necessary.

4. Do *not* give potassium chloride when the Mobitz type II SA block or complete AV block is present, because potassium salts and digitalis have a synergistic effect on the AV node. The combination of the two drugs may further depress conduction through the AV node and may cause cardiac arrest. However, potassium chloride can be given to patients with PAT with block (Chapter 6).

Tachyarrhythmias associated with digitalis toxicity

Nonparoxysmal AV junctional tachycardia. When an AV junctional tachycardia occurs as a result of digitalis toxicity, it is usually the nonparoxysmal type, unlike the paroxysmal AV junctional tachycardia that may occur (Chapter 6). Nonparoxysmal AV junctional tachycardia due to digitalis toxicity usually occurs in patients who have a basic rhythm of atrial fibrillation. It can be suspected when the ventricular rate suddenly becomes regular with a rate between 60 and 100 per min (although the ventricular rate can be as fast as 150 per min) (see Fig. 6-7).

Paroxysmal atrial tachycardia with AV block. This is discussed in Chapter 6.

Ventricular premature contractions. A major arrhythmia.

Ventricular premature contractions are the most common and often the earliest cardiac sign of digitalis toxicity. Ventricular premature contractions often occur in patients who are not taking digitalis. However, when digitalis toxicity is present, the ECG usually shows other signs of digitalis effects (RS-T and T changes). In addition, the ventricular premature contractions may occur alternately after normal QRS complexes, producing a bigeminal rhythm. A bigeminal rhythm is particularly suggestive of digitalis toxicity if the patient's basic rhythm is atrial fibrillation (Fig. 8-10).

Ventricular tachycardia and ventricular fibrillation. A major or life-threatening arrhythmia.

Ventricular tachycardia due to digitalis toxicity is usually preceded by premature ventricular contractions. The tachycardia may consist of a short run of ventricular premature contractions at first; later, a sustained ventricular tachycardia may develop. The ECG is not characteristic unless a bidirectional tachycardia (see below) is present. If the digitalis toxicity continues, ventricular fibrillation and death will occur.

Bidirectional tachycardia. A major or life-threatening arrhythmia.

Bidirectional tachycardia is a form of paroxysmal tachyarrhythmia in which alternate QRS complexes point in opposite directions. The QRS width may be normal or widened (Fig. 8-11). It is almost always due to digitalis toxicity.

Most cardiologists believe that a bidirectional tachycardia is supraventricular rather than ventricular. The ectopic stimuli may arise from either two alternating foci in the AV junction or in the bundle of His or from one focus that produces alternating aberration of the QRS complexes.

Carotid sinus pressure may cause one set of the alternate QRS complexes to disappear. However, carotid sinus pressure is very dangerous if digitalis toxicity is present because it may induce lethal ventricular fibrillation. Therefore, it should never be done for more than 5 sec when digitalis toxicity is suspected, and resuscitative drugs and equipment must be immediately available.

Emergency treatment

1. Potassium chloride is probably the most effective drug for abolishing supraventricular and ventricular tachyarrhythmias due to digitalis toxicity, particularly if hypokalemia is present. It can also be used to treat PAT with block due to digitalis toxicity (Chapter 6).

The amount of potassium chloride and the route of administration depend on the seriousness of the patient's condition and on the degree and chronicity of the potassium loss. It can be given orally in a dose of 4 to 6 gm/day or IV, 40 mEq in 500 ml 5% dextrose in water, in a period of 1 to 2 hours.

When potassium chloride is given IV, the patient must be continually monitored with the ECG. If the ECG shows signs of hyperkalemia, such as the development of peaked, tented T waves or widening of the QRS complex, or if the serum potassium concentration rises to an abnormal level (above 5.5 mEq/L), the patient can be given an infusion of 50 ml 50% dextrose with 5 units of regular insulin, or sodium bicarbonate IV to lower the serum potassium concentration.

2. If potassium chloride is not effective, diphenylhydantoin, (Dilantin) is the next drug of choice. It is effective because it

Table 3. Effect of drugs on digitalis-induced tachyarrhythmias*

Arrhythmia	Potassium chloride	Diphenyl-hydantoin	Lidocaine	Propranolol	Quinidine	Procain-amide
Supraventricular tachy-arrhythmias, including PAT with block	excellent	excellent	excellent	good	fair	good
Ventricular tachyarrhythmias	excellent	excellent	excellent	fair†	fair†	fair†

*Adapted from Bigger and Heissenbuttel: Postgrad Med **47:**119, 1970.
†Significant side effects limit the effectiveness of the drug in the condition noted.

depresses the automaticity of both the atrial and ventricular muscle fibers. In addition, it does not decrease the positive inotropic effects of digitalis.

Diphenylhydantoin can be given IV in a dose of 100 mg slowly every 5 min, for a total dose of 250 mg. A further dose can be given after 20 min, if necessary. Most patients will respond within a few seconds to a few minutes. However, the tachyarrhythmia may reappear in 4 to 6 hours. When the tachyarrhythmia has been abolished, the diphenylhydantoin can be continued orally in a dose of 100 mg every 6 hours.

3. Lidocaine (Xylocaine) is the next drug of choice for the treatment of digitalis-induced tachyarrhythmias.

4. Propranolol (Inderal) is also very effective for supraventricular tachyarrhythmias, including PAT with block or ventricular premature contractions, due to digitalis toxicity. It is not very effective in digitalis-induced ventricular tachycardia and should not be used for this purpose, because it can induce serious bradyarrhythmias.

5. Either quinidine or procainamide (Pronestyl) can be used to abolish a digitalis-induced supraventricular tachyarrhythmia only if potassium chloride, diphenylhydantoin, propranolol, or lidocaine is not effective or is contraindicated and if the patient is seriously ill. Quinidine or procainamide should *not* be used to abolish a digitalis-induced *ventricular* tachycardia, because each drug prolongs conduction through the ventricular muscle and may cause lethal ventricular fibrillation in these patients.

6. Synchronized DC shock should *not* be used for a digitalis-induced tachyarrhythmia because of the danger of inducing lethal ventricular fibrillation. However, if digitalis-induced ventricular tachycardia or ventricular fibrillation is present and if the patient is critically ill and drug therapy has not been helpful, it can be used as a des-perate treatment after the patient is pretreated with an IV bolus of 100 mg lidocaine or 100 mg diphenylhydantoin IV.

7. A transvenous cardiac pacemaker can be used to overdrive a digitalis-induced tachyarrhythmia if drug therapy is ineffective (p. 223).

REFERENCES
Bradyarrhythmia-tachyarrhythmia syndromes

Bradlow BA: Supraventricular paroxysmal tachycardia interrupted by repeated episodes of total cardiac standstill with syncopal attacks, Chest **58:**122, 1970.

Cheng TO: Transvenous ventricular pacing in the treatment of paroxysmal atrial tachyarrhythmias alternating with sinus bradycardia and standstill, Am J Cardiol **22:**874, 1968.

Cohen JF, Kahn M, Donoso E: Treatment of supraventricular tachycardia with catheter and permanent pacemakers, Am J Cardiol **20:**735, 1967.

Conde C, et al: The effectiveness of pacemaker insertion in management of the bradycardia-tachycardia syndrome, Am J Cardiol **31:**127, 1973.

Epstein S, Frieden J, Furman S: Alternating supraventricular tachycardia and sinus bradycardia treated with digoxin, propranolol, and transvenous pacemaker, NY State J Med **68:**3066, 1968.

Lange H: A case of paroxysmal auricular tachycardia with sino-auricular and atrioventricular block, Acta Med Scand **124:**52, 1946.

Pick A, Langendorf R, Katz LN: Depression of cardiac pacemakers by premature impulses, Am Heart J **41:**49, 1951.

Short DS: The syndrome of alternating bradycardia and tachycardia, Br Heart J **16:**208, 1954.

Arrhythmias associated with the Wolff-Parkinson-White syndrome

Bellet S: Clinical disorders of the heart beat, ed 3, Philadelphia, 1971, Lea & Febiger.

Castellanos A Jr, et al: Electrical conversion of paroxysmal atrial fibrillation in the Wolff-Parkinson-White (pre-excitation) syndrome, Am J Cardiol **10:**657, 1966.

Cobb FR, et al: Successful surgical interruption of the bundle of Kent in a patient with W-P-W syndrome, Circulation **38:**1018, 1968.

Cole JS, et al: The Wolff-Parkinson-White syndrome; problems in evaluation and surgical therapy, Circulation **42:**111, 1970.

Dreifus LS, et al: Control of recurrent tachycardia of W-P-W syndrome by surgical ligature of the A-V bundle, Circulation **38:**1030, 1968.

Dye CL: Atrial tachycardia in the Wolff-Parkinson-White syndrome; conversion to normal sinus rhythm with lidocaine, Am J. Cardiol 24:265, 1969.

Gettes LS, Surawicz B: Long-term prevention of paroxysmal arrhythmias with propranolol therapy, Am J Med Sci 254:257, 1967.

Hejtmancik MR: Treatment of arrhythmias, particularly paroxysmal tachycardia, associated with the Wolff-Parkinson-White syndrome, Am J Cardiol 17:104, 1966.

Hellman E, Altchek MR: Paroxysmal pseudoventricular tachycardia with ventricular rate of 290 in a patient with accelerated A-V conduction, NY State J Med 58:2427, 1958.

Herrmann GR, et al.: Paroxysmal pseudoventricular tachycardia and pseudoventricular fibrillation in patients with accelerated A-V conduction, Am Heart J 53:254, 1957.

James TN: The Wolff-Parkinson-White syndrome, Ann Intern Med 71:399, 1969.

Kaplan MA, Cohen KL: Ventricular fibrillation in the Wolff-Parkinson-White syndrome, Am J Cardiol 24:259, 1969.

Kossmann CE, et al: Anomalous atrioventricular excitation produced by catheterization of the normal human heart, Circulation 1:902, 1950.

Lindsay AE, et al: Attempted surgical division of the preexcitation pathway in the Wolff-Parkinson-White syndrome, Am J Cardiol 28:581, 1971.

Lown B, Ganong WF, Levine SA: Syndrome of short P-R interval, normal QRS complex and paroxysmal rapid heart action, Circulation 5:693, 1952.

Mark H, Luna LS: Treatment of Wolff-Parkinson-White syndrome, Am Heart J 83:565, 1972.

Massumi RA, Vera Z: Patterns and mechanisms of QRS normalization in patients with Wolff-Parkinson-White syndrome, Am J Cardiol 28:541, 1971.

Narula OS: Wolff-Parkinson-White syndrome; a review, Circulation 47:872, 1973.

Newman BJ, Donoso E, Friedberg CK: Arrhythmias in the W-P-W syndrome, Prog Cardiovasc Dis 9:147, 1966.

Okel BB: The Wolff-Parkinson-White syndrome, Am Heart J 75:673, 1968.

Preston TA, Kirsch MM: Permanent pacing of the left atrium for treatment of WPW tachycardia, Circulation 42:1073, 1970.

Spritz N, et al: Electrocardiographic interrelationship of the pre-excitation (Wolff-Parkinson-White) syndrome and myocardial infarction, Am Heart J 56:715, 1958.

Wallace AG, et al: Wolff-Parkinson-White syndrome; a new look, Am J Cardiol 28:509, 1971.

Wolff L: Wolff-Parkinson-White syndrome; historical and clinical features, Prog Cardiovasc Dis 2:677, 1960.

Wolff L, Richman JL: The diagnosis of myocardial infarction in patients with atrioventricular excitation (Wolff-Parkinson-White syndrome), Am Heart J 45:545, 1953.

Yahini JH, Zahavi I, Neufeld HN: Paroxysmal atrial fibrillation in Wolff-Parkinson-White syndrome simulating ventricular tachycardia, Am J Cardiol 14:248, 1964.

Arrhythmias associated with digitalis toxicity

Alexander S, Ping WC: Fatal ventricular fibrillation during carotid sinus stimulation, Am J Cardiol 18:289, 1966.

Bazzano G, Bazzano GS: Digitalis intoxication; treatment with a new steroid-binding resin, JAMA 220:828, 1972.

Castellanos A, Lemberg L, et al: Concealed digitalis induced arrhythmias unmasked by electrical stimulation of the heart, Am Heart J 73:484, 1967.

Chung EK: Digitalis-induced multifocal ectopic beats and rhythms, Postgrad Med 50:245, 1971.

Ewy GA, Marcus FI: Digoxin metabolism in the elderly, Circulation 39:449, 1969.

Fisch C: Digitalis-induced rhythm change; improvement or life-threatening arrhythmia? Consultant, Oct-Nov 1970, p 7.

Fisch C, Martz BL, Priebe FH: Enhancement of potassium-induced atrioventricular block by toxic doses of digitalis drugs, J Clin Invest 39:1885, 1960.

Helfant RH, Scherlag BJ, Damato AN: Protection from digitalis toxicity with the prophylactic use of diphenylhydantoin sodium, Circulation 36:119, 1967.

Katz MJ, Zitnik RS: Direct current shock and lidocaine in the treatment of digitalis-induced ventricular tachycardia, Am J Cardiol 18:552, 1966.

Kleiger R, Lown B: Cardioversion and digitalis. II. Clinical studies, Circulation 33:878, 1966.

Neff MS, Mendelssohn S, et al: Magnesium sulfate in digitalis toxicity, Am J Cardiol 29:377, 1972.

Ogilvie RI, Ruedy J: An educational program in digitalis therapy, JAMA 222:50, 1972.

Pick A, Dominguez P: Non-paroxysmal A-V nodal tachycardia, Circulation 16:1022, 1957.

Reynolds EW Jr: The use of potassium in the treatment of heart disease, Am Heart J 70:1, 1965.

Rios JC, Dziok CA, Ali NA: Digitalis-induced arrhythmias; recognition and management, Cardiovasc Clin 2 (2):262, 1970.

Rosenbaum JL, et al: The effect of disodium EDTA on digitalis intoxication, Am J Med Sci 240:111, 1960.

Rosenbaum M, Elizari M, Lazzari J: The mechanism of bidirectional tachycardia, Am Heart J 78:4, 1969.

Seller RH: The role of magnesium in digitalis toxicity, Am Heart J **82:**551, 1971.

Shapiro W, et al: Nonradioactive serum digoxin and digitoxin levels, Arch Intern Med **130:**31, 1972.

Soffer A, et al: Clinical applications and untoward reactions of chelation in cardiac arrhythmias, Arch Intern Med **106:**824, 1960.

Somylo AP: The toxicology of digitalis, Am J Cardiol **5:**523, 1960.

Turgen JRB: Propranolol in the treatment of digitalis-induced and digitalis-resistant tachycardias, Am J Cardiol **18:**450, 1966.

Weinstein WJ, Jick S: Bidirectional tachycardia, Am J Cardiol **3:**343, 1959.

9 / Acute myocardial infarction

The term acute myocardial infarction describes the development of ischemia and necrosis of a portion of the myocardium. It is associated with coronary atherosclerosis in approximately 90% of cases. However, it is not necessarily associated with coronary artery thrombosis. (There is evidence that the coronary artery thrombosis may occur after the infarction has developed. The exact mechanism by which the infarction occurs in these patients is not known.) In addition, acute myocardial infarction has been found in a small group of patients who have normal coronary arteries as shown by coronary arteriography. (Some of these patients showed a somewhat slower rate of oxygen release from hemoglobin solutions. At first it was thought that this was due to cigarette smoking, which can raise the carbon monoxide level in the blood and decrease the oxygen release rate of hemoglobin. However, the exact mechanism by which myocardial infarction occurs in these patients is unknown.)

When surgery is done on patients who have been given general anesthesia and who have had a myocardial infarction less than 3 months previously, more than one third develop a new myocardial infarct (particularly during the third postoperative day). Similarly, acute myocardial infarction is not unusual following saphenous vein bypass operations on the coronary arteries. Rarer causes of acute myocardial infarction include acute dissecting aneurysm of the aorta, coronary artery embolism, polyarteritis nodosa, radiation therapy, and neoplastic invasion. Acute myocardial infarction can also occur after sudden severe hemorrhage; with acute hypoxia, such as carbon monoxide poisoning; or when excessive doses of catecholamines, such as epinephrine or isoproterenol (Isuprel), have been administered. Although angina pectoris is also due to coronary artery disease, many patients with acute myocardial infarction do not have a history of angina.

Pathology

Two basic types of acute myocardial infarction have been described: transmural myocardial infarction and subendocardial infarction.

Transmural myocardial infarction is associated with atherosclerosis involving a major coronary artery. It can be subclassified into anterior, inferior (diaphragmatic), or posterior, particularly on the basis of electrocardiographic patterns.

Subendocardial infarction involves small areas, particularly in the subendocardial wall of the left ventricle, the ventricular septum, and the papillary muscles. The factors that determine whether subendocardial infarction rather than transmural myocardial infarction will occur are not known.

Atrial infarction can also occur, but it generally does not affect treatment or prognosis.

Clinical aspects

Most patients with acute myocardial infarction seek medical treatment because of chest pain. However, the clinical picture may vary from that of a patient who walks into the office for a routine examination, to a patient who develops severe substernal oppression and quickly develops shock and pulmonary edema, or to a previously healthy person who dies suddenly.

The onset of myocardial infarction is usually acute, with anginalike pain; but unlike ordinary angina, there is excruciating pressure in the chest, or a premonition of impending doom. If the patient has previously suffered from angina, he is aware that something different from his former attacks of angina is happening. Also, in contrast to ordinary angina, acute myocardial infarction usually occurs when the patient is at rest, often in the early hours of the morning. Nitroglycerin does not relieve the pain, which may wax and wane and may last hours and even days. Nausea and vomiting are frequent accompaniments of the pain and may be severe, particularly if morphine is given for the pain.

The pain has a diffuse constricting, choking, viselike, or boring quality. It is most marked in the substernal region, from which it may spread to both arms, the throat or jaw, or to the upper abdomen (so that it may simulate the pain of a gallbladder colic, acute cholecystitis, acute peptic ulcer, or acute pancreatitis).

Cases of myocardial infarction without pain have been reported. However, when these patients are questioned closely, they usually describe "indigestion" or a vague "lump in the chest," which was only slightly uncomfortable. Occasionally, patients experience breathlessness instead of substernal pressure. Hiccup due to irritation of the diaphragm by an inferior wall infarction, may occasionally occur.

The patient usually remains conscious, but he may be restless, excited, or confused. Syncope is rare. Unconsciousness due to cerebral ischemia resulting from the decreased cardiac output may also occur.

When patients are questioned carefully, they often state that for a varying time before the attack (from 1 day to 2 weeks)

their anginal pain had become increasingly more severe and was not responding well to nitroglycerin or that they had begun to develop vague substernal distress or "indigestion" *(premonitory symptoms)*. It has been suggested that, when angina begins to be more severe, the patient be put to bed for a week to prevent an attack of myocardial infarction. However, in my experience this has not helped prevent acute myocardial infarction.

When examined, the patient often shows an ashen-gray pallor, with profuse perspiration and cold skin, even if clinical signs of shock (Chapter 3) are absent. The pulse is usually rapid, unless incomplete or complete AV block is present. Within a few hours the patient's clinical condition begins to improve, but fever often develops. The temperature rises for a few days, even to 102 F or higher, and then slowly falls, returning to normal by the end of a week.

The blood pressure falls. This may occur abruptly, or gradually in the first 24 hours after the attack. Less commonly, the blood pressure continues to fall for approximately 1 week. At this point, the blood pressure may remain stable or may slowly begin to rise again.

A pericardial friction rub may occur. It is usually transient and is due to a localized pericardial reaction over the epicardial surface of the infarct. Less frequently, a generalized serosanguinous pericarditis may occur. Pericardial effusion is rare.

An atrial (S_4) gallop, ventricular (S_3) gallop, and other physical signs have been described in association with uncomplicated acute myocardial infarction. However, they are not diagnostic.

Moderate basal rales develop in approximately one third of patients. They usually disappear by the end of the first week without specific treatment. (Also see p. 139.)

Electrocardiogram

The acute electrocardiographic changes of myocardial infarction consist of abnor-

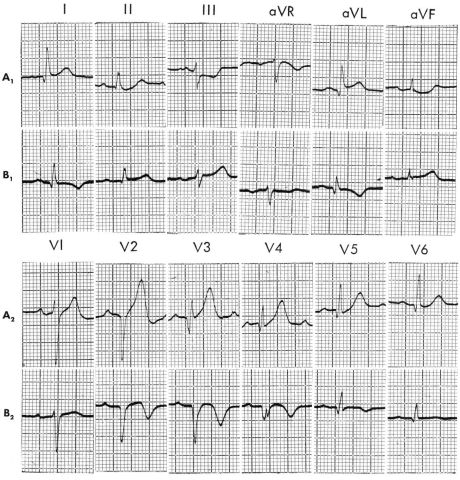

Fig. 9-1. Hyperacute T waves in acute myocardial infraction. $A_{1,2}$, Taken on patient's admission to the hospital. $B_{1,2}$, Eight days later. $A_{1,2}$, Precordial leads show tall, hyperacute T waves. Q waves have already developed in leads V_2, V_3, and V_4. (The patient's symptoms had started the evening before admission.) Extremity leads show characteristic elevation of the RS-T in lead aV_L, with reciprocal depression of the RS-T in lead aV_F and leads II and III. Lead I shows a tall T wave. $B_{1,2}$, Characteristic symmetrical downward T waves have developed in the precordial leads and in leads I and aV_L. (These changes had started 24 hours after admission.)

mal Q waves and a characteristic progression of RS-T and T wave changes. In general, these patterns are almost pathognomonic of acute myocardial infarction, with important exceptions, described below.

"Hyperacute" T waves. These are tall, prominent T waves, which often appear as the earliest electrocardiographic sign of acute myocardial infarction (Fig. 9-1). They are followed by the more familiar RS-T

elevations within 24 hours. (Similar tall, prominent T waves may also be a normal variant, especially in young men.)

RS-T elevations. The RS-T segment in acute myocardial infarction becomes elevated in one or more leads, and in addition, its shape becomes abnormal. It may be straightened and fuse with the T, or it may rise obliquely and fuse with the T, or it may show a dome-shaped convexity

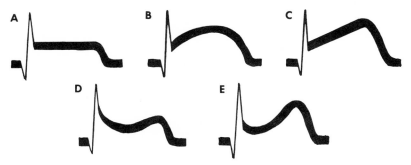

Fig. 9-2. Diagrams showing abnormally shaped, elevated RS-T segments. **A,** Plateau RS-T. **B,** Dome-shaped RS-T. **C,** Obliquely elevated RS-T. **D,** Crescent RS-T. **E,** Abnormally elevated RS-T with a normal upward convexity and a hyperacute T. (From Goldberger E: Unipolar lead electrocardiography and vectorcardiography, ed. 3, Philadelphia, 1953, Lea & Febiger.)

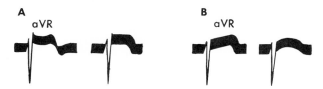

Fig. 9-3. Diagrams showing abnormal RS-T elevations in lead aV_R. **A,** Subendocardial ischemia (acute coronary insufficiency or subendocardial infarction). **B,** Digitalis effects. (From Goldberger E: Unipolar lead electrocardiography and vectorcardiography, ed. 3, Philadelphia, 1953, Lea & Febiger.)

(Figs. 9-2 and 9-3). Occasionally, the RS-T shows a normal contour but is elevated 2 mm or more above the base line.

Although these abnormal elevated RS-T segments are relatively specific for acute myocardial infarction, they also occur in two other ischemic conditions: atypical (Prinzmetal) angina with transient RS-T elevations (see below), and ventricular aneurysm, in which persistent RS-T elevations may occur (p. 142).

Pericarditis may also produce RS-T elevations that must be distinguished from those seen in acute myocardial infarction. In pericarditis, RS-T elevations *without* abnormal Q waves occur in one or more of the precordial leads, in leads aV_L and aV_F, and in one or more of the standard limb leads. (Later, T wave inversions develop in these leads.) The reciprocal changes in leads aV_L and aV_F and in leads I and III,

which are characteristic of acute myocardial infarction, do not appear in pericarditis.

RS-T elevations with abnormal Q waves occur rarely in myocarditis. In such patients, the electrocardiographic differentiation from acute myocardial infarction is not possible.

Marked RS-T elevations (up to 4 mm in the precordial leads) may also occur normally, probably due to early repolarization of the heart muscle. The elevated RS-T segments retain their normal upward concavity. This pattern is characteristically most marked in the left precordial leads and is especially common in young normal adults, although it has been reported in older people as well.

RS-T elevation in the right precordial leads is also commonly seen with left ventricular hypertrophy and with left bundle branch block.

T wave changes. As evolution of the infarct occurs, the elevated RS-T segments return to the base line, and deep symmetrical T waves appear in these leads. Tall, symmetrical, upright T waves will appear in reciprocal leads at the same time.

A diagnosis of acute myocardial infarction should not be made because of the presence of abnormal T waves alone. Numerous conditions can produce T wave changes, including eating; changes in posture; malnutrition; fear; drugs such as digitalis, quinidine, procainamide, diphenylhydantoin, epinephrine, deoxycorticosterone; tobacco; diseases such as myocarditis, pericarditis, and cardiomyopathies; acute infections of any etiology; uremia; endocrine disturbances, such as adrenocortical insufficiency; diabetic acidosis; and electrolyte disturbances, particularly hypokalemia.

In addition, T wave inversion in the right precordial leads is a normal variant in children. This juvenile pattern may also occur in young adults. Finally, patients with cerebral hemorrhage, meningitis, or head injury may show giant, wide T wave inversion (rarely giant tall T waves), often associated with a prolonged Q-T interval and prominent or inverted U waves. Autopsies of some of these patients have shown microscopic signs of myocardial damage. However, the significance of these giant inverted T waves is poorly understood.

Abnormal Q waves. A Q wave is not necessarily abnormal. However, the sudden development of Q waves may indicate an acute myocardial infarction. A Q wave is abnormal—that is, it is due to myocardial infarction (or destruction of muscle cells by any other process)—if it shows the following criteria.

1. Abnormal Q waves in precordial lead V_1 or in leads V_1 and V_2
2. Abnormal Q waves in precordial leads V_3, V_4, V_5, and V_6
3. Abnormal Q wave in lead aV_F

Abnormal Q waves in precordial lead V_1 or in leads V_1 and V_2. An abnormal QS due to acute anteroseptal myocardial infarction may appear in lead V_1 or in leads V_1 and V_2. However, lead V_1 often shows a QS normally. In such a case, the precordial lead immediately to the left shows an rS pattern. Once an rS pattern appears in a precordial lead, a QS in a precordial lead to the left is always abnormal, even if it occurs in lead V_2. An abnormal QS in leads V_1 and V_2 is usually notched or slurred, in contrast to a normal QS in these leads.

When left bundle branch block or left ventricular hypertrophy is present, a QS may appear in leads V_1, V_2, and V_3 in the absence of myocardial infarction. Also, in such cases the precordial lead immediately to the left shows an rS.

Precordial lead V_1 and rarely leads V_1 and V_2 may also show a QR pattern in the absence of myocardial infarction, particularly when right ventricular hypertrophy or acute or chronic pulmonary disease is present. In such patients, the precordial lead immediately to the left shows an rS or a tall R. In addition, right axis deviation is usually present.

Abnormal Q waves in precordial leads V_3, V_4, V_5, and V_6. (1) The depth of the Q wave is 25% or more the amplitude of the R wave in that lead, or the entire QRS complex consists of a QS deflection; and/or (2) the width of the Q wave is 0.04 sec or more. (The width of Q is measured on the upper level of the base line from the point where Q begins to the point where it returns to the base line.)

In right ventricular hypertrophy, abnormal Q waves may appear in leads V_5 and V_6 in the absence of myocardial infarction. Leads V_1 and V_2 in such patients show tall R waves or a QR pattern, characteristic of right ventricular hypertrophy. In addition, right axis deviation is usually present, with peaked P waves in leads II and III (P pulmonale pattern).

Idiopathic hypertrophic subaortic stenosis may also show abnormal Q waves in the lateral precordial leads (due to hypertrophy of the interventricular septum).

Abnormal Q wave in lead aV_F. The following three criteria are present.

1. The depth of the Q wave in lead aV_F is 25% or more the amplitude of the R wave in lead aV_F. A QS wave in lead aV_F may also be present.

2. The width of the Q wave in lead aV_F is 0.04 sec or more.

3. Lead aV_R shows a QS or an rS, but not a Qr, QR, or qR.

The abnormal Q wave in lead aV_F causes the abnormal Q waves in leads II and III.

The following other conditions may produce a Q wave in lead aV_F that resembles an abnormal Q. Massive pulmonary embolism may produce a deep, wide Q in lead aV_F, associated with an elevated RS-T, suggestive of acute inferior myocardial infarction. However, an acute right axis shift is present in the standard leads, with an S_1Q_3 pattern; lead aV_R shows a QR type of pattern; and in the precordial leads, the T wave may be downward in leads V_1 through V_3 or V_4. In the Wolff-Parkinson-White syndrome, a QS pattern may be present in leads II, III, and aV_F. In left bundle branch block, a QS pattern may be present in lead aV_F. In idiopathic hypertrophic subaortic stenosis, the abnormal Q wave is due to hypertrophy of the interventricular septum. In addition, abnormal Q waves, due to diffuse myocardial damage resulting from amyloidosis of the heart, scleroderma, and so on, may appear in any lead.

Progressive electrocardiographic changes of acute myocardial infarction

The abnormal Q and RS-T changes may appear in one or more leads as early as $\frac{1}{2}$ hour after an attack. However, maximal changes may not develop for several days. As the evolution of the electrocardiographic changes occurs, the RS-T deviations slowly return to the base line. Leads that showed elevated RS-T segments develop deep symmetrical T waves. Leads that showed depressed RS-T segments develop tall symmetrical T waves. Still later, the abnormal T waves shrink and become normal in size and shape, leaving only the abnormal Q waves as signs of an old healed myocardial infarction. Even the abnormal Q waves may disappear.

The time relations of these sequential changes are variable, and a pattern may remain at any stage indefinitely. For example, if a ventricular aneurysm develops, marked deviations of the RS-T segments may persist for years. More commonly, the RS-T segments begin to return to the base line in a week or two. The progression of T wave changes continues for several months. Therefore, by 6 months or 1 year, the ECG has returned to normal, with the exception of abnormal Q waves.

Localization of the electrocardiographic patterns of acute myocardial infarction

The electrocardiographic changes are the most reliable signs of acute myocardial infarction. Innumerable electrocardiographic patterns may develop, depending on the location and size of the infarct, the presence of previous infarctions, and the presence of pericarditis, bundle branch block, or other fascicular blocks. Generally, the electrocardiographic patterns can be described as anterior, inferior (diaphragmatic), posterior (dorsal), or subendocardial. (Atrial infarction, which produces elevation and depression of the P-Ta wave, will not be discussed.)

Anterior myocardial infarction. In a typical case of acute anterior infarction, abnormal Q waves and abnormal, elevated RS-T segments appear in one or more of the precordial leads, in lead aV_L, and usually in lead I. Leads aV_R, aV_F, and III show reciprocal RS-T depression (Fig. 9-4). Anterior wall infarction can be further localized as anteroseptal (changes in leads

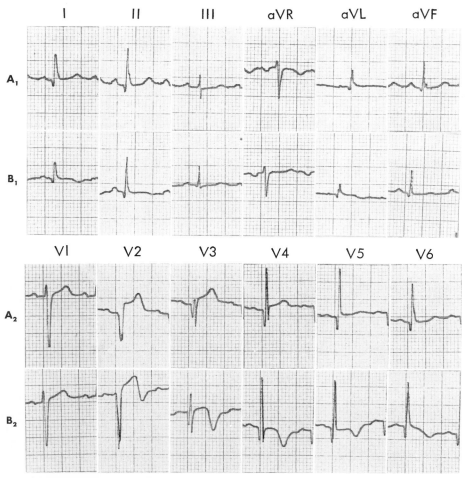

Fig. 9-4. Acute anterior myocardial infarction. $A_{1,2}$, Day after the attack occurred; abnormal RS-T elevations in precordial leads V_2, V_3, and V_4, and in lead AV_L, associated with abnormal Q waves in leads V_2, V_3, V_4, and V_5. $B_{1,2}$, Following day; development of deep symmetrical T waves in the precordial leads and in leads I and aV_L. It is unusual for a patient to show such abnormal Q waves in association with early RS-T changes after acute myocardial infarction. The patient did not give a history of a previous myocardial infarction, and an ECG taken a year previously was normal.

V_1 and V_2), strictly anterior (changes in leads V_3 and V_4), or anterolateral (changes in leads V_5 and V_6).

As the progressive changes occur, the elevated RS-T segments return to the base line, and deep symmetrical T waves appear in one or more of the precordial leads and in leads aV_L and I, and tall symmetrical T waves appear in leads aV_R, aV_F, and III.

Inferior (diaphragmatic) myocardial infarction. Abnormal deep wide Q waves and RS-T elevations occur in leads aV_F, II, and III (Fig. 9-5). Later, deep symmetrical T waves appear in these leads. Depressed RS-T segments and, later, tall symmetrical T waves appear in leads aV_L and aV_R, in one or more of the precordial leads, and in lead I.

Posterior (dorsal) myocardial infarction.

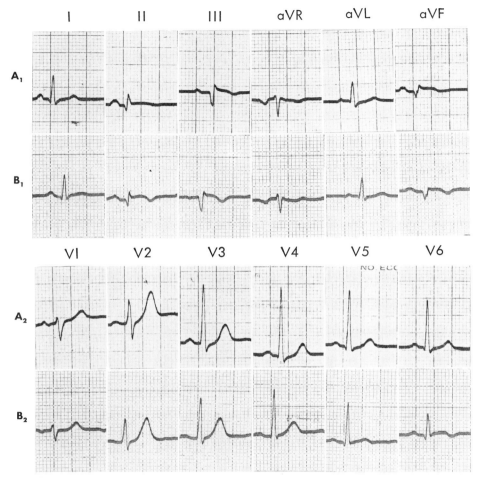

Fig. 9-5. Acute inferior myocardial infarction. **A**$_{1,2}$, Day after the attack occurred; characteristic abnormal Q and elevated RS-T in leads aV$_F$, II, and III. The precordial leads show tall T waves, which are not pathognomonic of myocardial infarction. **B**$_{1,2}$, Week after **A** was taken. Deep symmetrical T waves have developed in leads aV$_F$, II, and III. In addition, an abnormal RS-T and T has developed in lead V$_6$, indicating that the infarct had spread to the anterolateral wall of the left ventricle. This patient had suffered an attack of acute inferior wall myocardial infarction 9 years prior to this attack. His ECG had completely returned to normal.

This involves the posterior basal or infra-atrial wall of the left ventricle, rather than the diaphragmatic wall of the left ventricle.

When localized posterior infarction occurs, dorsal leads (such as low esophageal leads) show the characteristic RS-T elevations. Reciprocal leads, especially the right precordial leads, show RS-T depression. However, none of the conventional leads

show characteristic abnormal Q waves or RS-T elevations, unless the infarct extends either to the lateral or inferior wall of the left ventricle. However, tall R waves appear in precordial leads, such as V$_1$ or V$_2$, near the sternum. These tall R waves actually represent reciprocal changes to the deep Q waves that occur posteriorly.

Subendocardial infarction. When subendocardial infarction is present, the ele-

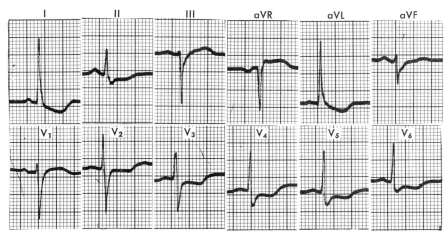

Fig. 9-6. Acute subendocardial myocardial infarction. Characteristic elevation of the RS-T occurs in lead aV$_R$ in association with depression of the RS-T in precordial leads V$_2$ through V$_6$ and in leads I, II, aV$_L$, and aV$_F$. The RS-T and T pattern in leads I and aV$_L$ is not due to the subendocardial infarction but to left ventricular hypertrophy and strain, which had been present before the subendocardial infarct occurred.

vated RS-T occurs in lead aV$_R$ because it reflects subendocardial potentials. Reciprocal depression of the RS-T occurs in one or more of the other leads, such as one or more of the precordial leads, aV$_L$, aV$_F$, or the standard leads (Fig. 9-6). As the progressive changes occur, these RS-T deviations return to the base line without abnormal T waves developing. Occasionally, the RS-T deviations persist indefinitely.

Deep T wave inversion, without Q waves, in the precordial and limb leads have also been described as a sign of subendocardial infarction. However, I believe that when such T wave changes occur, they indicate that there is also some degree of transmural ischemia.

Acute myocardial infarction complicated by bundle branch block

When acute myocardial infarction is complicated by right bundle branch block, the ECG shows both the patterns of the right bundle branch block and of the myocardial infarction. When acute myocardial infarction is complicated by left bundle branch block or by the Wolff-Parkinson-White syndrome, or in patients with a transvenous

pacemaker, the ECG does not usually show typical patterns of myocardial infarction. It may be necessary to treat such patients on the basis of the clinical signs and changing enzyme values. If a pacemaker can be turned off temporarily or if the Wolff-Parkinson-White pattern disappears temporarily, the patterns of acute myocardial infarction will appear. (Patients with the Wolff-Parkinson-White syndrome often show a deep, wide Q wave in leads aV$_F$, II, and III, which simulates the abnormal Q of inferior myocardial infarction, in spite of the fact that myocardial infarction is absent; see above.)

Laboratory tests
Serum enzyme tests

When acute myocardial infarction occurs, myocardial enzymes are released into the general circulation. Presence of these enzymes can be quantitated and used to determine the evolution and extent of myocardial necrosis. The following enzyme tests are most commonly employed.

1. Creatinine phosphokinase
2. Serum glutamic oxaloacetic transaminase
3. Lactic dehydrogenase

Creatine phosphokinase (CPK). Highest levels are found in skeletal muscle, myocardium, and brain tissue. CPK levels become elevated 2 to 4 hours after acute myocardial infarction, peak at 24 to 36 hours, and return to normal in approximately 3 days. Peak CPK levels may reach 10 times normal values. (In general, tenfold elevations in any of these enzyme levels is associated with a high mortality.) CPK levels may also be elevated by primary muscle disease, various types of acute cerebral accidents including cerebral infarction, diabetic acidosis, surgery, acute alcoholism, hypothyroidism, and IM injections. CPK elevations also occur with myocarditis, pericarditis (slight increase occasionally), coronary angiography, and cardiac catheterization. Recently, CPK isoenzyme determinations have been used to differentiate myocardial damage from enzyme elevation due to surgery and IM injections.

Serum glutamic oxaloacetic transaminase (SGOT). SGOT levels generally become elevated 8 to 12 hours after acute myocardial infarction, peak at values up to 10 times normal at 18 to 36 hours, and fall to normal in about 3 to 5 days. SGOT levels may be increased in myocarditis, occasionally in pericarditis, following DC shock (up to threefold increase), after tachyarrhythmias persisting for at least 30 min with rates over 140 per min, and after cardiac catheterization. High SGOT levels may occur in primary liver disease, shock, pulmonary infarction, with liver dysfunction secondary to passive congestion, and in muscle disease or injury. Certain drugs, including birth control pills, clofibrate (Atromid-S), and narcotics used in patients with biliary disease, may also lead to increased SGOT levels.

Lactic dehydrogenase (LDH). LDH is found in many types of tissue. LDH levels generally become elevated 8 to 48 hours after myocardial infarction, peak up to ten times normal values in 3 to 6 days, and return to normal in 8 to 14 days. LDH levels may also be increased with myocarditis, cardiac catheterization, pulmonary infarction, hepatic disease, renal infarction, megaloblastic anemia, and leukemia. Spurious elevation of LDH levels may be caused by hemolysis of the blood sample. LDH isoenzyme studies may be useful in determining the source of an increased LDH concentration.

Elevated serum enzyme levels have no significance in the first 5 days after a surgical operation.

Other laboratory tests

The sedimentation rate often increases following acute myocardial infarction. However, it is nonspecific.

A leukocytosis is often present, with white blood cell counts up to 20,000/ml.

Transient hyperglycemia may occur. In some patients, acute myocardial infarction unmasks latent diabetes mellitus, which may become manifest later on. Diabetic acidosis can be precipitated.

Finally, cholesterol levels may decrease and triglyceride levels may increase with an acute myocardial infarction. These values usually return to the base line in a few months.

Differential diagnosis

A severe anginal attack, acute nonspecific pericarditis, acute dissecting aneurysm of the aorta, massive pulmonary embolism, spontaneous emphysema, and acute abdominal conditions, such as acute cholecystitis, acute peptic ulcer, or acute pancreatitis, are common conditions that can simulate acute myocardial infarction.

Angina pectoris. The terms acute coronary insufficiency, coronary failure, intermediate coronary syndrome, and preinfarction angina have been used to describe patients whose symptoms and course are more severe than the usual anginal attack but less severe than the usual attack of acute myocardial infarction.

Although the substernal pain of such patients lasts at least 30 min and is unrelated to the usual precipitating factors, such as exertion or arrhythmias, serial ECGs for at least 2 days do not show the progressive changes of acute myocardial infarction, and serum enzyme tests remain normal in this period of time.

Variant angina pectoris (Prinzmetal's angina) describes patients whose anginal pain is typical. However, the pain usually occurs without any precipitating factor when the patient is at rest. It tends to recur in a cyclic waxing and waning fashion and often occurs at approximately the same time each day. The ECG during the anginal episodes characteristically shows abnormal elevated RS-T segments, suggestive of acute myocardial infarction, rather than the RS-T depressions that often occur with a usual anginal attack. These RS-T elevations, however, are transient and return to the base line when the pain disappears. The patient may also develop ventricular tachyarrhythmias or AV block during the anginal pain.

Variant angina is often due to obstruction of a single major coronary artery (corresponding to the site indicated by the electrocardiographic changes). The immediate treatment is the same as for the usual angina pectoris. However, saphenous vein graft bypass may be indicated if coronary arteriography confirms a localized stenotic lesion of a coronary artery.

Acute nonspecific pericarditis. The onset may be as severe as an attack of acute myocardial infarction and may include intense precordial pain and shock. However, fever is maximal on the first day, when a loud pericardial friction rub can also be heard. (In myocardial infarction, the peak of the fever does not occur for several days, and a pericardial friction rub is transient or delayed.)

The ECG is helpful in the differential diagnosis. In pericarditis, RS-T elevations without abnormal Q waves occur in one or more of the precordial leads, in leads aV_L and aV_F, and in one or more of the standard limb leads. (Later, downward T waves develop in these leads.) In addition, the reciprocal changes in leads aV_L and aV_F and in leads I and III, which occur after myocardial infarction, do not appear after pericarditis.

Enzyme changes may occur in pericarditis because of injury to the subepicardial layer of the myocardium. Therefore, these changes cannot be used for differential diagnosis.

Acute abdominal conditions. Epigastric pain, vomiting, upper abdominal tenderness, rigidity, shock, and even slight jaundice can occur with acute myocardial infarction and can simulate an attack of acute cholecystitis, gallbladder colic, ruptured peptic ulcer, acute pancreatitis, or other abdominal emergencies.

The differential diagnosis is usually not difficult, except in cases of acute pancreatitis, which can be associated with abnormal Q waves and RS-T elevations identical to those that occur with acute myocardial infarction. The cause of these changes is unknown. In acute pancreatitis, serum and urinary amylase concentrations are abnormally high.

Dissecting aneurysm of the aorta. The pain of a dissecting aneurysm may simulate the pain of acute myocardial infarction, but it does not commonly radiate into the shoulders, arms, or neck, as occurs with severe angina or acute myocardial infarction (Chapter 13). Similarly, the ECG of acute dissecting aneurysm shows nonspecific changes, unlike the characteristic Q waves, RS-T segment deviations, and T wave changes of acute myocardial infarction. However, if the dissection involves one of the coronary ostia, characteristic electrocardiographic patterns of acute myocardial infarction may appear.

Spontaneous mediastinal emphysema. Severe substernal pressure, which may radiate to the back, neck, shoulders, and rarely to the arms, may develop. However, the ECG remains normal, blood pressure remains normal, and constitutional signs, including the temperature, remain normal. Auscultation reveals a peculiar crunching sound, usually systolic, and occasionally also diastolic, due to the presence of air in the anterior mediastinum. Partial pneumothorax, usually involving the left upper chest, may also develop. The diagnosis is confirmed by x-ray examination of the chest.

Massive pulmonary embolism. See Chapter 11.

Other conditions that can simulate acute myocardial infarction. Abnormal ECGs that can simulate acute myocardial infarction can occur in the following conditions.

1. *Cerebral hemorrhage* or *head injury.* Deep, abnormal T waves or RS-T deviations with prominent U waves and a prolonged Q-T interval may develop. However, autopsy may show signs of subendocardial injury or diffuse injury to the heart muscle cells in some of these patients.

2. *Diffuse myocardial disease,* such as amyloidosis of the heart or scleroderma. Abnormal Q waves may be present, but the serial changes of acute myocardial infarction do not appear.

3. *Ventricular hypertrophy.* Patients with left ventricular hypertrophy may show a QS pattern in leads V_1 and V_2 or even in lead V_3, associated with RS-T elevations. In these patients, precordial leads, such as V_5 and V_6, usually show a reciprocal pattern, namely a tall R wave with depressed RS-T segment and downward T wave, characteristic of left ventricular strain rather than of myocardial infarction.

Patients with right ventricular hypertrophy show a tall R in precordial lead V_1 or in leads V_1 and V_2. Rarely, precordial lead V_5 or leads V_5 and V_6 show an abnormal Q wave. However, in these patients, also, the sequential changes of acute myocardial infarction do not appear.

4. *Digitalis* causes RS-T depressions associated with a shortened Q-T interval in the standard limb leads, in one or more of the precordial leads, and in lead aV_L and or aV_F, with an elevation in lead aV_R. These changes are not associated with the development of abnormal Q waves and should not be confused with the patterns of acute myocardial infarction.

5. *Severe acidosis* or *paroxysmal tachyarrhythmias* may occasionally be associated with abnormal RS-T deviations or transient abnormal Q waves. The mechanism of these changes is not known.

Treatment

All patients with an acute myocardial infarction or suspected myocardial infarction should be admitted to a coronary care unit (CCU). Approximately one half of the deaths from acute myocardial infarction occur within the first hour—often before the patient reaches the hospital. The death rate sharply declines after this; and if the patient survives for about a week, his chances of leaving the hospital alive are excellent. Treatment in the CCU should be directed to the highest-priority measures first: starting oxygen therapy, establishing an IV line, administering an analgesic, drawing blood for routine tests, taking an ECG and attaching the patient to a monitor, and, of course, treating serious arrhythmias or shock. In addition, orders must be written for general care, including diet, sedation, and bowel care. These matters are discussed in detail below.

Intravenous therapy and blood samples. An IV line is essential and should be started with an intracath, with 500 ml 5% dextrose in water flowing through a *microdrip bulb* at minimal flow rate. If an ordinary drip bulb is used, the patient may receive more than a liter of IV fluids in a 24-hour period. This can be deleterious for several reasons. Patients in acute stress often secrete increased amounts of ADH, thus producing an antidiuretic state with decreased water excretion. In addition, the patient with an acute myocardial infarction usually does not eat normally and instead drinks (mostly sodium-free) fluids. As a result, a significant dilution of the extracellular fluids in association with a decreased serum sodium concentration and a decreased cardiac output can occur. When a microdrip bulb is used with a minimal flow rate, a patient will receive approximately 300 ml of fluids in 24 hours.

While IV therapy is being started, admission blood samples can be obtained for the following tests: CBC, glucose, BUN, creatinine, CPK, LDH, and SGOT. In addition, clotting studies (including prothrombin time and platelet count), urinalysis, and stool guaiac (on voided specimen —avoid rectal exam) should also be obtained as a base line if anticoagulation therapy is administered.

Oxygen therapy. Administer oxygen by nasal catheter at 6 to 8 L/min. In general, oxygen is indicated for pain, cyanosis, dyspnea, left-sided failure, or cardiogenic shock. It should be used routinely for the first 24 to 48 hours after the attack and should be continued as long as significant pain is present. The conventional use of oxygen by nasal catheter rarely produces an inspired oxygen concentration greater than 40%. However, uncontrolled use of 100% oxygen by closed circuit methods is not indicated in uncomplicated acute myocardial infarction, because such a high oxygen concentration may actually decrease coronary blood flow and may also have a negative inotropic effect.

Monitor leads (Chapter 19). Set the high rate alarm signal at 110 beats per min and the low rate alarm signal at 50 beats per min.

Emergency treatment of arrhythmias and shock. Definitive therapy of these emergencies is discussed in Chapters 10 and 3, respectively. However, the following standing orders for CCU nurses can be written.

Tachyarrhythmias. If ventricular premature contractions occur more often than five per min, occur in groups of two or more, are multifocal, or occur at the apex of the T wave, give lidocaine (Xylocaine)* IV as a 75-mg bolus. This can be repeated in 5 min, if necessary. Then continue to give the lidocaine as a constant IV infusion, with a microdrip bulb, in a solution of 100 ml (2 gm) added to 400 ml 5% dextrose in water, at a rate of 15 to 60 microdrops per min (1 to 4 mg/min).

If ventricular tachycardia occurs, thump chest, give lidocaine bolus IV, as above. Continue with a lidocaine drip. If the patient's condition appears critical, prepare the DC shock apparatus. Call for medical help.

Bradyarrhythmias. If sinus bradycardia, AV junctional rhythm, or AV block occurs and the ventricular rate decreases below 50 per min, raise the patient's legs 45°, and give atropine, 0.6 mg IV.

If the ventricular rate does not rise above 50 per min after 10 min, start an IV drip of isoproterenol, one 5-ml ampul (1 mg) in 500 ml 5% dextrose in water. Adjust the flow rate to maintain a ventricular rate between 60 and 70 per min.

Cardiac arrest. If cardiac arrest occurs, start cardiopulmonary resuscitation and external cardiac compression. Call for medical help. In addition, give the following therapy.

If the monitor screen shows ventricular fibrillation, defibrillate the patient with a 400-ws DC shock. (In many hospitals, CCU nurses are permitted to defibrillate a patient if a physician is not present.)

If the monitor screen shows ventricular standstill, give the following drugs.

1. Epinephrine (1:10,000), 5 ml IV. A solution of 1:10,000 epinephrine can be made by adding 1 ml (1:1,000) epinephrine to 9 ml isotonic saline. However, prefilled syringes of 1:10,000 epinephrine (with or without an intracardiac needle) are available.
2. Sodium bicarbonate (7.5%). Give 2 ampuls (100 ml) IV.

Cardiogenic shock. Start an emergency infusion of levarterenol (Levophed), 1 ampul in 1,000 ml of 5% dextrose in water or

---

*This and other drugs are described in Part three.

dextrose in saline; or metaraminol (Aramine), 10 ml (100 mg) in 500 ml 5% dextrose in water or in saline, to raise the systolic blood pressure to 90 to 100 mg Hg, until definitive therapy (Chapter 3) can be started.

Analgesia. Severe pain must be treated promptly. The following drugs can be used.

1. Morphine sulfate
2. Meperidine (Demerol)
3. Codeine (phosphate or sulfate)

Morphine sulfate can be given subcutaneously, IM, or IV. Following subcutaneous injection, a peak analgesic effect results within 60 to 90 min; following IM injection, within 30 to 60 min; following IV injection, within 20 min.

One of the dangers of morphine is respiratory depression. Maximum respiratory depression occurs 90 min after subcutaneous injection and approximately 7 min after IV injection.

Average dosages of morphine sulfate in acute myocardial infarction are:

1. Subcutaneously or IM: initial dose of 8 to 15 mg. Smaller doses can be repeated every 3 to 4 hours, but not more than 60 mg should be given in a 12-hour period.
2. IV: the usual dose is 3 to 5 mg, although as much as 15 mg can be given. However, it is preferable to use the smaller doses to prevent respiratory depression and hypotension.

Because of its hypotensive action, morphine is contraindicated if shock is present.

Meperidine (Demerol) may be preferable to morphine because it is less constipating. However, it may cause as much respiratory depression and may be slightly less effective for pain relief. Meperidine can be given orally but is more effective when given IM. Its peak analgesic effect occurs within 30 to 40 min after IM injection. It should *not* be given IV to a patient with acute myocardial infarction, because it has a vagolytic effect and can increase the heart rate. The average dose of meperidine is 50 to 150 mg IM every 3 to 4 hours.

Codeine (phosphate or sulfate) in a dose of 30 to 60 mg subcutaneously or orally every 8 hours can also be given. It may produce severe constipation as a side effect.

Nitroglycerin should *not* be used for pain in the first week after an acute myocardial infarction. It is usually ineffective and may cause marked vasodilatation with decreased blood pressure.

Nausea. Nausea may be a symptom of the acute myocardial infarction or may be due to opiates or other medication. Diphenhydramine (Benadryl) can be given in a dose of 25 to 50 mg orally three to four times a day. It should *not* be given IV to a patient with acute myocardial infarction, because it can cause changes in blood pressure (elevation or lowering) and can also cause T wave changes.

Bed rest. For the first 48 hours, I prefer to keep the patient flat in bed with the head elevated slightly on one pillow. If left-sided heart failure is present, it will be necessary to raise the patient's head and shoulders. If shock is present, the patient should lie supine. After 48 hours, the patient can be propped up with pillows at an angle of approximately 30° to 45°. Side rails should be up at all times.

A patient with an acute myocardial infarction should have as much bed rest as possible. However, if a patient bears down excessively while on a bedpan, excessive vagal stimulation and sudden death may occur. Therefore, a bedside commode is preferable. (See also Bowel Care, below.)

Most male patients can urinate in bed. However, if prostatism is present, the patient may have to stand to void. If this is necessary, he must wear Ace bandages or antiembolism stockings to prevent postural hypotension.

Dangling should not be allowed. When a patient dangles his legs from the side of the bed, acute pooling of blood into the lower extremities occurs, and the patient may develop hypotension.

Armchair treatment. Many physicians believe that after the first 48 hours, a patient with uncomplicated myocardial infarction can sit in a chair at the bedside for a short period (5 to 15 min) several times a day, unless shock is present. This can be done even when IV tubing and cardiac monitor wires are connected to the patient. Armchair treatment often makes the patient less anxious. In addition, the physical effort of moving from bed to chair decreases the tendency to thromboembolism.

An alternative to the armchair treatment is to have the patient propped up in bed and to give instructions that he move the lower extremities frequently.

Diet. A liquid diet is preferable for the first day after the attack. A soft diet can then be ordered when the patient is able to tolerate food. The sodium content can be moderately restricted (2 gm a day). However, if congestive heart failure is present, a 1-gm sodium diet may be necessary. A rigid low-sodium (500-mg) diet may be detrimental to the patient with an uncomplicated acute myocardial infarction for many reasons. The patient may already have some degree of sodium depletion because of previous diuretic therapy. Further sodium depletion may then develop if the patient is given a diuretic because of congestive heart failure. Still further sodium depletion may develop if the patient is anorectic, eats little, but drinks (sodium-free) liquids. (Also see note above on IV fluids.)

When sodium depletion occurs, the osmotic pressure of the blood and extracellular fluid falls below the osmotic pressure of the cells. This is followed by a movement of fluid from the blood and extracellular tissues into the cells. As a result, the circulating blood volume decreases, systemic blood pressure falls, and shock may develop.

Decaffeinated coffee, such as Sanka and Decaf, is permitted. Coffee, tea, very hot or cold liquids, which may cause vagal overstimulation, and alcoholic beverages are not permitted, unless specifically ordered.

Sedation. Patients are usually very tense and anxious and should be routinely sedated. Phenobarbital in oral doses of 30 mg three times a day, a short-acting barbiturate such as butabarbital (Butisol) 30 mg three times a day or diazepam (Valium) in oral doses of 5 mg three times a day, or chlordiazepoxide (Librium) in oral doses of 10 mg three times a day are all effective. The barbiturates may decrease sensitivity to warfarin. For insomnia, one of the above sedatives can be given. Chloral hydrate, 0.5 gm at night, is also effective. Chloral hydrate may increase sensitivity to warfarin.

Bowel care. Constipation may become a problem, particularly if opiates have been used for pain. A bowel movement is not necessary for the first 3 to 5 days. However, the patient should routinely be given a stool softener, such as dioctyl sodium sulfosuccinate (Colace). The dosage for adults varies from 100 to 300 mg or more daily.

If the patient has a history of constipation, milk of magnesia, 1 to 3 tablespoonfuls at night, or mineral oil, 1 to 2 tablespoonfuls at night, may be helpful.

General care. *Vital signs,* such as blood pressure, pulse, respiration, and oral temperature, should be checked regularly; for example, every 4 hours, or as indicated. The physician should be alerted when the blood pressure falls to 90 mm Hg. However, a fall in systolic blood pressure to 90 mm Hg or lower after acute myocardial infarction is not uncommon. Opiates may also decrease the blood pressure. If the patient is comfortable and if there are no signs of shock, the patient should merely be watched carefully.

A 12-lead ECG should be taken daily for 3 days; thereafter, as indicated.

Ace bandages or antiembolism stockings should be placed on both lower extremities from the toes to just below the knees. If Ace bandages are rolled above the knee, there is a danger that they may compress a popliteal artery, particularly if the bandage becomes bunched and if peripheral vascular disease is present. The bandages should be removed and rerolled every 12 hours. If the patient has peripheral vascular disease, the bandages should be inspected to make certain that they do not impede the arterial circulation, because many patients with acute myocardial infarction also have diabetes or peripheral vascular disease or both.

Temperatures should not be taken rectally. Inserting a rectal thermometer theoretically can stimulate vagal reflexes. Therefore, *oral temperatures* should be taken of patients with acute myocardial infarction. If shock is present, marked vasoconstriction may be associated with coldness of the skin and mucous membranes of the mouth. In such a case, rectal temperatures may be needed. In addition, a rectal examination should be deferred unless necessary (for example, to diagnose a fecal impaction).

Visitors should be limited to the immediate family. No more than one visitor at a time should be allowed in the patient's room, and visits should be limited to 5 min in each hour for the first 48 hours or until the patient's condition is stable.

There should be *no radio* or *TV* in the patient's room; there should be *no telephone* at the bedside.

REFERENCES

Abelmann W, Cashion WR: Third thoughts on the therapy of myocardial infarction, Med Counterpoint, March 1972, p 31.

Adgey AAJ, et al: Acute phase of myocardial infarction, Lancet 2:501, 1971.

Bourassa M, et al: The effects of inhalation of 100% oxygen on myocardial lactate metabolism in coronary heart disease, Am J Cardiol 24:172, 1969.

Brewer DL, Bilbro RH, Bartel AG: Myocardial infarction as a complication of coronary bypass surgery, Circulation 47:58, 1973.

Cohen MH, et al: Electrocardiographic changes in acute pancreatitis resembling acute myocardial infarction, Am Heart J 82:672, 1971.

Cook RN, Edwards JE, Pruitt RD: Electrocardiographic changes in acute subendocardial infarction. I. Large subendocardial and large nontransmural infarcts, Circulation 18:603, 1958; II. Small subendocardial infarcts, Circulation 18:613, 1958.

Earnest O, Fletcher G: Danger of rectal examination in patients with acute myocardial infarction, N Engl J Med 281:238, 1969.

Eddy JD, Singh SP: Nursing posture after acute myocardial infarction, Lancet 2:1378, 1969.

Eliot RS, Bratt G: The paradox of myocardial ischemia and necrosis in young women with normal coronary arteriograms; relation to abnormal hemoglobin-oxygen dissociation, Am J Cardiol 23:633, 1969.

Friedberg CK: Diseases of the heart, ed 3, Philadelphia, 1966, WB Saunders Co.

Fulton MC, Marriott HJL: Acute pancreatitis simulating myocardial infarction in the electrocardiogram, Ann Intern Med 59:730, 1963.

Georas CS, Dahlquist E, Cutts FB: Subendocardial infarction, Arch Intern Med 111:488, 1963.

Goldberger E: Unipolar lead electrocardiography and vectorcardiography, ed 3, Philadelphia, 1953, Lea & Febiger.

Goldberger E: How to interpret electrocardiograms in terms of vectors, Springfield, Ill, 1968, Charles C Thomas, Publisher.

Goldberger E: A primer of water, electrolyte and acid-base syndromes, ed 4, Philadelphia, 1970, Lea & Febiger.

Goldberger E, Alesio J, Woll F: The significance of hyperglycemia in myocardial infarction, NY State J Med 45:391, 1945.

Goldfinger P: Recurrent electrocardiogram changes in subarachnoid hemorrhage, NY State J Med 72:2771, 1972.

Goldman AG, Gross H, Rubin IL: Transitory Q waves simulating the Q wave of myocardial infarction, Am Heart J 60:61, 1960.

Guy C, Eliot RS: The subendocardium of the left ventricle; a physiologic enigma, Editorial, Chest 58:555, 1970.

Hersch C: Electrocardiographic changes in head injuries, Circulation 23:853, 1961.

Horan LG, et al: The significance of diagnostic Q waves in the presence of bundle branch block, Chest 58:214, 1970.

Horan LG, et al: Significance of the diagnostic Q wave of myocardial infarction, Circulation 43:428, 1971.

Hunt D, Gore I: Myocardial lesions following experimental intracranial hemorrhage; prevention with propranolol, Am Heart J 83:232, 1972.

Klein MS, et al: Differentiation between CPK elevations after myocardial infarction from those due to injections or surgery, Circulation 46 (Suppl 2):25, 1972.

Koskelo P, et al: Subendocardial hemorrhage and ECG changes in intracranial bleeding, Br Med J 1:1479, 1964.

Krauss KR, et al: Acute coronary insufficiency;

course and follow-up, Arch Intern Med **129**:808, 1972.

Levine SA, Lown B: "Armchair" treatment of acute coronary thrombosis, JAMA **148**:1365, 1952.

Linhard JW, Beller BM, Talley RC: Preinfarction angina; clinical, hemodynamic and angiographic evaluation, Chest **61**:313, 1970.

Lovell RRH, Prineas RJ: Mechanisms of sudden death and their implication for prevention and management, Prog. Cardiovasc Dis **13**:482, 1971.

Marriott HJL, Slonim R: False patterns of myocardial infarction, Heart Bull **16**:71, 1967.

Mather HG, et al: Acute myocardial infarction; home and hospital treatment, Br Med J **3**:334, 1971.

Merrill SL: An autopsy study of the accuracy of the electrocardiogram in the diagnosis of recurrent myocardial infarction, Am Heart J **81**:48, 1971.

Morris J, et al: The negative inotropic effects of oxygen, Circulation **42**:111, 1971.

Nevins MA, Lyon LJ: Second thoughts on the therapy of myocardial infarction, Med Counterpoint, March 1972, p 30.

Perloff JK: The recognition of strictly posterior myocardial infarction by conventional scalar electrocardiography, Circulation **30**:706, 1964.

Pfister CW, dePando B: Cerebral hemorrhage simulating acute myocardial infarction, Dis Chest **42**:206, 1962.

Piscatelli RL, Fox LM: Myocardial injury from epinephrine overdosage, Am J Cardiol **21**:735, 1968.

Prinzmetal M, et al: Variant form of angina pectoris, JAMA **174**:1794, 1960.

Ravel R: Clinical laboratory medicine, Chicago, 1969, Year Book Medical Publishers, Inc.

Roberts WC: Coronary arteries in fatal acute myocardial infarction, Circulation **45**:215, 1972.

Rose G: Early mobilization and discharge after myocardial infarction, Mod Concepts Cardiovasc Dis **41**:59, 1972.

Short D, Stowers M: Earliest symptoms of coronary heart disease and their recognition, Br Med J **2**:387, 1972.

Silverman ME, Flamm MD Jr: Variant angina pectoris; anatomic findings and prognostic implications, Ann Intern Med **75**:339, 1971.

Silverman ME, Hurst JW: Abnormal physical findings associated with myocardial infarction, Mod Concepts Cardiovasc Dis **38**:69, 1969.

Sobel BE, Shell WE: Serum enzyme determinations in the diagnosis and assessment of myocardial infarction, Circulation **45**:471, 1972.

Tarhan S, et al: Myocardial infarction after general anesthesia, JAMA **220**:1451, 1972.

Thomas M, et al: Hemodynamic effects of morphine in patients with acute myocardial infarction, Br Heart J **27**:863, 1965.

Verani MS, Baron H, Maia IG: Myocardial infarction associated with Wolff-Parkinson-White syndrome, Am Heart J **83**:684, 1972.

Wasserburger RH, Corliss RJ: Prominent precordial T waves as an expression of coronary insufficiency, Am J Cardiol **16**:195, 1965.

Watkins SM, Lewis A: Serum enzyme levels in diagnosis of postoperative myocardial infarction, Br Med J **3**:733, 1972.

10 / Complications of acute myocardial infarction

The following complications of acute myocardial infarction are discussed in this chapter: acute left-sided congestive heart failure with or without acute pulmonary edema, thromboembolic complications, papillary muscle dysfunction and rupture, rupture of the interventricular septum, rupture of the heart, ventricular aneurysm, postmyocardial infarction syndrome (Dressler's syndrome), and bradyarrhythmias and tachyarrhythmias. Cardiogenic shock has been described in Chapter 3.

ACUTE LEFT-SIDED CONGESTIVE HEART FAILURE

Acute left-sided congestive heart failure occurring after acute myocardial infarction is characterized by moist rales at the lung bases that persist after vigorous coughing. In addition, a third heart sound is often present and is associated with a sinus tachycardia, dyspnea, or tachypnea. X-ray examination of the chest may or may not show hilar congestion or other signs of pulmonary edema.

Acute left-sided congestive heart failure complicating acute myocardial infarction can be classified into three types.

1. Mild or moderate congestive heart failure; rales involve less than one-half both lung fields
2. Acute pulmonary edema; rales involve more than one-half both lung fields
3. Acute pulmonary edema associated with cardiogenic shock

Basal rales (mild congestive left-sided heart failure) commonly are present for the first few days after an acute myocardial in-farction. They usually disappear before the end of the first week. However, if they persist after this, the patient should be digitalized.

Emergency treatment. Patients with moderate congestive heart failure should be digitalized. There is some evidence that patients with acute myocardial infarction are excessively sensitive to digitalis for the first 24 hours after the infarction. If congestive heart failure develops during these first 24 hours, three-fourths the usual digitalizing dose can be given. Thereafter, the usual doses of digitalis can be given. If the condition is not critical, the patient can be digitalized over a period of 24 hours, or an initial dose can be given IM or IV, and the remainder orally.

Acute pulmonary edema complicating acute myocardial infarction should be treated as follows.

1. The effect of IV digitalization, with a rapid-acting digitalis preparation, such as digoxin (Lanoxin) or deslanoside (Cedilanid-D),* is noted in 5 to 10 min.

2. Morphine sulfate, 5 to 10 mg IV, decreases the venous return, lowers pulmonary capillary pressure, and relieves anxiety. Its effect is noted in 15 to 30 min.

3. Rotating tourniquets should be applied (p. 158).

4. IV doses of diuretics, such as furosemide (Lasix), 40 to 80 mg, or ethacrynic acid, 50 to 100 mg, are also effective in approximately 15 to 30 min.

5. If this treatment is not effective and

---

*These and other drugs are described in Part three.

if the patient appears moribund, a phlebotomy of 250 to 500 ml blood can be cautiously tried. However, it may precipitate cardiogenic shock or sudden death.

Because of its ability to produce pulmonary and peripheral vasodilatation, sublingual administration of nitroglycerin has recently been used in patients with acute pulmonary edema complicating acute myocardial infarction who do not respond to conventional therapy (Gold and others).

The treatment of acute pulmonary edema associated with cardiogenic shock is described on p. 44.

THROMBOEMBOLIC COMPLICATIONS

Thromboembolic complications of acute myocardial infarction can occur in several ways. The bed rest promotes stasis of blood and phlebothrombosis in the veins of the lower extremities, particularly if the patient has varicose veins; or a thrombus may form in either the wall of the right or left ventricle, usually at the endocardial site of the infarct. (A thrombus of the right ventricle can occur if the interventricular septum is infarcted.) Thrombi can also form in the left or right atrium, particularly if atrial infarction occurs. When these thrombi break off, both pulmonary and systemic embolization may occur, resulting in emboli in the lungs, brain, spleen, kidneys, intestines, upper and lower extremities, and so on.

Prophylaxis and treatment. Thromboembolic complications are much less frequent now, since patients with acute myocardial infarction ambulate early. (Some physicians keep patients resting in bed for only 1 week. I prefer to keep a patient resting in bed for 2 weeks.) In addition, Ace bandages from the toes to just below the knees or antiembolism stockings, and anticoagulants have been used to prevent thromboembolism.

There is still controversy about the value of prophylactic anticoagulant therapy in patients with acute myocardial infarction. For this reason, patients have been divided into "good risk" and "poor risk" categories. A poor risk patient has one or more of the following characteristics: a previous myocardial infarction; intractable pain; extreme or persistent shock; significant enlargement of the heart; gallop rhythm or congestive heart failure; tachyarrhythmias such as atrial fibrillation, atrial flutter, or ventricular tachycardia; AV block; intraventricular block; diabetic acidosis; or other conditions (such as polycythemia) predisposing to thrombosis. A good risk patient has none of these characteristics.

Many physicians give anticoagulants to poor risk patients but not to good risk patients because the possible complications of anticoagulants outweigh any possible benefits. However, I have seen embolic phenomena occur in so-called good risk patients. Therefore, I routinely give anticoagulant therapy to patients with acute myocardial infarction at least until they ambulate (unless contraindicated by peptic ulcer, and so on).

If embolization has occurred or if a condition such as polycythemia, which predisposes to thromboembolism, is present, longterm anticoagulation is indicated.

If reaction to a control prothrombin time test is normal, warfarin sodium (Coumadin) can be ordered in a daily dose of 10 mg until the prothrombin time (tested daily) rises to approximately 18 to 20 sec. This usually occurs in approximately 72 hours. Then the dose is adjusted to the rise in the prothrombin time, which is maintained at approximately 23 to 25 sec (twice the control value). If the patient enters the hospital more than 48 hours after the myocardial infarction has developed or if signs of thromboembolic complications develop, the patient should be given heparin and warfarin sodium simultaneously.

PAPILLARY MUSCLE DYSFUNCTION AND RUPTURE

Papillary muscle dysfunction is commonly caused by myocardial ischemia.

However, actual rupture of a papillary muscle is a rare complication of acute myocardial infarction. Papillary muscle dysfunction secondary to ischemia may occur transiently during an anginal attack (with a transient murmur), with acute myocardial infarction involving the papillary muscle and subjacent myocardium, and with left ventricular dilatation or a ventricular aneurysm that distorts the papillary muscle–chordae tendineae area.

The major physical finding in papillary muscle dysfunction is an apical systolic murmur that is highly variable. It may be either holosystolic, midsystolic (sometimes with an associated click), or early or late systolic. The murmur may change in intensity and quality in the same patient. A loud first heart sound is often associated with the murmur. In severe cases, papillary muscle dysfunction without rupture may lead to severe congestive heart failure, refractory to medical treatment.

Actual rupture of a papillary muscle is a rare and usually lethal complication, usually occurring 2 to 10 days after the acute infarction. (The term papillary muscle rupture refers to rupture of one of the apical heads of the papillary muscle. Rupture of the entire trunk is incompatible with life.) In general, the posterior papillary muscle is most commonly affected and is associated with electrocardiographic signs of inferior myocardial infarction. Clinically, the patient usually develops a loud pansystolic apical murmur, usually without a thrill (in contrast to rupture of the interventricular septum, in which the murmur is usually loudest at the left sternal border and is often associated with a thrill). Rupture of the anterior papillary muscle may produce a murmur with radiation to the right of the sternum, so that definitive differentiation of papillary muscle rupture and rupture of the interventricular septum may require catheterization.

There is a 90% 2-week mortality associated with papillary muscle rupture, and many patients die with severe failure in the first 24 hours. Although successful mitral valve replacement has been reported in the first week following the acute infarct, the mortality of early surgical intervention is very high. If possible, the patient's condition should be stabilized with maximal medical therapy for at least a few weeks, and preferably a few months, before open heart valve replacement is attempted. However, Cheng and associates have reported successful mitral valve replacement and saphenous vein bypass grafting in a patient with severe papillary muscle dysfunction 5 days after the acute infarction.

RUPTURE OF THE INTERVENTRICULAR SEPTUM

Rupture of the interventricular septum is less common than rupture of the heart, but more common than rupture of a papillary muscle. It usually occurs within the first week after the acute myocardial infarction. It is associated with the development of intense dyspnea due to acute left-sided congestive heart failure or pulmonary edema and with signs of cardiogenic shock. Chest pain may or may not reappear. (Right-sided congestive heart failure may develop later.)

A loud holosystolic murmur develops. It is usually loudest in the third, fourth, or fifth intercostal space, near the left sternal border, and extends to the apex. A systolic thrill is usually present.

Various arrhythmias may also develop, including various types of AV block, AV junctional rhythm, and right or left bundle branch block. The ECG shows signs of anteroseptal infarction and often inferior or anterolateral myocardial infarction.

The symptoms and signs of a ruptured interventricular septum are similar to those of a ruptured papillary muscle (see above). Differential diagnosis can be made by angiocardiography, if the patient is well enough, or by bedside catheterization of the heart, using a Swan-Ganz flow-directed catheter (p. 46). If an interventricular septal defect is present, angiocardiography will show the passage of dye through the septal defect; and cardiac catheterization will reveal a step-up of 1 volume percent or greater in blood oxygen content between the right atrium and the right ventricle. (If a ruptured papillary muscle is present, catherization will show a giant *v* wave in the pulmonary wedge tracing.)

Death often occurs within a week. However, if the patient can be treated medically for about 2 months, repair of the septal defect during open heart surgery can be done.

RUPTURE OF THE HEART

Rupture of the heart usually occurs between the first and twelfth day after the onset of the myocardial infarction. It rarely occurs after the fourteenth day. It is common in patients who have hypertension that persists after the infarction develops and who do not show signs of congestive heart failure. It occurs in the absence of previous myocardial infarction and is rare after isolated inferior myocardial infarction. Physical strain or continued activity after the infarct develops may be a precipitating factor. Anticoagulant therapy is probably not a factor.

The patient may develop severe substernal pressure and then becomes unconscious. Signs of cardiac tamponade, such as distended neck veins and marked cyanosis, may be present. Some patients may show a pericardial friction rub or a continuous low-pitched rumbling murmur. The ECG will continue to show signs of myocardial infarction, even when the heart apparently stops beating (*electromechanical dissociation*). Bradycardia is usually present. Total electrical alternans (of P, QRS, and T) due to the cardiac tamponade may also be present. In addition, downward precordial T waves may become upward, due to blood in the pericardial sac. Low voltage of the QRS complexes in the limb leads may be present.

When cardiac rupture is suspected and is associated with cardiac tamponade, pericardiocentesis should be done immediately with a relatively large-bore IV catheter. (Also see p. 191.) To prevent recurrent cardiac tamponade, the catheter can be left in the pericardial space while the patient is brought to the operating room.

Cobbs and associates recommend that in addition to the pericardiocentesis, the following should be done prior to emergency cardiac surgery: administration of IV fluids (preferably with colloidal solutions), correction of metabolic acidosis, and the administration of an inotropic amine (such as isoproterenol, metaraminol, or levarterenol). Large doses of atropine can be given for the bradycardia.

VENTRICULAR ANEURYSM

Acute myocardial infarction may be followed by the development of a ventricular aneurysm (usually involving the wall of the left ventricle). Although the diagnosis is usually made months after the myocardial infarction has occurred, the aneurysm can develop shortly after the onset of the myocardial infarction. Ordinarily, the life expectancy of a patient with a ventricular aneurysm is the same as that of a patient with a postmyocardial infarction without an aneurysm. However, when a ventricular aneurysm develops, it may be associated with complications, such as exacerbation of congestive heart failure, embolizations from a thrombus within the aneurysm wall, pericarditis with or without pericardial effusion (which may be bloody), or recurrent ventricular tachycardia.

The diagnosis of a ventricular aneurysm occurring during the acute myocardial infarction can be best made by means of x-ray examination of the chest. Electrocardiographic signs suggestive of a ventricular aneurysm are persistent elevation of the RS-T segments 3 weeks or more after the infarction.

No specific treatment is ordinarily indicated for the aneurysm. However, surgical excision of the aneurysm has been performed when it is associated with recurrent ventricular tachycardia, intractable congestive heart failure, recurrent embolizations, or persistent angina that does not respond to medical treatment. (Also see p. 151.) (To allow adequate healing of the wall of the myocardium, aneurysmectomy should not be done for at least 3 months after the myocardial infarct.)

POSTMYOCARDIAL INFARCTION SYNDROME (DRESSLER'S SYNDROME)

Postmyocardial infarction syndrome is characterized by a generalized pericarditis, with or without a pericardial effusion, which may be hemorrhagic. In addition, pleuritis or pneumonitis may be present. There is some evidence that the syndrome is due to an autoimmune reaction with development of antibodies to heart muscle. The syndrome usually appears 2 to 6 weeks after acute myocardial infarction but may occur as early as the first week.

Symptoms and signs include fever and pleuropericardial chest pain. The pain is substernal and may extend to the neck, the shoulders, or the interscapular area, but not down the arms. The diagnosis of the postmyocardial infarction syndrome is often suggested by the increased pain during deep inspiration. The pain often decreases when the patient sits.

The ECG may or may not show signs of generalized pericarditis.

The white blood cell count and the sedimentation rate increase.

The major importance of the postmyocardial infarction syndrome is that it may simulate pulmonary embolism (particularly if pneumonitis is present and if the patient is expectorating blood-streaked sputum) or an extension of the myocardial infarction.

Often the diagnosis is not certain until the patient responds with a rapid decrease of symptoms and signs within 24 hours after administration of prednisone or a similar corticosteroid has been started.

Prednisone can be given in a dose of 60 mg orally daily for 7 to 10 days. Then the drug can be abruptly stopped. If symptoms and signs reappear, the prednisone should be given again in a smaller dose—15 to 20 mg daily. The duration of corticosteroid therapy is variable because the syndrome may last for months. The best way to determine the effectiveness of therapy is to taper and stop administration of the prednisone periodically.

Because of the risk of a hemorrhagic pericarditis, anticoagulants are contraindicated and must be stopped if the patient has received them. Analgesics can be used when symptoms are not severe.

ARRHYTHMIAS

When patients with acute myocardial infarction are continuously monitored in a CCU, 75% to 95% will show some arrhythmias. Many factors contribute to the development of these arrhythmias; the location and size of the infarct may determine whether the AV node or the bundle of His or its branches are involved. Pain, anxiety, hypoxia, acidosis, electrolyte disturbances (particularly hypokalemia), congestive heart failure, shock, and straining at the stool may also induce arrhythmias. In addition, pericarditis associated with acute myocardial infarction may involve the SA node, and drugs such as morphine, digitalis, antiarrhythmic drugs, and sympathomimetic drugs can cause arrhythmias.

Cardiogenic shock is usually associated with serious arrhythmias. Life-threatening arrhythmias occur in more than 90% of patients with acute myocardial infarction and cardiogenic shock and in only about one-half of patients without shock. Similarly, AV block is three times more frequent and ventricular fibrillation is twice as frequent after acute myocardial infarction if shock is present. However, ventricular tachycardia occurs equally in patients with myocardial infarction with or without shock.

Most supraventricular tachyarrhythmias associated with acute myocardial infarc-

Table 4. Cardiac arrhythmias and conduction disturbances complicating acute myocardial infarction

Minor (Usually do not need treatment)	Major (Should be treated as soon as possible)	Life-threatening (Emergency treatment must be given)
Sinus arrhythmia	SA block	Ventricular tachycardia
Sinus bradycardia	AV junctional rhythm	Ventricular flutter
Wandering pacemaker	Mobitz type II AV block§	Ventricular fibrillation
AV junctional rhythm*	Complete AV block§	Ventricular standstill
AV dissociation*	Bifascicular or trifascicular	
First-degree AV block	heart block§	
Wenckebach type of AV block*	Multiple APCs†	
Sinus tachycardia	Paroxysmal atrial fibrillation	
Occasional atrial premature contractions APCs)†	Paroxysmal atrial flutter	
	Paroxysmal atrial tachycardia	
Occasional ventricular premature contractions (VPCs)‡	Paroxysmal AV junctional tachycardia	
Idioventricular tachycardia	Multiple VPCs‡	

*Treatment is needed if arrhythmia is associated with worsening of patient's condition.
†Treatment is needed if more than 6 APCs occur per min, or produce a bigeminal or trigeminal rhythm, or if associated with worsening of patient's condition.
‡Treatment is needed if more than 5 VPCs occur per min, or in salvos, or if they show an R on T pattern.
§The condition is serious, but specific treatment may not be indicated.

tion are benign. However, any ventricular tachyarrhythmia is potentially lethal because either ventricular premature contractions or ventricular tachycardia may be a precursor of ventricular fibrillation or cardiac standstill. However, ventricular fibrillation may occur without any previous arrhythmias.

The cardiac arrhythmias usually appear within the first hours after the acute myocardial infarction. The heart is then particularly susceptible to ventricular fibrillation for about 1 week thereafter. This may be due partly to the increased sympathetic stimulation and the increased secretion of catecholamines that occur.

Cardiac arrhythmias due to acute myocardial infarction can be classified as:

1. Bradyarrhythmias due to a disturbance in the sinus node or AV junction
2. Fascicular heart blocks, due to a disturbance in the spread of the stimulus from the AV node through the bundle of His and its branches
3. Tachyarrhythmias due to increased stimula-

tion of normal or ectopic pacemaker tissues or to reentry phenomena

Cardiac arrhythmias due to acute myocardial infarction can also be described in terms of prognosis (Table 4). For example:

1. *Minor arrhythmias* do not usually need treatment.
2. *Major arrhythmias* should be treated as soon as possible.
3. *Life-threatening arrhythmias* require immediate and emergency treatment.

Bradyarrhythmias (Table 5)
Sinus bradycardia

Sinus bradycardia occurs in approximately 20% of patients with acute myocardial infarction. It may be due to a decreased blood supply to the sinus node, which is usually supplied by the right coronary artery. However, it may simply be a sign of increased vagal tone, which often occurs in acute myocardial infarction.

Many patients with acute myocardial infarction show no symptoms referable to the sinus bradycardia. Others may develop a

Table 5. Treatment of bradyarrhythmias complicating acute myocardial infarction

Arrhythmia	First-choice emergency treatment	Second-choice emergency treatment	Comments
Sinus arrhythmia	No treatment needed		If the ventricular rate slows to 50 per min or less and the patient's clinical condition worsens, treatment should be started; in addition, the patient's legs should be raised 45° to increase the venous return and the heart rate
Wandering pacemaker	No treatment needed		
Sinus bradycardia	No treatment needed if patient is asymptomatic	Atropine Isoproterenol Cardiac pacing*	
AV junctional rhythm	No treatment needed if patient is asymptomatic	Atropine Isoproterenol Cardiac pacing*	
AV dissociation	No treatment needed if patient is asymptomatic	Atropine Isoproterenol	
First-degree AV block	No treatment needed		
Wenckebach type of AV block	No treatment needed if patient is asymptomatic	Atropine Isoproterenol Cardiac pacing*	It may be produced by morphine or digitalis
Mobitz type II AV block	No treatment needed if patient is asymptomatic	Atropine Isoproterenol Cardiac pacing*	Cardiac pacing is not needed unless shock, syncope, or severe congestive heart failure develops
Complete AV block with inferior myocardial infarction	No treatment needed if patient is asymptomatic	Atropine Isoproterenol Cardiac pacing*	
Complete AV block with anterior myocardial infarction	Cardiac pacing*		These patients are critically ill and usually die even when cardiac pacing is used
Ventricular standstill	Immediate cardiopulmonary resuscitation (see Chapter 2)		

*Indications for cardiac pacing include poor response to drug therapy, frequent ventricular premature contractions, progressive congestive heart failure, or shock.

decreased cardiac output and hypotension. In addition, the sinus bradycardia may be a precursor to more serious arrhythmias, such as AV block or sinus arrest. In addition, the prolonged period of ventricular diastole associated with the sinus bradycardia increases the possibility of nodal or ventricular escape beats, accelerated idioventricular tachycardia, ventricular premature contractions, or ventricular tachycardia or fibrillation.

No treatment is needed for asymptomatic sinus bradycardia. However, if the heart rate falls below 50 per min and if the patient's clinical condition worsens, the patient's legs can be raised 45°. This will increase the venous return and may increase the ventricular rate, so that drug therapy is not needed. If this is not effective, atropine sulfate can be given.

Atropine can be given orally in a dose of 0.4 mg (gr 1/150) three times a day. It can also be given IV in a dose of 0.4 to 0.8 mg every 4 to 6 hours. Treatment is usually not needed for more than 24 hours. (When atropine is used for more than 1 day, it may cause side effects such as dryness of the mucous membranes, urinary retention, and aggravation of glaucoma, and it may precipitate mental confusion and delirium.)

If atropine does not increase the heart rate, isoproterenol can be given IV at a flow rate to increase and maintain the ventricular rate between 60 and 70 beats per min. However, isoproterenol can cause atrial or ventricular tachyarrhythmias. It can also cause vasodilatation and a fall in blood pressure (p. 301).

Temporary atrial or ventricular transvenous cardiac pacing has been used in patients with acute myocardial infarction when sinus bradycardia lasts longer than 24 hours. However, I do not consider sinus bradycardia to be an indication for cardiac pacing unless the slow heart rate produces syncope or hypotension and does not respond to medication.

Sinus arrhythmia or wandering pacemaker

No treatment is needed.

SA block

If the patient is taking cardiac-depressant drugs, administration of the drugs should be stopped immediately. Atropine or isoproterenol should be used if the pauses last more than two successive heartbeats or if the patient's clinical condition worsens. Cardiac pacing should be performed only if drug therapy is not effective.

AV junctional rhythm

AV junctional rhythm does not produce any significant hemodynamic changes in circulation unless the ventricular rate decreases to 40 per min or less and is associated with hypotension or congestive heart failure. If this occurs, atropine, isoproterenol, or temporary transvenous cardiac pacing may be needed. Cardiac pacing should be used only if drug therapy is not effective.

AV dissociation

No treatment is needed.

First-degree AV block

No treatment is needed.

Second-degree AV block

Wenckebach type. The Wenckebach type of AV block is usually transitory, and no specific treatment is needed. It may be precipitated by morphine or digitalis. If this occurs, administration of the drug should be stopped.

Mobitz type II AV block. The Mobitz type II AV block is more common after inferior myocardial infarction than after anterior myocardial infarction. It is often a precursor of complete AV block or sinus arrest. Therefore, many cardiologists believe that a temporary transvenous demand pacemaker should be inserted prophylactically when this occurs. However, if the patient is asymptomatic and if inferior myocardial infarction is present, the patient can be treated with either atropine or an isoproterenol infusion.

When the Mobitz type II AV block occurs in a patient with anterior myocardial infarction, the situation is much more serious because there is a greater danger of sinus arrest. However, atropine or isoproterenol should be used before a pacemaker is inserted because the prognosis is poor even when cardiac pacing is used.

Complete AV block

Complete AV block occurs in about 6% of patients with acute myocardial infarction. In about one third of these patients, it occurs within a few hours after the onset of the infarction and in almost all patients within 48 hours. It rarely occurs after the fourth day.

When acute myocardial infarction is complicated by complete AV block, the prognosis is serious. Clinical studies show that from 50% to 80% of these patients will die. However, when these cases are separated into inferior (diaphragmatic) and anterior myocardial infarction it becomes obvious that when complete AV block complicates anterior myocardial infarction, it is much more serious than when it complicates inferior myocardial infarction.

When a temporary demand type of pacemaker is inserted in a patient with acute myocardial infarction, sinus rhythm usually reappears after a few days. When this occurs, the pacemaker should be left in place for 3 to 4 more weeks if the patient continues to show persistent bradycardia or a fascicular block. If regular sinus rhythm returns and there is no fascicular block, the pacemaker can be removed in less than 3 weeks.

Atkins and associates have pointed out that when a patient with right bundle branch block, left axis deviation, and acute myocardial infarction develops complete AV block, there is a high risk of sudden death after the patient has been discharged from the hospital, even if the complete AV block is only transient during the attack of acute myocardial infarction. They therefore suggest that a temporary transvenous pacemaker should be inserted when the complete AV block occurs in these patients and that a long-term pacemaker should be implanted before the patient is discharged from the hospital.

Complete AV block complicating inferior (diaphragmatic) myocardial infarction.

Most patients with acute myocardial infarction with complete AV block show inferior myocardial infarction. One of the reasons for this is that the right coronary artery that supplies the inferior wall of the left ventricle almost always supplies the AV node. However, at autopsy the area of inflammation of the inferior wall of the left ventricle is often comparatively small and the AV node may be normal, even when complete AV block had been present.

When complete AV block develops after an acute inferior myocardial infarction, it is almost never permanent and usually disappears in the first week. It rarely develops suddenly and is usually preceded by lesser degrees of AV block. It can be precipitated by morphine, digitalis, or the antiarrhythmic drugs.

Since the location of the AV block is in the AV node, idioventricular stimuli arise high in the bundle of His, with a relatively rapid rate, usually more than 50 per min. In addition, the QRS complexes are a normal width.

Complete AV block occurring as a complication of inferior myocardial infarction is not associated with an increased mortality unless cardiac decompensation, shock, syncope, asystole, or an idioventricular rhythm with wide, aberrant QRS complexes develop. Therefore, cardiac pacing is not necessary, unless the above complications develop. However, if these complications occur, the prognosis is very poor even when cardiac pacing is used. Thus it is questionable whether cardiac pacing is valuable in these patients.

Complete AV block complicating anterior myocardial infarction. Complete AV block complicating anterior myocardial infarction is usually due to extensive infarction of the ventricular septum, usually with complete destruction of the right main bundle of His and partial destruction of the left bundle of His. Because of this, the idioventricular rhythm that develops is slow and shows wide, aberrant QRS complexes.

This type of complete AV block occurs suddenly and is usually not preceded by lesser degress of AV block. However, if the Mobitz type II block develops, it may be a precursor of complete AV block or asystole.

Because these patients with anterior myocardial infarction and complete AV block have extensive myocardial injury, they usually show hypotension and cardiac decompensation, and the survival rate is very low, even when cardiac pacing is used.

Use of corticosteroids. Although corticosteroids may be beneficial in noncoronary patients with complete AV block, they have little or no value when the complete AV block is due to myocardial infarction.

Ventricular standstill

Ventricular standstill is a most serious complication. Cardiopulmonary resuscitation must be started immediately (Chapter 2).

Fascicular blocks

When acute myocardial infarction occurs in a patient with an antecedent right or left bundle branch block, or if bifascicular or trifascicular block develops, the mortality is increased because the Mobitz type II AV block, or complete AV block and cardiac arrest may occur. Because of this, some cardiologists have recommended that a temporary transvenous ventricular demand pacemaker be inserted prophylactically in such patients. Unfortunately, even if this is done, the mortality remains high. One should remember that the insertion of a cardiac pacemaker in a patient with acute myocardial infarction may further increase the irritability of the ventricles and may induce ventricular tachycardia or ventricular fibrillation. In addition, numerous other complications may develop from the insertion of a transvenous pacemaker (Chapter 15).

The development of left anterior hemiblock after acute myocardial infarction does not increase mortality. The development of left anterior hemiblock and right bundle branch block is more serious (p. 147), as is left posterior hemiblock and right bundle branch block, because if either of these two patterns develop, there is increased danger of complete AV block and cardiac arrest.

Tachyarrhythmias (Table 6)
Supraventricular tachyarrhythmias

Treatment depends on the patient's clinical condition and the type of tachyarrhythmia. Supraventricular tachyarrhythmias tend to recur during the first week after an acute myocardial infarction. Therefore, synchronized DC shock is usually not indicated unless the tachyarrhythmia is associated with sudden worsening of the patient's clinical condition, such as the development of severe congestive heart failure or shock.

The primary goal of treatment of all the supraventricular tachyarrhythmias, therefore, is to slow the ventricular rate. Digitalis is the drug of choice. It can be given orally or parenterally. However, since patients with acute myocardial infarction may be excessively sensitive to digitalis (because of hypoxia) during the first 24 hours after the infarction, only three fourths of the usual therapeutic doses of digitalis should be used.

Atrial premature contractions. The atrial premature contractions are frequently precursors of atrial fibrillation, atrial flutter, or paroxysmal atrial tachycardia. No treatment is needed for occasional atrial premature contractions. However, if they occur more frequently than 6 per min, if they produce a bigeminal or trigeminal rhythm, or if the patient's clinical condition worsens, they should be treated with digitalization.

Paroxysmal atrial fibrillation. This occurs in about 10% of patients with acute

Table 6. Treatment of tachyarrhythmias complicating acute myocardial infarction*

Arrhythmia	First-choice emergency treatment	Second-choice emergency treatment	Comments
Atrial premature contractions	Digitalis	Quinidine	If more than 6 APCs per min occur, or with bigeminy or trigeminy, or if the patient's condition worsens, emergency treatment should be started; patients with acute myocardial infarction may be excessively sensitive to digitalis for the first 24 hours; therefore, three-fourths the usual therapeutic doses should be used
Paroxysmal atrial fibrillation	Digitalis	Synchronized DC shock	DC shock should be avoided if possible, because the atrial fibrillation tends to recur; it is more important to slow the ventricular rate with digitalis (see note above)
Paroxysmal atrial tachycardia	Digitalis	Synchronized DC shock	See note above
Paroxysmal atrial flutter	Digitalis	Synchronized DC shock	See note above; some cardiologists recommend immediate synchronized DC shock for atrial flutter
AV junctional premature contractions	Digitalis	Quinidine	
Paroxysmal AV junctional tachycardia	Digitalis	Synchronized DC shock	
Nonparoxysmal AV junctional tachycardia	No treatment		If caused by digitalis toxicity, stop the digitalis, and give potassium chloride; diphenylhydantoin can also be used
Ventricular premature contractions	Lidocaine	Procainamide Quinidine Diphenylhydantoin	Isolated VPCs do not need treatment; however, if more than 5 per min occur, or in salvos, or if they show an R on T pattern, or are multifocal, emergency treatment should be started; when the VPCs disappear, prophylactic oral treatment with procainamide or quinidine should be given
Accelerated idioventricular tachycardia	No treatment		If VPCs also occur, lidocaine can be given
Ventricular tachycardia	Thump over sternum Lidocaine or synchronized DC shock	Synchronized DC shock or Lidocaine Quinidine Procainamide Diphenylhydantoin Overdriving with pacemaker	If the situation is urgent (for example, the patient has become unconscious), DC shock rather than lidocaine should be used; ventricular tachycardia occurring in acute myocardial infarction is often a precursor of ventricular fibrillation; therefore, drug treatment or DC shock should be followed by long-term oral administration of second-choice antiarrhythmic drugs
Ventricular fibrillation	Thump over sternum Unsynchronized DC shock	Cardiopulmonary resuscitation (Chapter 2)	Unsynchronized DC shock must be given immediately; a delay of more than 1 min will greatly decrease the chances for survival

*Adapted from Killip T: Hosp Practice, April 1972, p. 131.

myocardial infarction. The patient should be digitalized (see above).

Paroxysmal atrial flutter. This occurs about one half as frequently as atrial fibrillation. Treatment is the same. However, some cardiologists prefer to use immediate synchronized DC shock.

Paroxysmal atrial tachycardia. This is an uncommon complication of acute myocardial infarction. The patient is treated by digitalization (see above).

AV junctional premature contractions. These have the same significance as atrial premature contractions (see above).

Paroxysmal AV junctional tachycardia. Paroxysmal AV junctional tachycardia occurs about one half as frequently as atrial fibrillation after acute myocardial infarction. Treatment is the same.

Nonparoxysmal AV junctional tachycardia. No treatment is needed, because the heart rate is comparatively slow. However, if the nonparoxysmal AV junctional tachycardia is due to digitalis, the digitalis must be stopped immediately. Potassium chloride can be given. If this is not effective, diphenylhydantoin can be given.

Ventricular tachyarrhythmias

Ventricular premature contractions. These are the most common arrhythmia after acute myocardial infarction and occur in about three fourths of patients. They are often a precursor of ventricular tachycardia and ventricular fibrillation, particularly when the premature QRS complex occurs simultaneously with the apex of the T wave of the previous heartbeat (R on T phenomenon).

Isolated ventricular premature contractions do not require any specific treatment. However, when more than five ventricular premature contractions per min occur, or if they occur in groups of two or more or are multifocal, or when they occur simultaneously with the apex of the preceding T wave, an intravenous bolus of 75 mg lidocaine (Xylocaine) should be given.

This can be repeated in 5 min, if necessary. The lidocaine should then be continued as a constant IV infusion to prevent recurrence of the ventricular premature contractions. The lidocaine infusion should be continued for 48 to 72 hours. The dosage is gradually reduced until the patient is weaned from the drug.

Ventricular tachycardia. This can be divided into three groups for treatment.

Group I.   Short runs of three or more successive ventricular premature contractions occur. However, there are no symptoms or any significant changes in the patient's clinical condition.

Group II.   A sustained ventricular tachycardia is present, but there are no symptoms or any significant changes in the patient's clinical condition.

Group III. A sustained ventricular tachycardia is present, with signs of inadequate cardiac output, such as increasing congestive heart failure, hypotension, or shock.

Treatment. Groups I and II ventricular tachycardia are treated by an IV lidocaine bolus followed by a continuous lidocaine infusion (see Ventricular Premature Contractions, above).

Group III ventricular tachycardia must be treated with immediate synchronized DC shock. Premedicate with lidocaine, if possible. If the ventricular rate is very rapid and the QRS complexes wide and bizarre, it may not be possible to synchronize the electrical discharge with the peak of the R wave. This is not too important, because even if ventricular fibrillation occurs due to an unsynchronized shock, an additional DC shock will convert the ventricular fibrillation to sinus rhythm. A continuous lidocaine infusion should be started immediately after the DC shock.

One should always remember that a chest thump may terminate a ventricular tachycardia.

Maintenance therapy. The patient who has had an attack of ventricular tachycardia should be given long-term treatment with an antiarrhythmic drug, such as procainamide or quinidine, administered orally after the ventricular tachycardia has been abolished but while the patient is still receiving the lidocaine infusion.

Many cardiologists recommend maintenance treatment with an antiarrhythmic drug for 3 weeks to 3 months after the attack of ventricular tachycardia complicating acute myocardial infarction. I believe that oral maintenance treatment should be continued indefinitely in a patient who has had ventricular tachycardia complicating acute myocardial infarction.

Patients who develop recurrent ventricular tachycardia in association with a ventricular aneurysm after myocardial infarction have been successfully treated by surgical excision of the ventricular aneurysm. However, I have not had experience with this type of surgical therapy for recurrent ventricular tachycardia. An alternative treatment is long-term cardiac pacing (p. 238).

Idioventricular tachycardia (accelerated idioventricular rhythm). This is usually transient and does not need treatment (p. 99). However, if there are associated ventricular premature contractions, lidocaine can be given. If the idioventricular tachycardia is due to digitalis, stop administration of the digitalis.

Ventricular fibrillation. This may occur as a result of a ventricular tachycardia but may also occur without prior arrhythmias. Immediate unsynchronized DC shock must be given with a charge of 400 ws. If ventricular fibrillation complicating acute myocardial infarction is treated within 1 min, the prognosis is good.

Prophylaxis of ventricular tachyarrhythmias. The prophylactic use of antiarrhythmic drugs such as lidocaine, procainamide, or quinidine to prevent ventricular tachyarrhythmias has been advocated by some cardiologists. However, such prophylactic therapy has not been associated with any reduction in mortality from myocardial infarction in spite of the reduced incidence of ventricular premature contractions and ventricular tachycardia. I therefore do not recommend the prophylactic use of antiarrhythmic drugs in patients with acute myocardial infarction. In addition, if lidocaine is given prophylactically and if the patient develops paroxysmal atrial fibrillation, the lidocaine can cause a 1:1 ventricular response with a very rapid ventricular rate, by increasing conduction through the AV node.

REFERENCES
Complications of acute myocardial infarction (excluding arrhythmias)

Björck G, et al: Studies of myocardial rupture with cardiac tamponade in acute myocardial infarction. 1. Clinical features, Chest **61**:4, 1972.

Burch GE, DePasquale NP, Phillips JH: Clinical manifestations of papillary muscle dysfunction, Arch Intern Med **112**:112, 1963.

Bures AR, Karr RM, Iseri LT: Reliability of the electrocardiographic signs of ventricular aneurysm, Circulation **46** (Suppl 2):135, 1972.

Cheng TO, et al: Acute severe mitral regurgitation from papillary muscle dysfunction in acute myocardial infarction; successful early surgical treatment by combined mitral valve replacement and aorto-coronary saphenous vein bypass graft, Circulation **46**:491, 1972.

Clark WH, Russel M: Recurrent ventricular tachycardia in association with ventricular aneurysm, Letter, Am J Cardiol **31**:529, 1973.

Cobbs BW Jr, Hatcher CR Jr, Robinson PH: Cardiac rupture; three operations with two long-term survivals, JAMA **223**:532, 1973.

Daicoff GR: Rupture in and of the heart. In Eliot RS, editor: The acute cardiac emergency, Mount Kisco, NY, 1972, Futura Publishing Co, Inc.

Dressler W: The post-myocardial infarction syndrome, Arch Intern Med **102**:28, 1959.

Friedman HS, et al: Clinical and electrocardiographic features of cardiac rupture following acute myocardial infarction, Am J Med **50**:709, 1971.

Gold HK, et al: Use of sublingual nitroglycerin in congestive failure following acute myocardial infarction, Circulation **46**:839, 1972.

Goldberger E, Schwartz SP: The electrocardiographic patterns of ventricular aneurysm, Am J Med **21**:243, 1948.

Heikkila J: Electrocardiography in acute papillary muscle dysfunction and infarction, Chest **57**:510, 1970.

Hodges M, et al: Effects of intravenously administered digoxin on mild left ventricular failure in acute myocardial infarction in man, Am J Cardiol 29:749, 1972.

Karliner JS, Braunwald E: Present status of digitalis treatment in acute myocardial infarction, Circulation 45:891, 1972.

Kiely J, et al: Role of furosemide in the therapy of left ventricular failure due to acute myocardial infarction, Circulation 46(Suppl 2):175, 1972.

London RE, London SB: The electrocardiographic sign of acute hemopericardium, Circulation 25:780, 1962.

Lovell RRH, Prineas RJ: Mechanisms of sudden death and their implications for prevention and management, Prog Cardiovasc Dis 13:482, 1971.

Malach M: Peritoneal dialysis for intractable heart failure in acute myocardial infarction, Am J. Cardiol 29:61, 1972.

Meister SG, Helfant RH: Rapid bedside differentiation of ruptured interventricular septum from acute mitral insufficiency, N Engl J Med 287:1024, 1972.

Morrison J, Donnelly W, Killip T: Digitalis and myocardial infarction, Circulation 46 (Suppl 2):113, 1972.

Morrison J, Killip T: Serial serum digitalis levels in patients with acute myocardial infarction (abstr), Clin Res 19:353, 1971.

Roberts WC, Cohen LS: Left ventricular papillary muscles; description of the normal and a survey of conditions causing them to be abnormal, Circulation 41:138, 1972.

Ronan JA Jr, Roberts WC, Harvey WP: Rupture of the ventricular septum in acute myocardial infarction, Circulation 46(Suppl 2):213, 1972.

Rosen KM: Junctional tachycardia, Circulation 47:654, 1973.

Stock E: Furosemide after recent myocardial infarction, Med J Aust 2:480, 1970.

Stock E: Cardiac slowing, not cardiac irritability, major problem in prehospital phase of myocardial infarction, Med J Aust 2:747, 1971.

Wolk MJ, Scheidt S, Killip T: Heart failure complicating acute myocardial infarction, Circulation 45:1125, 1972.

Wanderman KL, et al: Perforation of the interventricular septum in a 71-year-old woman; successful repair nine days following acute myocardial infarction, Chest 63:632, 1973.

Yatteau RF, Orgain ES: Bedside diagnosis of post-infarction ventricular septal defect using the hydrogen-sensitive platinum-tipped wire electrode, Annotation, Am Heart J 84:712, 1972.

Arrhythmias associated with acute myocardial infarction

Atkins JM, Leshin SJ, Blomqvist G, Mullins GB: Ventricular conduction blocks and sudden death in acute myocardial infarction, N Engl J Med 288:281, 1973.

Barry WH, et al: Diagnosis and treatment of a case of recurrent ventricular tachycardia, Am Heart J 84:235, 1972.

Bergovitch J, et al: Management of acute myocardial infarction complicated by advanced atrioventricular block; role of artificial pacing, Am J Cardiol 23:54, 1969.

Bilitch M: A manual of cardiac arrhythmias, Boston, 1971, Little, Brown and Co.

Christiansen I, et al: Complete heart block in acute myocardial infarction; drug therapy, Am Heart J 85:162, 1972.

Church G, Biern R: Prophylactic lidocaine in acute myocardial infarction, Circulation 46(Suppl 2):139, 1972.

D'Ambrosio U, Czarnecki SW: Treatment of arrhythmias in acute myocardial infarction, Hosp Med, Sept 1971, p 141.

Gould L, et al: Prognosis of right bundle branch block in acute myocardial infarction, JAMA 219:502, 1972.

Graham AF, et al: Surgical treatment for life-threatening ventricular arrhythmias, Am J Cardiol 31:136, 1973.

Killip T: Management of arrhythmias in acute myocardial infarction, Hosp Practice, April 1972, p 131.

Kimball JT, Killip T: Aggressive treatment of arrhythmias in acute myocardial infarction, Prog Cardiovasc Dis 10:483, 1968.

Kinkaid DT, Botti RE: Significance of isolated left anterior hemiblock and left axis deviation during acute myocardial infarction, Am J Cardiol 30:797, 1972.

Koch-Weser J: Antiarrhythmic prophylaxis in acute myocardial infarction, Editorial, N Engl J Med 285:1024, 1971.

Langendorf R, Pick A: Atrioventricular block, type 2 (Mobitz); its nature and clinical significance, Circulation 38:819, 1968.

Müller OF, Schelbert H: Management of acute emergencies associated with myocardial infarction, Hosp Med, April 1972, p. 88.

Rothfield EL, et al: Idioventricular rhythm in acute myocardial infarction, Circulation 37:203, 1968.

Scheidt S, Killip T: Bundle branch block complicating acute myocardial infarction, JAMA 222:919, 1972.

Shillingford J, Thomas M: Treatment of bradycardia and hypotension syndrome in patients with acute myocardial infarction, Am Heart J 75:843, 1968.

Simon AB, Steinke WE, Curry JJ: Atrioventricular block in acute myocardial infarction, Chest 62:156, 1972.

Smirk FH, Palmer DG: A myocardial syndrome with particular reference to the occurrence of sudden death and of premature systoles interrupting antecedent T waves, Am J Cardiol **6:** 620, 1960.

Stock E: Arrhythmias after myocardial infarction, Am Heart J **75:**435, 1968.

Wardekar A, et al: Recurrent ventricular tachycardia successfully treated by excision of ventricular aneurysm, Chest **62:**505, 1972.

White BB: Therapy in acute coronary care, Chicago, 1971, Year Book Medical Publishers, Inc.

Zipes DP: Treatment of arrhythmias in myocardial infarction, Arch Intern Med **124:**101, 1969.

11 / Cardiopulmonary emergencies

In this chapter acute pulmonary edema and acute cor pulmonale are discussed.

ACUTE PULMONARY EDEMA

Pulmonary edema is characterized by an excessive transudation of serous fluid first in the interstitial tissues of the lungs and later in the alveolar spaces. Pulmonary edema is usually acute, but it may be sub-acute or chronic.

Classification of acute pulmonary edema

Acute pulmonary edema is usually a sign of severe left-sided congestive heart failure. However, it can also occur in the absence of heart disease. Acute pulmonary edema can be classified according to the mechanism producing it (after Robin and associates).

Acute pulmonary edema due to:
1. Increased pulmonary capillary pressure
2. Altered permeability
3. Decreased oncotic pressure
4. Lymphatic insufficiency
5. Increased negative interstitial pressure
6. Mixed or unknown mechanisms

Increased pulmonary capillary pressure. Acute pulmonary edema due to increased pulmonary capillary pressure can be caused by *cardiogenic factors,* such as left-sided congestive heart failure or mitral stenosis. Acute left-sided congestive heart failure is associated with an increased left ventricular end-diastolic pressure, increased left atrial pressure, increased pulmonary venous pressure, and increased pulmonary capillary pressure, because the weakened left ven-

tricle is unable to empty adequately during systole. Since the right ventricle continues to function efficiently, it pumps more blood into the lungs (and left atrium) than the left ventricle can expel. This results in marked pulmonary congestion, or acute pulmonary edema. The clinical spectrum of acute left-sided congestive heart failure therefore can range from mild orthopnea and paroxysmal nocturnal dyspnea to fulminant pulmonary edema. (Paroxysmal nocturnal dyspnea describes attacks of acute left-sided congestive heart failure that may waken the patient from sleep. There are many reasons for the attacks: the patient may slide down in bed during sleep and may not be able to tolerate a supine position; the patient may be disturbed by a frightening dream; bronchial secretions may accumulate during the night so that a paroxysm of coughing occurs.)

Acute left-sided congestive heart failure (or acute pulmonary edema) can occur in the following conditions.

1. It can occur in hypertensive cardiovascular disease, aortic valvular disease, coronary artery disease, or cardiomyopathies. The left-sided heart failure or pulmonary edema can be precipitated by strenuous exercise, excitement, sexual intercourse, intercurrent infections, and so on, all of which can put stress on an already weakened left ventricle. It can also be precipitated in a similar way by a transfusion of whole blood or by the administration of excessive IV fluids to a patient with minimal cardiac reserve. Tachyarrhythmias

can also precipitate acute left-sided congestive heart failure or acute pulmonary edema.

2. Acute pulmonary edema can also occur in patients with mitral stenosis. Here the mechanism is slightly different. When right ventricular output suddenly increases, because of exercise, pregnancy, tachyarrhythmias, and so on, the efficient right ventricle propels more blood into the lungs (and left atrium) than can pass into the left ventricle through the stenosed mitral valve, resulting in acute pulmonary edema.

3. Recently, Dodek and associates have described several patients who had coronary artery disease and recurrent pulmonary edema but who did not show radiological signs of cardiomegaly on x-ray examination. These patients apparently had a restrictive type of ischemic cardiomyopathy.

Acute pulmonary edema due to increased pulmonary capillary pressure can also be caused by *noncardiogenic factors,* such as: (1) overinfusion or overtransfusion (with whole blood) or (2) less common conditions, such as pulmonary venous disease due to pulmonary veno-occlusive disease, pulmonary venous fibrosis with high pulmonary blood flow, and pulmonary venous stenosis (due to mediastinal granuloma, fibrosing mediastinitis, and mediastinal masses).

Altered permeability. Acute pulmonary edema due to altered permeability can be caused by uremia, radiation pneumonia, aspiration pneumonia, infectious pulmonary edema (due to bacterial or viral agents), drowning or near-drowning, smoke inhalation, and inhaled toxic agents, such as phosgene, ozone, and oxides of nitrogen. It can also be caused by less common conditions, including adult respiratory distress syndromes (due to posttraumatic pulmonary insufficiency, shock, prolonged positive pressure ventilation, pulmonary embolism, cardiac pulmonary edema, overinfusion, and so on); by reactions to vasoactive substances such as histamine, kinins,

and prostaglandins; by diffuse capillary leak syndrome due to diffuse injury of the capillaries by endotoxins or due to other, unknown mechanisms; by disseminated intravascular coagulation due to disorders of the clotting mechanism (this occurs in conditions such as malaria, postinfectious immune-complex disease, heat stroke, eclampsia, and amniotic fluid embolism, and as a reaction to endotoxins); and by immunological reactions to drugs such as nitrofurantoin, sulfonamides, hydralazine, hexamethonium, methotrexate, and busulfan.

Decreased oncotic pressure. Acute pulmonary edema due to decreased oncotic pressure occurs with hypoalbuminemia due to renal or hepatic disease, protein-losing enteropathy, or malnutrition.

Lymphatic insufficiency. Acute pulmonary edema due to lymphatic insufficiency occurs in silicosis, for example.

Increased negative interstitial pressure. Acute pulmonary edema due to increased negative interstitial pressure occurs, for example, after rapid removal by suction of a large pleural effusion or pneumothorax.

Mixed or unknown mechanisms. Acute pulmonary edema due to mixed or unknown mechanisms includes high-altitude pulmonary edema, which occurs when a person rapidly ascends to an altitude higher than 9,000 feet and does strenuous physical exercise before acclimatization occurs; neurogenic pulmonary edema, which may occur after skull fracture, intracranial hemorrhage, or brain tumor; an overdose of a narcotic (heroin or methadone); pulmonary parenchymal disease; pulmonary embolism; eclampsia; or uremia, in which left-sided congestive heart failure may also be present in addition to increased capillary permeability. Acute pulmonary edema can also occur after cardioversion, after an anesthetic has been administered to the patient, or after cardiopulmonary bypass surgery.

Clinical aspects

The patient is usually found sitting upright or bending forward, in intense respiratory distress. He may be cyanotic and is often covered by a cold sweat. Cough is present, and light pink frothy sputum may literally pour out of the mouth. As much as a pint or more can be coughed up in an hour or two. Coarse moist rales are heard posteriorly over more than one half of both lung fields. Occasionally, only asthmatic wheezes and expiratory squeaks are present *(cardiac asthma)*. The pulmonary second sound may be accentuated, and an S_3 gallop rhythm may be present in association with a tachycardia. The blood pressure is often elevated. The systolic blood pressure may exceed 300 mm Hg (with a high diastolic pressure) if the patient is hypertensive. (A fall in blood pressure during acute pulmonary edema, before treatment is given, is suggestive of acute myocardial infarction.)

When a patient suffers a mild attack of paroxysmal nocturnal dyspnea, he may have few symptoms. He may awake with cough and a feeling of anxiety and may constantly clear his throat. Some viscid muscus may be coughed up; the patient will feel relieved, and he may fall asleep again in a few minutes. If the patient has coronary artery disease, the attack of dyspnea may be associated with angina.

The differentiation of cardiac asthma from bronchial asthma is important because morphine is contraindicated in bronchial asthma and epinephrine is contraindicated in cardiac asthma. Rales heard at the lung bases indicate cardiac asthma. A patient with bronchial asthma usually gives a history of cough over a period of years, occurrence of attacks during the day as well as at night, seasonal variations, and relief with epinephrine or ephedrine. Similarly, x-ray examination of the chest will reveal emphysema or nonspecific findings in bronchial asthma but will show signs of pulmonary congestion in left-sided congestive heart failure. The circulation time will be normal during a bronchial asthmatic attack but will be prolonged with left-sided congestive heart failure.

If one is not certain whether cardiac or bronchial asthma is present, the patient can be given aminophylline (p. 159) because it is effective in both conditions. In addition, oxygen (24% to 28%) can be given, using a Ventimask. This avoids giving excessive oxygen, in case the patient has severe pulmonary disease.

X-ray examination

The hilar regions show increased width and density, and their outlines are indistinct due to interstitial pulmonary edema. The lung fields also appear indistinct, due to the pulmonary congestion and to the dilatation of the pulmonary vessels. In addition, pleural effusion and Kerley B lines may be present. The pulmonary veins are characteristically distended in the upper lung fields but are relatively constricted in the lower lung fields.

When acute pulmonary edema occurs in uremia, the chest x-ray film often shows characteristic symmetrical opacities that radiate from both hilar areas like the wings of a bat. This is due to alveolar edema. (It can also occur in pulmonary edema due to other causes.)

Lung scan may reveal areas of underperfusion, simulating pulmonary embolism.

The shape and size of the cardiac silhouette depends on the presence of cardiac dilatation, the presence of heart disease, and the type of heart disease (mitral valvular, aortic valvular, coronary, and so on).

Electrocardiogram

There are no characteristic electrocardiographic changes associated with acute pulmonary edema.

Blood gas findings

Pulmonary edema may produce variable arterial blood gas findings. Hypoxemia is present, so that the arterial oxygen content (Pa_{O_2}) is slightly or moderately reduced (normal range, 95 to 100 mm Hg). Respiratory and metabolic acid-base disturbances may also be present. Many patients hyperventilate and develop a respiratory alkalosis (Pco_2 below 35 mm Hg) and a high pH. However, when the pulmonary edema is extensive, and particularly if the patient has been given morphine (which depresses respiration), hypoventilation may occur, and the patient may develop a respiratory acidosis (Pco_2 greater than 45 mm Hg) and a low pH. The respiratory acidosis can be further complicated by a simultaneous metabolic acidosis. In addition, a metabolic acidosis, including a lactic acidosis, may develop, due to tissue hypoxia, particularly in the liver, associated with the decreased cardiac output that is usually present. The combination of a respiratory and metabolic acidosis is very serious and may be lethal. If oxygen does not control the respiratory acidosis, sodium bicarbonate* can be used cautiously. However, sodium bicarbonate may aggravate the pulmonary edema by causing retention of fluid.

Respiratory alkalosis does not need specific treatment.

Emergency treatment

The emergency treatment of acute pulmonary edema depends on the etiology.

Emergency treatment of cardiogenic acute pulmonary edema

1. Place the patient in a sitting position, even in a chair, or with his feet dangling from the side of the bed (unless acute myocardial infarction or shock is present). Some patients get relief by standing.

2. Morphine sulfate can be given as the drug of first choice. It decreases the tachypnea, decreases the pulmonary edema by its peripheral dilating effect and also

---

*This and other drugs are described in Part three.

alleviates the patient's intense anxiety. It can be given subcutaneously or IM in a dose of 10 to 15 mg (gr 1/6 to gr 1/4) or IV in a dose of 5 mg every 4 to 6 hours. (Morphine should be avoided if acute pulmonary edema is associated with intracranial bleeding, chronic pulmonary disease, or bronchial asthma.)

3. Digitalis, administered IV, can also be used as the drug of first choice. A rapid-acting preparation such as digoxin (Lanoxin) or deslanoside (Cedilanid-D) can be used. If the patient has not had digitalis in the past 2 weeks, an initial "loading" dose of 2 to 4 ml (0.5 to 1.0 mg) digoxin can be given IV. Further doses of 1 ml (0.25 mg) can then be given every 2 to 4 hours until a full digitalizing dose of 6 ml (1.5 mg) has been reached; or deslanoside can be given IV in an initial dose of 4 ml (0.8 mg), repeated in 2 to 4 hours to obtain full digitalization.

When a patient who is taking digitalis develops acute pulmonary edema, one should suspect that decreased cardiac output due to digitalis toxicity may be one of the causes of the pulmonary edema, particularly if the patient is nauseated or has been vomiting, or if paroxysmal atrial tachycardia with AV block, nonparoxysmal AV junctional tachycardia, ventricular premature contractions with a bigeminal rhythm, or ventricular tachycardia is present.

If there are no signs of digitalis toxicity, a test dose, such as 1 ml (0.2 mg) deslanoside or 0.5 ml (0.125 mg) digoxin, can be given IV. Further small doses can be given IV every 1 or 2 hours, as indicated.

4. Administer humidified oxygen to prevent excessive drying of the mucous membranes. It can be given in several ways.

First, when a nasal catheter is used at an oxygen flow rate of 8 L/min, it provides an oxygen concentration of approximately 40%. The concentration will be less if the patient breathes through his mouth.

Second, if a higher concentration of oxygen is needed, a well-fitting oronasal mask should be used. When oxygen is administered at a flow rate of 5 to 6 L/min with such a mask, approximately 50% to 60% oxygen concentrations can be attained; and when 12 L/min are given, a concentration of almost 100% oxygen can be attained. When a very high concentration (75% to 100%) of oxygen is given, the flow should be stopped for a few minutes at least every 12 hours to prevent oxygen toxicity. (Pulmonary oxygen toxicity should be suspected when a patient who is receiving a rich oxygen mixture develops severe burning or aching chest pain, aggravated by breathing, nonproductive cough, increased difficulty in oxygenating the arterial blood, and unexplained patchy pulmonary infiltrates. These changes can occur within 72 hours after administration of a very high concentration of oxygen is started. Cerebral signs, including generalized convulsions due to oxygen toxicity, can also occur.)

If desired, oxygen can be bubbled through an antifoaming agent, such as 50% ethyl alcohol or 2-ethyl-1-hexanol.

Third, oxygen can also be administered under positive pressure when pulmonary edema is present. This method of administration not only provides oxygen, but helps alleviate pulmonary edema by decreasing venous return and by forcing the edema fluid out of the alveoli and the interstitial tissues. Oxygen under positive pressure can be given in three ways.

  a. A special face mask with an adjustable valve that determines the caliber of the exit airway can be used. The airway exits are calibrated so that *expiration* under a positive pressure of 1 to 4 or even 6 cm water can be obtained.

  b. A Bird (or similar) positive pressure respirator can also be used to alleviate the pulmonary edema. The setting should be adjusted to provide an *inspiratory* pressure of 15 to 20 cm water.

  c. When overwhelming pulmonary edema of noncardiac origin is present, even intermittent positive pressure breathing may not relieve the hypoxemia. Such patients have recently been treated with positive end-expiratory pressure (PEEP) breathing, with the end-tidal positive pressure maintained at approximately 5 to 20 cm water. However, continuous positive pressure breathing of this type can cause a marked decrease in cardiac output and may result in coronary insufficiency and shock.

5. Apply tourniquets or blood pressure cuffs to the extremities. Wide soft rubber tubing should be used for the tourniquets. The tourniquets should be placed approximately 6 inches below the groins and approximately 4 inches below the shoulders.

Compress only three extremities at one time. Every 15 to 20 min release one of the tourniquets and apply it to the free extremity. Apply the tourniquets (or blood pressure cuffs) at a pressure less than that of the systolic blood pressure. (The arterial pulse must be palpable distal to each tourniquet or blood pressure cuff.)

6. A rapid-acting diuretic, such as furosemide (Lasix) or ethacrynic acid (Edecrin), can be given IV.

Furosemide is given in a dose of 2 ampuls (40 mg) slowly (over a 1- to 2-min period). An additional dose of 2 ampuls (40 mg) can be given IV 1 to 1½ hours later, if indicated.

Ethacrynic acid is given in a dose of 50 mg IV (or 0.5 to 1 mg/kg body weight). If necessary, a second dose can be given IV at another injection site (to avoid thrombophlebitis) in approximately 2 hours. (If the patient is critically ill, a single IV dose not exceeding 100 mg can be given.)

Since these diuretics can cause massive diuresis and a decreased circulating blood volume, the patient must be carefully watched for the development of hypotension.

All six steps described above can be done concomitantly.

7. If the patient fails to respond to the above treatment, a phlebotomy of 250 to 500 ml can be done. (If shock is present, phlebotomy is contraindicated.) The blood should be collected in a vacuum bottle under sterile conditions so that, if necessary, the red blood cells can be removed and reinfused into the patient (plasmapheresis).

8. Aminophylline can be given IV if there are signs of bronchospasm, such as wheezing. A dose of 250 to 500 mg is given slowly at a rate of 1 ml (25 mg) per min to avoid side effects, such as headache, flushing, palpitation, dizziness, precordial pain, hypotension, or cardiac arrest due to ventricular fibrillation. (Aminophylline is available for IV use in 10- and 20-ml ampuls in a concentration of 25 mg/ml. The ampul should be warmed to body temperature before the injection is given.) Aminophylline can also be given as a slow IV drip over a period of 4 to 6 hours by diluting 250 or 500 mg in 100 to 250 ml 5% dextrose in water.

Aminophylline can also be given IM in a dose of 250 to 500 mg. (For this purpose, it is supplied in 2-ml ampuls in a concentration of 250 mg/ml.) It can also be given by suppository.

9. If the patient shows signs of bronchospasm (expiratory wheezes and squeaks) but no rales, and it is not certain whether the attack is due to bronchial asthma or cardiac asthma, aminophylline can be given because it is effective in both conditions. (Morphine is contraindicated in bronchial asthma, and epinephrine is contraindicated in cardiac asthma.)

10. When acute pulmonary edema occurs in a patient with uremia, the methods described above can be used. However, digitalis will not be helpful unless left-sided congestive heart failure is one of the causes of the pulmonary edema. Either furosemide or ethacrynic acid can be used in the presence of azotemia.

The treatment of pulmonary edema associated with the following conditions is described elsewhere: with a hypertensive crisis, p. 174; complicating acute myocardial infarction, p. 139; complicating cardiogenic shock, p. 44; complicating massive pulmonary embolism, p. 165.

Emergency treatment of noncardiogenic acute pulmonary edema

Treatment differs from that of cardiogenic acute pulmonary edema, because digitalis and diuretics are not used. In addition, morphine should not be used if bronchial asthma, chronic pulmonary disease, or intracranial bleeding is present. If the pulmonary edema is associated with an allergic reaction, corticosteroids can be used. Acute pulmonary edema due to heroin toxicity can be treated with oxygen. The heroin (or methadone) overdose can be treated with Naloxone (Narcan). High-altitude pulmonary edema is treated by bed rest, 100% oxygen, and prompt removal of the patient to a lower altitude. When pulmonary edema is associated with shock caused by gram-negative bacteria, massive doses of corticosteroids may be needed (p. 166). When pulmonary edema is associated with disseminated intravascular coagulation, dextran 40 and heparin may be effective.

Prophylaxis

A patient who shows signs of even minimal congestive heart failure should be treated with diuretics, digitalis, a sodium-restricted diet, a weight-reducing program, and so on, as indicated.

When a patient with heart disease requires a transfusion, resuspended (packed) red blood cells rather than whole blood should be transfused. Similarly, excessive infusions of either saline or dextrose in water should be avoided in a patient with heart disease. The patient should be examined daily to detect enlargement of the liver, edema of the lower extremities, increased respiratory rate, rales at the lung bases, sudden gain in weight, and so on.

Acute pulmonary edema occurring in a patient with mitral stenosis is an indication for mitral valve surgery. Similarly, acute pulmonary edema in a patient with aortic stenosis is an indication for aortic valve replacement.

ACUTE COR PULMONALE

Massive pulmonary embolism is the most common cause of acute cor pulmonale. Acute cor pulmonale can also occur after fat embolism (p. 165) or after pulmonary arterial air embolism (p. 166). Rarer causes of acute cor pulmonale include rupture of an aortic aneurysm into the pulmonary artery, spontaneous pneumothorax, massive pulmonary atelectasis, or extensive pneumonitis.

Massive pulmonary embolism

Acute cor pulmonale is characterized by acute dilatation of the right ventricle and of the pulmonary artery. It is usually due to massive embolism of the main pulmonary artery or of one of its major branches. However, it may also occur when only a secondary branch of the pulmonary artery is occluded, especially if underlying cardiac or pulmonary disease is present.

Pulmonary thrombosis associated with embolism of one or more of the smaller pulmonary arteries is a common finding of routine autopsies. In many of these patients, the diagnosis had not been made clinically, because signs of the embolism or thrombosis were minimal. However, massive pulmonary embolism usually produces characteristic clinical, electrocardiographic, and laboratory signs of acute cor pulmonale.

When approximately 60% or more of the pulmonary circulation is occluded, the right ventricle is unable to pump out the blood it is receiving from the systemic veins, and acute right ventricular dilatation occurs in an attempt to overcome the obstruction. This is followed by signs of right-sided congestive heart failure (di-

lated neck veins, engorgement of the liver, and so on). Some degree of shock is also usually present because of the sudden drop in cardiac output.

Acute pulmonary edema may also occur as a result of massive pulmonary embolism. The reason for the pulmonary edema is not completely understood. It may be due to overperfusion of the unobstructed portions of the pulmonary vascular bed and a resulting rise in pulmonary capillary pressure.

Etiology

Pulmonary emboli develop when a portion of a thrombus in a systemic vein or in the right atrial appendage or right ventricle breaks off. Common etiological factors include acute myocardial infarction, chronic congestive heart failure, cardiomyopathies, immobilization for cerebrovascular insufficiency, malignancy (particularly pancreatic), and fractures of the lower extremity (particularly of the hip). Pulmonary emboli also occur after parturition, in postoperative patients, especially after pelvic operations or prostatectomy, and after operations for varicose veins. Other factors include polycythemia, obesity, age above 50 years, and a history of deep vein thrombosis. Occasionally, pulmonary embolism occurs when a person sits for several hours in a cramped position, as in an automobile or airplane, particularly if varicose veins are present.

Patients with acute myocardial infarction may develop pulmonary embolism from a thrombus in the right ventricle if the ventricular septum has been infarcted. Similarly, patients with a cardiomyopathy may develop a pulmonary embolus from a thrombus in the right ventricle. Both these groups of patients may also develop systemic emboli from a thrombus in the left ventricle. Patients with rheumatic heart disease may develop pulmonary embolism from a thrombus in the right atrial appendage, particularly if atrial fibrillation is present. If a thrombus in the left atrial appendage is present, systemic embolism may also occur.

Clinical aspects

The most common symptom is sudden dyspnea. In addition, the patient may complain of crushing substernal pressure, identical to the pain of acute myocardial infarction. Tachypnea, cough, and wheezing may also be present. If pulmonary infarction has occurred, pleuritic chest pain may be present. Less frequently, hemoptysis occurs. Nonspecific symptoms, such as nausea, vomiting, abdominal pain, dizziness, mental confusion, syncope, and even a convulsive seizure due to cerebral underperfusion, may obscure the primary diagnosis.

Physical examination may reveal low blood pressure, with or without other signs of shock. Cyanosis due to shock or inadequate pulmonary perfusion is often present. The patient's temperature may be elevated to 101 F. The dilated pulmonary artery may produce a forceful pulsation that may be seen as well as felt. The pulmonic component of the second heart sound (P_2) is usually accentuated, and a systolic pulmonic murmur may be present as well. A rough friction rub over the pulmonary area may appear. This is probably produced by rubbing of the dilated pulmonary artery against the pericardium. A pleural friction rub may be present if pulmonary infarction has occurred. The acute right ventricular dilatation and right-sided congestive heart failure may be associated with a right ventricular heave and a right ventricular gallop (S_3).

Mild jaundice may appear, due to lysis of blood in the lungs or acute congestion of the liver, associated with severe right-sided congestive heart failure.

The patient should also be examined for signs of peripheral thrombophlebitis.

Electrocardiogram

Acute cor pulmonale due to massive pulmonary embolism can be associated with any of the following electrocardiographic patterns (Fig. 11-1).

1. Right ventricular strain. The T waves in the right precordial leads (V_1 through V_5 or V_6) may become inverted, often with a cove shape, simulating acute myocardial infarction.

2. Clockwise rotation. Acute dilatation of the right ventricle and anatomical rotation of the heart may produce a delayed transition zone in the precordial leads, with an rS or RS pattern in leads V_1 through V_5 or V_6. In addition, a qR pattern may develop in lead V_1 or leads V_1 and V_2.

3. An S_1Q_3 pattern may appear. This is associated with the development of a Qr or QR pattern in lead aV_R. In addition, leads aV_F and III may develop a QR pattern and an elevated RS-T segment, simulating acute inferior myocardial infarction.

4. Transient (complete or incomplete) right bundle branch block may develop.

5. A P pulmonale pattern (tall, peaked P waves) may appear in leads II, III, and aV_F.

6. Signs of subendocardial ischemia (p. 129) may also develop.

7. Frontal plane axis shifts. The frontal plane electrical axis of the QRS complex may shift acutely to the right. Recently, acute left axis shift has also been described in cases of acute pulmonary embolism.

8. Arrhythmias. Sinus tachycardia is the most common arrhythmia. Atrial arrhythmias, especially atrial flutter, may also appear suddenly.

X-ray examination and laboratory tests

Even with massive pulmonary embolism, the x-ray films may show only minor or nonspecific changes. Elevation of the diaphragm on the affected side is often an early radiological sign of massive pulmonary embolism. In addition, the x-ray film should be examined for signs of infiltrates, pleural effusion, and pulmonary artery dilatation.

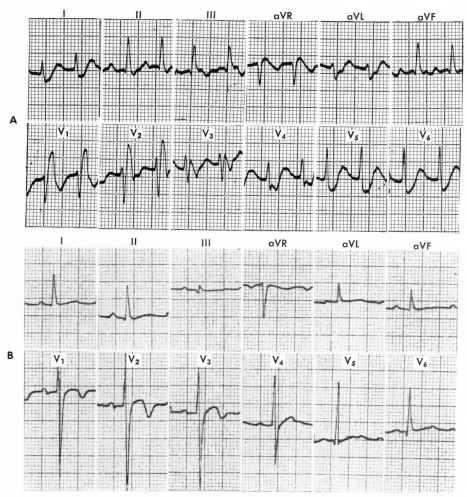

Fig. 11-1. Massive pulmonary embolism. **A,** ECG taken shortly after the embolism occurred; shows characteristic changes of massive pulmonary embolism, including an S_1Q_3 pattern, right bundle branch block (rSR′ pattern in lead VI with a prolonged QRS of 0.12 sec), and subendo-cardial anoxia (elevated RS-T in lead aV_R, associated with depression of the RS-T in precordial leads V_4 to V_6, aV_L, and I). In addition, a supraventricular tachycardia is present, probably atrial flutter—best seen in aV_F. The ventricular rate is slightly faster than 150 per min. **B,** Same patient as in **A;** ECG taken 3 days later. The heart rate has slowed, and sinus rhythm has returned. The S_1Q_3 pattern and the right bundle branch block have disappeared. Now the precordial leads show typical changes of right ventricular strain (downward T waves in leads V_1 to V_3 and biphasic T waves in leads V_4 and V_5).

Lung scan. When ^{131}I-labeled macroaggregated albumin particles are injected IV, they will diffuse through the lung fields, but will not appear (or will be underperfused) in areas supplied by the occluded pulmonary artery. A normal lung scan excludes the possibility of massive pulmonary embolism. Unfortunately, an abnormal lung scan is compatible with, but not diagnostic of, massive pulmonary embolism, because numerous other pulmonary conditions, such as pneumonia, emphysema, bronchitis, pulmonary congestion, or lung carcinoma, can also produce abnormal lung scans. The lung scan is particularly useful in detecting areas of abnormal decreased perfusion that are not revealed by routine x-ray examination.

Pulmonary arteriography. This is the most accurate test for the diagnosis of massive pulmonary embolism. Right heart catheterization is required, with placement of the catheter tip in the outflow tract of the right ventricle or in the pulmonary artery. Dalen and associates have reported a 4% morbidity and 1 death in a series of 367 patients. Complications included cardiac perforation, pyrogen reactions and arrhythmias related to the catheterization, bronchospasm, angioneurotic edema, anaphylaxis, and cardiogenic shock related to the angiography.

There are two major angiographic signs of massive pulmonary embolism: intraluminal defects and cutoff of an artery. Oligemia and asymmetry of blood flow are relatively nonspecific signs that may be due to underlying pulmonary or cardiac disease.

Arterial blood gases. The classic blood gas findings with massive pulmonary embolism are a decreased Pa_{O_2} due to ventilation-perfusion defects, bronchoconstriction, and other causes, and a decreased Pco_2 secondary to compensatory hyperventilation. With massive pulmonary embolism the Pa_{O_2} is usually below 80 mm Hg (with the patient breathing room air), and the Pco_2 is usually below 40 mm Hg (un-

less the patient was a CO_2 retainer before the embolism occurred).

Similar blood gas findings can also occur with acute pulmonary edema. In addition, a Pa_{O_2} less than 80 mm Hg can occur in otherwise asymptomatic elderly patients.

Central venous pressure (CVP). The CVP is characteristically elevated, due to the acute right-sided congestive heart failure. (The presence of hypotension or shock along with a low CVP indicates that massive pulmonary embolism is not the cause of the shock or hypotension.)

Serum enzyme tests. It has been suggested that the triad high LDH, normal SGOT, and elevated bilirubin concentrations is diagnostic of massive pulmonary embolism. Unfortunately, this triad has been found in only a small percentage of patients with pulmonary embolism. Furthermore, these patients may also have elevated SGOT and CPK concentrations in addition to the LDH elevation that is usually present.

The presence of fibrin-split products has been described as a useful test for massive pulmonary embolism, but it is not widely used.

Differential diagnosis

Numerous conditions can simulate massive pulmonary embolism.

Acute myocardial infarction. The symptoms and signs of acute myocardial infarction and massive pulmonary embolism may be very similar. However, the patient with a pulmonary embolism often gives a history of having been bedridden for 1 week or longer because of an operation, fractured hip, congestive heart failure, or a chronic illness, such as cancer, and may have a history of a deep vein thrombosis.

The ECG of acute myocardial infarction is very characteristic (p. 123). If massive pulmonary embolism is present, the ECG may or may not show characteristic signs (see above). However, some patients with massive pulmonary embolism may show a

Q wave and an elevated RS-T segment in lead aV_F, simulating acute inferior myocardial infarction. When this occurs, lead aV_R is useful in differentiating the two conditions. When inferior myocardial infarction occurs, lead aV_R shows either an rS or a QS, but not a QR (unless anterior myocardial infarction is also present). In massive pulmonary embolism, lead aV_R typically shows a QR type of pattern.

Pulmonary embolism may also show RS-T depressions, due to subendocardial ischemia. However, in such patients, other electrocardiographic signs of pulmonary embolism are also present (see above).

In addition, deep T wave inversions in the precordial leads, secondary to acute right ventricular strain, may simulate anterior wall myocardial infarction. However, abnormal Q waves are not present in leads V_3, V_4, V_5, or V_6. In addition, these downward T waves may occur in association with a QR type of pattern in precordial lead V_1 or in leads V_1 and V_2, a characteristic that is virtually diagnostic of pulmonary embolism when these changes occur acutely.

The diagnosis of massive pulmonary embolism complicating acute myocardial infarction can be very difficult because the electrocardiographic patterns of the pulmonary embolism may be obscured by the pattern of the acute myocardial infarct. However, sudden severe chest pain, tachypnea, and fever suggest pulmonary embolism. In addition, the ECG may show a sudden shift of the electrical axis in the limb leads to the right (or to the left).

As mentioned above, a normal lung scan or normal blood gases also rule out massive pulmonary embolism. Angiography, of course, will give the most accurate diagnosis. However, if acute myocardial infarction has occurred, angiography may be dangerous. Similarly, if ventricular irritability is present, angiography is also contraindicated.

Pneumonia. The differential diagnosis between pneumonia and pulmonary embolism may be difficult if signs of shock (due to the pulmonary embolism) do not appear, because x-ray examination may show pulmonary infiltration in either case. However, if the pulmonary embolus produces a pulmonary infarct, the infarct will be located in the periphery of the lung fields and will be in contact with one or more pleural spaces. In pneumonia, the infiltration is often more centrally located in the lung fields.

In pulmonary embolism, the white blood cell count may be elevated as high as 15,000, but a polynuclear shift to the left is not present as occurs in pneumonia. The sputum in pulmonary embolism shows red blood cells; in pneumonia, white blood cells and bacteria are present.

Lung scan is also helpful in the differential diagnosis. In pulmonary embolism, decreased perfusion may occur in areas that are normal on x-ray examination. In pneumonia, the perfusion defects are limited to areas that are abnormal on x-ray examination.

Acute left-sided congestive heart failure with hemoptysis. Hemoptysis is rare except in mitral stenosis or unless the patient is receiving anticoagulants.

Emergency treatment

1. Oxygen is urgently needed. It can be given by mask at a rate of 10 to 15 L/min. However, even the inhalation of 100% oxygen may not correct the inadequate oxygenation.

2. Start IV administration of heparin immediately. Heparin is not only an anticoagulant, but it is also capable of quickly relieving the bronchospasm associated with massive pulmonary embolism.

3. Treat shock immediately. The drug of first choice is isoproterenol (Isuprel) because it dilates the pulmonary vasculature. The CVP must be monitored carefully, and extra fluids may be needed as the CVP falls (Chapter 3). It may not be possible to

give isoproterenol after massive pulmonary embolism if a tachycardia is present, because isoproterenol may increase the heart rate excessively.

If the patient does not respond to isoproterenol, give other vasopressors and the general treatment for shock described in Chapter 3.

4. Most patients with massive pulmonary embolism will respond to the emergency medical treatment described above. However, if the patient remains critically ill, pulmonary embolectomy may be lifesaving. However, the operative mortality from pulmonary embolectomy may be 60% or higher. Therefore, the operation should be done only when the following conditions are present: massive pulmonary embolism with obstruction of more than 60% of the pulmonary vasculature as revealed by angiography; right-sided heart failure with an elevated right ventricular end-diastolic pressure (p. 47) and an elevated CVP exceeding 15 cm water; or persistent shock unresponsive to treatment with fluids and vasopressor drugs.

Recently a national cooperative study was made of the value of urokinase administered IV in conjunction with heparin to help lyse pulmonary emboli. Preliminary studies indicate that this combination may be particularly valuable for patients with pulmonary embolism and shock who were previously considered candidates for emergency pulmonary embolectomy.

When acute pulmonary edema occurs in association with massive pulmonary embolism, treatment of the pulmonary embolism is primary (see above). Morphine or digitalis is probably not indicated. In addition, if the circulating blood volume is decreased (by tourniquets, phlebotomy, and so on) the patient may develop severe shock.

Prophylaxis

The majority of patients with massive pulmonary embolism have a predisposing condition, such as old age, recent operation, immobilizing fracture or other causes for immobilization or prolonged bed rest, chronic congestive heart failure, or malignant neoplasm. It is now rare to see massive pulmonary embolism following acute myocardial infarction because patients are ambulatory early, wear antiembolism stockings, and are often given anticoagulant therapy.

Excessive bed rest should be avoided in patients predisposed to pulmonary embolism. Ace bandages or antiembolism stockings should be routinely used, and anticoagulant therapy may be beneficial (if there are no contraindications).

In addition, in patients with massive pulmonary embolism who have had previous episodes of smaller emboli, the occurrence of sudden tachypnea or dyspnea, tachycardia, fever, or accentuated P_2 on auscultation of the heart should suggest that pulmonary emboli are occurring and that preventive or therapeutic measures should be taken immediately. Ligation or plication of the inferior vena cava in patients who are prone to recurrent pulmonary emboli does not necessarily prevent massive pulmonary embolization.

Fat embolism

Acute cor pulmonale due to fat embolism can occur when globules of liquid fat enter the systemic veins and are carried to the lungs. Common causes of fat embolism include severe fractures or extensive crushing injuries, amputations, osteomyelitis, and burns. It can also occur after cardiopulmonary bypass operations, and so on.

Since the fat globules are able to penetrate the lung capillaries and enter the general circulation, they may become lodged in the blood vessels of the brain. Therefore, pulmonary or cerebral symptoms and signs or both may develop, usually within 72 hours after an accident.

Patients with predominantly pulmonary symptoms show tachypnea and dyspnea.

Rales in the chest or pulmonary edema may be present. Patients with predominantly cerebral symptoms show restlessness, confusion, stupor, or coma. Fever is usually present. Petechial hemorrhage often appears on the skin, particularly on the neck, and on the anterior chest wall and conjunctiva. The eyegrounds may show papilledema, hemorrhages, or even fat emboli, which are diagnostic.

Laboratory tests are helpful in establishing the diagnosis. Arterial blood gases show a low Pa_{O_2} and a low Pa_{CO_2}. The hemoglobin and hematocrit values fall, and thrombocytopenia may also occur. The serum calcium concentration may be low, due to the interaction of calcium ions with fatty acids. Fat globules may appear in the urine, but this finding is not specific for fat embolism. When the Pa_{O_2} is less than 60 mm Hg, a cryostat-frozen section of clotted blood should be studied to detect the presence of neutral fat.

Emergency treatment

1. Administer oxygen—for example, 10 to 15 L/min by mask—to counteract the inadequate oxygenation of the lungs.

2. Administer heparin unless it is contraindicated because of the danger of bleeding from injured areas.

3. Massive doses of corticosteroids have also been found helpful. The following dosage can be given: 125 mg methylprednisolone sodium succinate (Solu-Medrol) IV, followed by 80 mg every 6 hours for 3 days. The patient should be protected from gastrointestinal bleeding with milk, antacids, or the use of continuous gastric suction (Fischer and associates).

Pulmonary arterial air embolism

Acute cor pulmonale can also be produced if a large amount of air enters the systemic veins and is carried to the right ventricle and the lungs. At least 100 to 150 ml or more is required to cause death. The air may remain in the right ventricle, where it acts as a trap, preventing the expulsion of blood into the lungs, or it may enter the lungs, where it obstructs the pulmonary arterioles. The air does not penetrate the pulmonary capillaries (unlike fat emboli).

Pulmonary arterial air embolism can be caused by many factors, including operations involving the neck veins, dural sinuses, or uterine mucosa; diagnostic perirenal, peritoneal, bladder, or joint air injections; pneumoperitoneum; angiography; angiocardiography; encephalography; vaginal insufflation of powders; and rarely from the accidental entrance of air during an IV infusion when the bottle becomes empty.

Cyanosis, dyspnea, and shock occur suddenly, and a characteristic churning waterwheel murmur appears over the heart, due to the air in the right ventricle.

Emergency treatment is to turn the patient onto the left lateral position (right side up). The inhalation of 100% oxygen may be helpful. Cardiopulmonary resuscitation and external cardiac compression should be done if necessary.

Pulmonary arterial air embolism should not be confused with pulmonary venous (systemic arterial) air embolism.

Pulmonary venous (systemic arterial) air embolism

In pulmonary venous (systemic arterial) air embolism, air enters the pulmonary veins and is carried to the left atrium and into the systemic circulation. This is in contrast to pulmonary arterial air embolism, where air enters a systemic vein and is carried to the right heart and into the lungs (see above).

Air can enter the pulmonary veins accidentally if one of the pulmonary veins is pierced during thoracic surgery or during artificial pneumothorax. (So-called pleural shock is probably due to pulmonary venous air embolism).

Symptoms and signs are due to the occlusion of systemic arteries by air bubbles.

The patient becomes dizzy and confused. A convulsive seizure may occur, with resulting monoplegia, hemoplegia, aphasia, or blindness. These signs may disappear or may persist. Shock and cyanosis may develop, along with Cheyne-Stokes respiration. If one of the coronary arteries is blocked, marked substernal pain may develop, with electrocardiographic signs of myocardial injury or infarction.

Ophthalmoscopic examination may reveal bubbles of air in the retinal arterioles. Later, retinal pallor develops. Marbling of the skin may occur, due to embolism of the skin arteries. If a large amount of air enters the systemic circulation, death may occur.

Emergency treatment is not completely satisfactory. Because air is buoyant, the patient should be kept in a head-down position to prevent cerebral embolism.

REFERENCES
Acute pulmonary edema

Aberman A, Fulop M: The metabolic and respiratory acidosis of acute pulmonary edema, Ann Intern Med **76**:173, 1972.

Avery WG, et al: The acidosis of pulmonary edema, Am J Med **48**:320, 1970.

Beiser, GD, et al: Studies on digitalis. XVII. Effects of ouabain on the hemodynamic response to exercise in patients with mitral stenosis in normal sinus rhythm, N Engl J Med **278**:131, 1968.

Bresnick E, et al: Fatal reaction of intravenous administration of aminophylline, JAMA **136**:397, 1948.

Burch GE, DePascuale NP: Congestive heart failure; acute pulmonary edema, JAMA **208**:1895, 1969.

Dodek A, Kassebaum DG, Bristow JD: Pulmonary edema in coronary artery disease without cardiomegaly, N Engl J Med **286**:1347, 1972.

Gibson DG: Hemodynamic factors in the development of acute pulmonary edema in renal failure, Lancet **2**:1217, 1966.

Goldman AL, Enquist RW: Methadone pulmonary edema, Chest **63**:275, 1973.

Hultgren HN, Flamm MD: Pulmonary edema, Mod Concepts Cardiovasc Dis **38**:1, 1969.

Karliner JS: Noncardiogenic forms of pulmonary edema, Circulation **46**:212, 1972.

Mazzullo JM, Sundaresan PR: Treatment of chronic obstructive pulmonary disease,, Rational Drug Therapy **7**(2), 1973.

Robin ED, Cross CE, Zelis R: Pulmonary edema, N Engl Med **288**:239, 1973.

Senior RM, Wessler S, Avioli LV: Pulmonary oxygen toxicity, JAMA **217**:1373, 1971.

Sugarman HJ, et al: Positive end-expiratory pressure (PEEP); indications and physiologic considerations, Chest **65**(Suppl 2): 86, 1972.

Acute cor pulmonale

Beveridge RJ: Fat embolism; is prophylaxis possible, Internist Observer **10**(5), 1972.

Bradley EC, et al: Hemodynamic studies on clinical shock following pulmonary embolization, Clin Res **14**:122, 1966.

Breckenridge RT, Ratnoff OD: Pulmonary embolism and unexpected death in supposedly normal individuals, N Engl J Med **270**:298, 1964.

Codley EL: Enzyme profiles in pulmonary infarction, Letter, JAMA **208**:1704, 1969.

Dalen JE, editor: Pulmonary embolism, New York, 1972, Medcom Press.

Dalen, JE, Dexter L: Pulmonary embolism, JAMA **207**:1505, 1969.

Dalen JE, et al: Pulmonary angiography in acute pulmonary embolism, Am Heart J **81**:175, 1971.

DelGuercio LRM, et al: Pulmonary embolism shock, JAMA **196**:751, 1966.

Dines DE, Linscheid RL, Didier EP: Fat embolism syndrome, Mayo Clin Proc **47**:237, 1972.

Fischer JE, et al: Massive steroid therapy in severe fat embolism, Surg Gynecol Obstet **132**:667, 1971.

Huaman A, Nice W, Young I: Fat embolism syndrome; premortem diagnosis by cryostat frozen sections, J Kans Med Soc **70**:487, 1969.

Johnson JC, et al: Unexplained atrial flutter; a frequent herald of pulmonary embolism, Chest **60**:29, 1971.

Lynch RE, et al: Leftward shift of frontal plane QRS as a frequent manifestation of acute pulmonary embolism, Chest **61**:443, 1972.

Mack I, Harris R, Katz LN: Acute cor pulmonale in the absence of pulmonary embolism, Am Heart J **39**:664, 1950.

McDonald IG, et al: Isoproterenol in massive pulmonary embolism; hemodynamic and clinical effects, Med J Aust **2**:201, 1968.

McIntyre KM, Sasahara AA, Littman D: Relation of the electrocardiogram to hemodynamic alterations in pulmonary embolism, Am J Cardiol **30**:205, 1972.

Modan B, Sharon E, Jelin N: Factors contributing to the incorrect diagnosis of pulmonary embolic disease, Chest **62**:388, 1972.

Quinn JL: Radioisotope lung scanning, Semin Roentgenol **2**:406, 1967.

Sasahara AA, et al: Diagnostic requirements and therapeutic decisions in pulmonary embolism, JAMA **202**:553, 1967.

Sasahara AA, Hyers TM, et al: The urokinase pulmonary embolism trial, Circulation 47(Suppl 2), 1973.

Scannel JG: The surgical management of acute massive pulmonary embolism, Prog Cardiovasc Dis 9:488, 1967.

Smith M, Ray CT: Electrocardiographic signs of early right ventricular enlargement in acute pulmonary embolism, Chest 205:58, 1970.

Spodick DH: Electrocardiographic responses to pulmonary embolism, Am J Cardiol 30:695, 1972.

Szucs MM, et al: Diagnostic sensitivity of laboratory findings in acute pulmonary embolism, Ann Intern Med 74:161, 1971.

Wagner HN Jr: Current status of lung scanning, Radiology 91:1235, 1968.

Wenger NK, Stein PD, Willis PW: Massive pulmonary embolism; the deceivingly nonspecific manifestations, JAMA 220:843, 1972.

Westcott JL: Air embolism complicating percutaneous needle biopsy of the lung, Chest 63:108, 1973.

12 / Hypertensive emergencies

Arterial hypertension can be divided into two types: (1) essential (benign) hypertension, in which the course is slow but progressive over a period of 10 to 20 years, and (2) accelerated (malignant) hypertension, which shows marked diastolic hypertension and causes renal necrotizing arteriolitis, uremia, and death in approximately 1 year if untreated. Accelerated hypertension can complicate any type of hypertension, but it is more common in hypertension associated with renal disease, especially chronic glomerulonephritis. It rarely occurs in hypertension associated with a pheochromocytoma or with primary hyperaldosteronism.

In accerated hypertension, the patient has a diastolic blood pressure usually higher than 120 mm Hg and shows advanced funduscopic findings, including retinal exudates, hemorrhages, and often papilledema. In the early stages, renal function tests, including BUN, may be normal. However, renal failure can occur in a period of weeks.

A hypertensive emergency (crisis) is characterized by a sudden rise in diastolic blood pressure to approximately 140 mm Hg or higher, with a corresponding rise in systolic pressure to approximately 250 mm Hg or higher.

Hypertensive emergencies can occur in patients who have either essential or accelerated hypertension and also in patients who have been previously normotensive. A hypertensive crisis in a previously normotensive patient suggests acute glomerulonephritis, a drug reaction to a monamine oxidase (MAO) inhibitor, pheochromocytoma, or toxemia of pregnancy. When the patient has had chronic hypertension, the most likely cause of the hypertensive crisis is chronic glomerulonephritis, pyelonephritis, or collagen vascular disease. Renovascular hypertension and pheochromocytoma may be present with either acute or chronic hypertension.

The following types of hypertensive emergencies can be described.

1. Hypertensive encephalopathy
2. Hypertensive emergencies due to the sudden release of catecholamines
3. Hypertensive emergencies associated with intracranial (intracerebral or subarachnoid) hemorrhage
4. Hypertensive emergencies associated with acute pulmonary edema
5. Hypertensive emergencies associated with renal disease (usually acute glomerulonephritis)
6. Acute dissecting aneurysm of the aorta (Chapter 13)
7. Eclampsia and preeclampsia (treatment of these conditions is outside the scope of this book)

GENERAL PRINCIPLES OF TREATING HYPERTENSIVE EMERGENCIES

The goal of treatment is to reduce the systolic (and diastolic) blood pressures as quickly and as safely as possible. The actual level to which the blood pressure should be lowered depends on the clinical situation.

If the patient has an acute dissecting aneurysm of the aorta or a pheochromocytoma with acute hypertension, or has been taking an MAO inhibitor and has developed a hypertensive crisis, the *systolic* blood pressure can be lowered to 110 to 120 mm Hg. Similarly, if renal function is normal and if there is no history of cerebral or coronary artery disease, the blood pressure can be lowered to normal.

However, if the patient has coronary or cerebral disease or has had a recent cerebral thrombosis (especially within 6 weeks), it may be dangerous to lower the blood pressure to normal because increased coronary insufficiency or cerebrovascular insufficiency may develop. In such patients, a safe blood pressure level is 160 to 180 mm Hg systolic, and 100 to 110 mm Hg diastolic.

When renal insufficiency is present, the blood BUN and creatinine levels can be used to determine the safe level to which the blood pressure can be lowered (p. 176).

The rapidity with which the blood pressure is lowered and the hypertensive drug or drugs used also depend on the patient's clinical condition.

If immediate lowering of the blood pressure is needed, the following drugs can be used: *diazoxide (Hyperstat),** for acute hypertensive encephalopathy, hypertensive emergencies associated with intracerebral bleeding, hypertensive emergencies associated with acute or chronic glomerulonephritis, or accelerated hypertension; *trimethaphan (Arfonad),* for acute hypertensive encephalopathy, hypertensive emergencies associated with acute pulmonary edema, hypertensive emergencies associated with intracerebral bleeding or acute dissecting aneurysm of the aorta; *sodium nitroprusside,* for acute hypertensive encephalopathy, hypertensive emergencies associated with acute or chronic glomerulonephritis, hypertensive emergencies associated with intracerebral bleeding, or accelerated hypertension; or *phentolamine (Regitine),* for hypertensive emergencies associated with the sudden release of catecholamines.

*This and other drugs are described in Part three.

If less rapid lowering of the blood pressure is needed—for example, within 1 to 2 hours, as in hypertensive encephalopathy, hypertensive crisis associated with acute glomerulonephritis, intracranial (intracerebral or subarachnoid) hemorrhage—the above drugs can also be used cautiously (to prevent excessive hypotension). In addition, the following drugs can also be used: *pentolinium (Ansolysen),* IM or subcutaneously; *reserpine,* IM; or *methyldopate hydrochloride (Aldomet Ester),* IM (used chiefly for hypertension associated with acute glomerulonephritis).

In the treatment of acute hypertensive emergencies, it is often preferable to use several drugs simultaneously or alternately to lower the blood pressure and maintain it at a low level. For example, reserpine administered IM is an excellent antihypertensive drug, but there is a delay of several hours before it becomes effective. In addition, it may have significant side effects, such as profound somnolence (but the patient can be awakened). Both these disadvantages can be overcome. One way is the concomitant use of pentolinium bitartrate administered IM or subcutaneously. This is effective within 30 to 60 min. Treatment can therefore be started with IM injections of both reserpine and pentolinium bitartrate simultaneously. Then the injections of the two drugs can be repeated either simultaneously or alternately to maintain the blood pressure at a desired level (for example, a diastolic blood pressure of 120 mm Hg). When this is done, smaller doses of each drug may be effective without producing excessive side effects of either drug.

Another combination is IM doses of reserpine with IV doses of trimethaphan (or IV doses of sodium nitroprusside) and with oral doses of guanethidine (Ismelin); or diazoxide can be used in conjunction with a diuretic, such as furosemide (Lasix) or ethacrynic acid (Edecrin).

If there is no immediate danger, as in a patient with accelerated hypertension who does not yet have any of the symptoms or signs of a hypertensive crisis, oral doses of one of the antihypertensive drug combinations mentioned below can be used.

Hypertensive emergencies require the use of antihypertensive drugs parenterally. However, oral administration of antihypertensive medication should be substituted for parenteral medication as soon as possible. Oral doses of antihypertensive drugs should be started before parenteral drug therapy is stopped if the patient requires continued antihypertensive treatment. The following antihypertensive drug combinations can be given orally: a diuretic plus reserpine plus mecamylamine (Inversine); a diuretic plus methyldopa; a diuretic plus guanethidine; a diuretic plus guanethidine plus methyldopa; or a diuretic plus hydralazine.

HYPERTENSIVE ENCEPHALOPATHY

Hypertensive encephalopathy is an acute neurological syndrome associated with an abrupt rise in systolic and diastolic blood pressure. Symptoms range from headache to coma and death. The most frequent cause of hypertensive encephalopathy is acute nephritis, but it may occur with hypertension from almost any cause. However, it rarely is associated with hyperaldosteronism or pheochromocytoma.

Pathophysiology

Severe vasoconstriction with secondary cerebral edema is probably the most important factor in the etiology of hypertensive encephalopathy. If the vasoconstriction continues, multiple cerebral thromboses and petechiae may develop.

Clinical aspects

Headache is the initial symptom. It may begin in the occipital region, but it quickly becomes generalized and may be associated with nausea and vomiting. Following the headache, the patient may show mental confusion, restlessness or somnolence, disorientation, and defective memory. Myoclonic twitching of the muscles, signs of transient hemiparesis with a positive Babinski reflex, hemianopic loss of vision, focal convulsions, and coma may develop.

These symptoms and signs are associated with a rise in *diastolic* blood pressure to 130 mm Hg or higher. The eyegrounds usually show exudates or hemorrhages and sometimes papilledema. Laboratory tests, including the BUN concentration, may be within normal. The pressure of the cerebrospinal fluid may be normal; in other patients it may be markedly elevated, even to 400 mm water, and the protein content may be increased (may exceed 100 mg/100 ml). The EEG will show varying abnormalities, depending on the severity of the symptoms and signs.

Acute hypertensive encephalopathy must be differentiated from several conditions, including subarachnoid hemorrhage, in which signs of meningeal irritation are usually present and the spinal fluid is bloody; and brain tumor, which may produce neurological signs and papilledema suggesting hypertensive encephalopathy. However, marked diastolic hypertension and funduscopic hemorrhages and exudates are not present.

Emergency treatment

Lower the blood pressure to approximately 170 to 190 mm Hg systolic and 105 to 115 mm Hg diastolic, in a period of 1 to 2 hours. The following drugs can be used: diazoxide, pentolinium, trimethaphan, or sodium nitroprusside. Pentolinium, given subcutaneously or IM, can be used simultaneously or concomitantly with IM doses of reserpine (see above). However, remember that reserpine produces somnolence, which may interfere with an assessment of the patient's neurological condition. Trimethaphan or sodium nitroprusside should be administered IV. However, avoid too rapid a reduction of blood pressure.

RELEASE OF CATECHOLAMINES

A hypertensive crisis due to the release of catecholamines can occur in two groups of patients: (1) patients who are taking an MAO inhibitor and (2) patients with pheochromocytoma.

MAO inhibitors

Etiology

MAO inhibitors include furazolidone (Furoxone), isocarboxazid (Marplan), nialamide (Niamid), pargyline (Eutonyl), phenelzine (Nardil), procarbazine (Matulane), and tranylcypromine (Parnate).

An acute release of catecholamines can occur in a patient who is taking an MAO inhibitor when the patient also receives a centrally acting sympathomimetic amine, such as amphetamine and its derivatives, or a peripherally acting sympathomimetic drug, such as ephedrine and its derivatives. Such drugs may be present in anorectal preparations, cold remedies, and hay fever preparations.

It can also occur when the patient eats aged and natural cheese, such as Cheddar, Camembert, and Stilton, or other food, such as pickled herring, Chianti wine, pods of broad beans, and chicken livers, which require the action of brewers' yeast, bacteria, or molds for their preparation or preservation. These foods contain tyramine (or other pressor substances), which produces a rise in blood pressure by releasing norepinephrine at nerve endings. However, cream cheese, processed cheese, and cottage cheese can be eaten because they have a negligible tyramine content.

If IM doses of reserpine or guanethidine are given to a patient who is receiving an MAO inhibitor or if either drug is given for at least 1 week following treatment with an MAO inhibitor, a severe hypertensive crisis may result due to the sudden release of catecholamines.

Clinical aspects

The hypertensive crisis induced by the release of tyramine is characterized by some or all of the following symptoms: occipital headache that may radiate frontally, palpitation, neck stiffness or soreness, nausea or vomiting, sweating (sometimes with fever and sometimes with cold, clammy skin), and photophobia. Either tachycardia or bradycardia may be present and may be associated with constricting chest pain and dilated pupils. Visual disturbances, intracranial bleeding, coma, and death may also occur.

Emergency treatment

When a hypertensive crisis occurs, stop administering the MAO inhibitor and start antihypertensive treatment immediately. Phenotolamine, 5 mg slowly IV, or pentolinium, 3 mg subcutaneously or IM, is very effective. Do *not* use reserpine parenterally to lower the blood pressure of these patients.

Pheochromocytoma

Pheochromocytoma is a tumor of chromaffin tissue. It causes hypertension because it can produce and release a large amount of catecholamines (norepinephrine or epinephrine or both). It is usually found in the adrenal medulla, but it may also occur at other sites, including the organ of Zuckerkandl (at the bifurcation of the aorta) and in abdominal or thoracic sympathetic paraganglia. In most cases it is benign.

Clinical aspects

The clinical signs vary and depend partly on the amount and type of catecholamine released. Norepinephrine produces hypertension. Epinephrine tends to produce both hypertension and hypermetabolism.

In a typical case, the patient, whose blood pressure has been normal, develops a marked rise in systolic pressure, even to 300 mm Hg or more, with usually a proportionate rise in diastolic pressure. There is sudden marked palpitation due to tachycardia; severe pounding headache; pallor, especially of the face; numbness, tingling, and coldness of the feet and hands; sometimes nausea and vomiting; and epigastric pain or a sense of constriction radiating into the precordial region. There is great anxiety and sometimes a feeling of impending doom.

During the attack, acute pulmonary edema may occur, as well as cardiac arrhythmias, such as paroxysmal atrial fibrillation, premature contractions, or AV dissociation. The ECG may show T wave changes of left ventricular strain. Transient hyperglycemia and glycosuria may also develop. The end of an attack is accompanied by profuse sweating.

An attack may last from several minutes to hours and may occur as often as several times a day to once a month or less. During the intervening periods the patient is usually asymptomatic. However, approximately one half of the patients show a fixed hypertension.

Diagnosis

A diagnosis of a pheochromocytoma can be made in several ways.

The urinary excretion of metanephrine and vanillylmandelic acid (VMA), which are metabolites of norepinephrine and epinephrine, are abnormally high in practically all patients with a functioning pheochromocytoma. A false-positive reaction to a VMA test can occur if the patient has had foods (for example, coffee, bananas, and substances such as cakes and ice cream, which contain vanilla) and medications that may cause phenoxy acid excretion in the urine. In addition, if the patient has been treated with an MAO inhibitor, phenoxybenzamine, methyldopa, tetracyclines, amphetamines, or even catecholamine-containing nasal decongestants, high levels of urinary catecholamine metabolites may result. High levels may also occur in patients with severe anxiety, neuroblastoma, or increased intracranial pressure.

IM or IV injection of phentolamine has been used as a diagnostic test for pheochromocytoma. However, false-positive and false-negative reactions can occur.

IV pyelography with laminography will show a suprarenal mass in approximately 20% of patients.

Treatment

A pheochromocytoma should be surgically removed, if possible.

To control or prevent an attack of paroxysmal hypertension prior to surgery, phentolamine hydrochloride can be given orally in a dose of 50 mg (1 tablet) 4 to 6 times a day for 3 days prior to surgery. These doses may need to be doubled when the attacks are severe.

Propranolol (Inderal) can also be given concomitantly in a dose of 30 mg daily. Propranolol must never be given alone to a patient with a pheochromocytoma, because it can cause severe hypertension.

Injections of phentolamine myselate are given during the surgical removal of the pheochromocytoma. To prevent a paroxysmal attack during surgery, 2 to 5 mg can be given IM or IV 1 to 2 hours before surgery. During the operation, 2 to 5 mg phentolamine can be given IV whenever the blood pressure begins to rise.

Postoperatively, hypotension often occurs. This can be prevented by giving the patient blood, plasma, or serum albumin (500 to 1,500 ml in addition to replacement needs) to counteract the reduced blood volume that often occurs after the pheochromocytoma is removed. If necessary, levarterenol (Levophed) can also be given.

INTRACRANIAL (INTRACEREBRAL OR SUBARACHNOID) HEMORRHAGE

The onset of *intracerebral hemorrhage* is usually abrupt, with severe headache, nausea and vomiting, and signs of hemiplegia or hemisensory defects. Many patients lose consciousness within a few minutes when the hemorrhage is large. Many of those who remain conscious eventually become comatose.

The most common initial symptoms of *subarachnoid hemorrhage* is violent headache. It is first localized but soon becomes generalized, due to the spread of blood into the subarachnoid space. The patient may become unconscious soon after the headache starts. If the hemorrhage is not extensive, consciousness returns in a few minutes to a few hours. The patient may later become lethargic or delirious.

The second most common symptom of subarachnoid hemorrhage is stiffness of the neck, also due to meningeal irritation caused by the bleeding. This is often associated with neurologic signs, such as inequality of the pupils, unilateral disturbances of function of the eye muscles, shifting hemiplegia, hemiparesis, hemisensory defects, or hemianopsia, depending on the site of the bleeding. Fever, due to an aseptic meningitis, may appear 1 to 3 days after the subarachnoid hemorrhage.

Most patients with intracranial bleeding are hypertensive, even if hypertension had not been present previously, because the increased intracranial pressure resulting from the bleeding may cause acute hypertension.

Diagnosis

The diagnosis of intracranial hemorrhage can be confirmed by examination of the cerebrospinal fluid. Within 1 to 24 hours it shows red blood cells, and when it is centrifuged, the supernatant fluid shows a pink color due to oxyhemoglobin and gives a positive reaction with benzidine. The protein content of the cerebrospinal fluid is characteristically elevated. After 24 hours the fluid shows a characteristic yellow coloration (xanthochromia).

Laboratory tests may show a leukocytosis, transient albuminurea, and glycosuria.

Clinically, it may be impossible to differentiate the conditions that can be asso-

ciated with intracranial hemorrhage. Arteriography should be done if subarachnoid hemorrhage due to a bleeding aneurysm is suspected and if the patient's condition is satisfactory.

Electrocardiogram

A characteristic electrocardiographic pattern consisting of giant T wave inversions, prominent U waves, a prolonged Q-T interval, and a sinus bradycardia has been described in many patients with intracranial (especially subarachnoid) hemorrhage.

Treatment

The elevated blood pressure should be treated with parenteral injections of antihypertensive drugs in the same way as hypertensive encephalopathy is treated (p. 171). However, if an intracerebral hemorrhage is present or if the patient has had a recent cerebral thrombosis and infarction, marked lowering of the blood pressure may further decrease cerebral blood flow and may worsen the neurological condition.

ACUTE PULMONARY EDEMA

Acute pulmonary edema can be associated with high systolic and diastolic blood pressures even if a hypertensive crisis is not present. In such patients, the high blood pressure falls when the pulmonary edema is treated. However, if the funduscopic examination of a patient with acute pulmonary edema shows exudates or hemorrhages, it can be assumed that a hypertensive crisis is also present.

The usual methods of treating acute pulmonary edema, such as having the patient sit with his feet dangling or on the floor, administering morphine sulfate, rotating tourniquets to the extremities, and administering digitalis IV, diuretics IV, and positive pressure oxygen, should be used (Chapter 11). If the blood pressure does not fall in a few minutes, a rapid-acting drug such as trimethaphan or sodium nitroprusside should be given IV. Pentolinium, given subcutaneously or IM, can also be used, but its peak action does not occur for approximately 2 hours.

ACUTE AND CHRONIC GLOMERULONEPHRITIS
Acute glomerulonephritis

Acute glomerulonephritis characteristically follows a group A streptococcal infection of the pharynx, skin, or other area after a latent period of 1 to 4 weeks (usually 10 to 14 days). Headache, malaise, anorexia, edema of the lower extremities, puffy eyes, and occasionally anasarca, oliguria, and hematuria are common findings. Moderate hypertension is often present. In most severe attacks, signs of congestive heart failure, such as dilatation of the heart along with a gallop rhythm, and retinal hemorrhages and papilledema may occur. The urine shows microscopic hematuria and characteristic red blood cell casts and may be obviously bloody or may show a smoky appearance. Proteinuria is present. The specific gravity is normal for the first few days, then tends to become fixed at 1.010. The BUN concentration may remain normal in approximately one half of the patients. However, when the glomerulonephritis is severe, results of the BUN and other kidney function tests, such as the serum creatinine concentration, may be abnormal.

A hypertensive emergency associated with acute glomerulonephritis should be treated with parenteral injections of antihypertensive drugs. The following can be used: diazoxide, given IV; reserpine, given IM; methyldopa hydrochloride; sodium nitroprusside, given IV; or hydralazine (Apresoline) hydrochloride, given IM or IV. Hydralazine increases renal blood flow. However, it also increases the cardiac output and is contraindicated if congestive heart failure or coronary artery disease is present. It also does not always effectively lower blood pressure, even when given parenterally.

Chronic renal disease

The development of accelerated hypertension may indicate the end stage of a chronic glomerulonephritis or chronic pyelonephritis or of other vascular diseases involving the kidneys, rather than the end stage of essential hypertension. Regardless of the pathogenesis of the hypertension, it is important to determine renal function.

A BUN concentration of more than 60 mg/100 ml and an elevated serum creatinine concentration, and particularly a BUN concentration higher than 100 mg/100 ml and a serum creatinine concentration higher than 10 mg/100 ml, are signs that antihypertensive treatment will probably not prolong the patient's life and that it may be dangerous to lower the blood pressure excessively. When the blood pressure falls in such patients, it may be associated with decreased renal blood flow and worsening of the azotemia. However, if a patient with hypertension and chronic renal disease develops acute pulmonary edema, hypertensive encephalopathy, or blurring of vision (due to retinal exudates, hemorrhages, or papilledema), moderate lowering of the blood pressure may be beneficial. The level to which the blood pressure can be safely lowered in these patients varies and depends partly on the BUN concentration (Table 7).

The rules given in Table 7 are not absolute. Some patients may not be able to tolerate even these reductions in blood pressure. Therefore, the BUN concentration must be checked periodically, and administration of antihypertensive drugs must be stopped or the dose reduced if the BUN concentration rises.

Most of the antihypertensive drugs decrease renal blood flow and therefore should be avoided. However, methyldopa increases renal blood flow and can be used. Similarly, reserpine given orally or parenterally is also satisfactory. However, hydralazine must be used cautiously in chronic renal disease.

Table 7. Approximate level to which blood pressure can be lowered*

BUN	Systolic†	Diastolic†
Normal	130-150 mm Hg	80-100 mm Hg
30-60 mg/100 ml	150-170 mm Hg	100-110 mm Hg
60-100 mg/100 ml	180-190 mm Hg	110-120 mm Hg
Over 100 mg/100 ml	Do not lower the blood pressure	Do not lower the blood pressure

*Adapted from Brest AN, Moyer JH: Treatment of the ambulatory patient with diastolic hypertension. In Hypertension, recent advances; Second Hahnemann Symposium on Hypertensive Disease, Philadelphia, 1961, Lea & Febiger.
†With the patient in the standing position.

Diuretics must also be given cautiously. They produce sodium depletion, which is associated with decreased renal blood flow, increased BUN concentration, and worsening of the azotemia.

REFERENCES

Breslin DJ: Hypertensive crisis, Med Clin North Am 53:351, 1969.

Brest AN, Moyer JH: Treatment of the ambulatory patient with diastolic hypertension. In Hypertension, recent advances; Second Hahnemann Symposium on Hypertensive Disease, Philadelphia, 1961, Lea & Febiger.

Earle DP: Glomerulonephritis. In Beeson PB, McDermott W, editors: Cecil-Loeb textbook of medicine, ed 12, Philadelphia, 1967, WB Saunders Co.

Fairbairn JF II: Drug management of hypertensive emergencies. In Brest AN, Moyer JH, editors: Cardiovascular drug therapy; Eleventh Hahnemann Symposium, New York, 1965, Grune & Stratton, Inc.

Finnerty FA: Hypertensive emergencies, Am J Cardiol 17:652, 1966.

Freis ED: Hypertensive crisis, JAMA 208:338, 1969.

Gifford RW Jr: The management of emergencies associated with essential hypertension. In The cyclopedia of medicine; surgery specialties, vol 4, Philadelphia, 1964, FA Davis Co, pp 191-203.

Gifford RW Jr: Management of hypertension complicated by cerebrovascular disease, Drug Therapy, April 1971, p 22.

Hoobler S, Julius S: Questions and answers on hypertension, Med Times 99:92, 1971.

Kirkendall WM: Management of the hypertensive patient with renal insufficiency. In Brest AN, Moyer JH, editors: Hypertension, recent advances; Second Hahnemann Symposium on Hypertensive Disease, Philadelphia, 1961, Lea & Febiger.

McDowell F: The treatment of hypertensive encephalopathy. In Spitzer S, Oaks WW, editors: Emergency medical management; Twenty-First Hahnemann Symposium, New York, 1971, Grune and Stratton, Inc.

Moser M: Treatment of hypertensive encephalopathy (accelerated hypertension), Am Heart J 77: 566, 1969, part 1; 77:704, 1969, part 2.

Palmer R: Extracardiac crises, Emergency Med 4:47, 1972.

Sheps SG: Hypertensive crisis, Postgrad Med, May 1971, p 95.

13 / Acute dissecting aneurysms of the aorta

Myron W. Wheat, Jr.

An acute dissecting aneurysm of the aorta is the most frequent catastrophe involving the aorta, occurs at a rate of about five to ten patients per million per year, and is approximately two to three times more common than the acutely rupturing abdominal aortic aneurysm (Sorensen and Olsen). In addition to being the most common catastrophe that involves the aorta, the acute dissecting aneurysm is also the most lethal. Fig. 13-1 illustrates the extreme lethality of the acute dissecting aneurysm without treatment (Anagnostopoulos and associates). As shown in Fig. 13-1, the mor-

tality is approximately 22% at 6 hours, 28% at 24 hours, and 50% within 48 hours. At the time of 1 week 70% of the patients have died, and at 3 months 90% have died. Of those 8% to 10% of patients who survive 3 months, essentially all of them (80%) will continue to survive for the next 1 to 3 years.

Pathogenesis

Most aortas in which a dissecting aneurysm develops show some type of medial degeneration most commonly described as cystic medial necrosis (Wheat and Palmer,

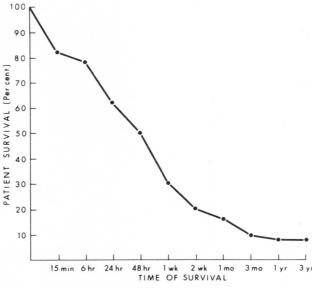

Fig. 13-1. Length of survival of 963 patients with acute dissecting aneurysms that were not treated. (Adapted from Anagnostopoulos CE, Prabhakar MJS, Kittle CF: Am J Cardiol **30:**263, 1972.)

1971). Atherosclerosis and syphilis are not significant factors in the etiology of aortic dissections. The intimal tear, which is the initiating factor in dissecting aneurysms of the aorta, probably is the end result of a number of forces acting upon the ascending aorta and the first portion of the descending thoracic aorta (Wheat and Palmer, 1971).

The heart, averaging over 37 million beats per year, is suspended like the pendulum of a clock by the great vessels of the neck and moves predominantly from side to side. This motion involves primarily the ascending aorta and the first portion of the descending thoracic aorta. As a result of the continuous motion in the first portion of the aorta, the underlying cystic medial necrosis in the aortic wall, plus the force of the blood ejected from the left ventricle, intimal tears occur most commonly in the ascending aorta in approximately two thirds of the cases and in the descending thoracic aorta just distal to the left subclavian artery in about another third of the cases.

As the intimal tear develops, blood at systemic arterial pressure levels is immediately directed into the underlying degenerated medial layer, producing an acute dissecting hematoma (Fig. 13-2). The dis-

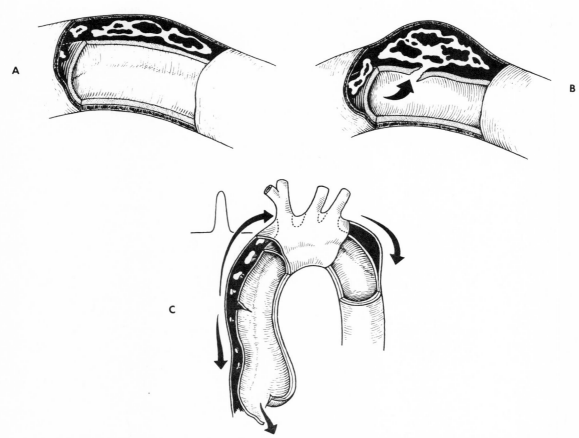

Fig. 13-2. Diagrammatic representation of pathogenesis of dissecting aneurysms. **A,** Cystic medial necrosis in aortic wall sets the stage. **B,** Combined forces acting on aortic bloodstream into diseased media. **C,** Resulting dissecting hematoma is propagated in both directions by pulse wave produced by each myocardial contraction.

secting hematoma, or dissecting aneurysm, is then propagated for varying distances throughout the aorta, the rapidity and extent of the dissection being directly related to the steepness of the pulse wave, or dp/dt_{max}, and the extent of the medial necrosis in the aortic wall (Fig. 13-2, *C*). The propagation of the dissecting hematoma is the process that leads to death in 90% to 95% of untreated patients with rupture into a pleural cavity—usually left—or the pericardium, with lethal tamponade, in most instances.

Clinical picture and diagnosis

Prompt diagnosis of the patient with an acute dissecting aneurysm is particularly important today because of the excellent methods now available for definitive diagnosis and treatment (Wheat and Palmer, 1971; Wheat, 1973).

Acute dissecting aneurysms of the aorta occur two to three times more commonly in men and are more common in black patients. Approximately 90% of the patients will either be hypertensive when seen in the emergency room or will have a history of hypertension in the past. A fairly common patient with an acute dissecting aneurysm would be a black man, aged 60 years, with known hypertension.

The diagnosis of acute dissecting aneurysm of the aorta should be considered in any patient who has severe back pain or anterior chest or epigastric pain. The diagnosis should also be considered in the patient who has possibly had a stroke, has an abrupt onset of a pulseless extremity, or has acute aortic valve insufficiency without previously known heart disease.

The patient frequently will be a middle-aged man with known hypertension who suddenly experiences excruciating pain. When the dissecting aneurysm occurs in younger individuals, it is usually in association with Marfan's syndrome, congenital heart disease such as aortic valve stenosis or coarctation, or a woman who is pregnant.

The onset of the pain is frequently catastrophic and is the most intense pain that the patient has ever experienced. The pain may be described as sharp, tearing, and knifelike or ripping in nature, and it is usually difficult or impossible to relieve the pain completely with opiates. A sudden pain that is very severe, subsides, and then suddenly recurs may be very ominous, indicating the impending lethal rupture of the dissecting hematoma either into the pleural cavity or the pericardium, with lethal pericardial tamponade.

The pain accompanying dissecting aneurysm has been described as originating in the chest and then spreading down the back into the abdomen or lower extremities. Such a pattern would be suggestive of the condition, but it occurs in such a characteristic fashion only rarely. The pain does not commonly radiate into the shoulders, arms, or neck as is typical of angina pectoris. The pain can occur primarily in the abdomen and involve either the back or the upper gastric region. When the pain is primarily abdominal, acute intra-abdominal problems must be differentiated from the diagnosis of dissecting aneurysm. Nausea and vomiting are unusual, as are bloody stools.

Precordial systolic murmurs are common, and the diastolic murmur of aortic valve insufficiency may be present. Murmurs may be present over major branches of the aorta, such as the carotid, the subclavian, and the femoral arteries. There may be a significant difference in blood pressure between the two upper extremities, indicating partial compression of one or both subclavian arteries by the dissecting hematoma. All areas where superficial pulses can be palpated or auscultated should be examined carefully, such as the radial pulses, the brachial pulses, the sounds over the sternoclavicular joints, the suprasternal notch, the cervical regions, the back, the abdomen just above the aortic bifurcation, and the common femoral arteries. The sudden onset of pain, with the loss of pulses or blood flow to one or both lower extremities, should always trigger the tentative diagnosis of acute dissecting aneurysm.

Signs and symptoms pointing toward central nervous system involvement can be confusing because patients with acute dissecting aneurysms can appear with a stroke-like picture with hemiplegia or paraplegia. The central nervous system symptoms and signs may be related to partial or complete occlusion of one or both carotid arteries or to the shearing off or compromise of the intercostal branches of the descending thoracic aorta. The patients may have paresthesias, paraplegia, hemiplegia, or monoplegia. Neurological signs and symptoms, as well as the blood flow to one or several extremities, may come and go as the pressure in the dissecting hematoma is increased or decreased. The occurrence of severe pain in the chest, suggestive of coronary artery occlusion, may point toward a dissecting aneurysm with the additional onset of neurological findings, since the neurological signs and symptoms are uncommon with a primary coronary artery occlusion.

The patient with an acute dissecting aneurysm is usually in acute distress and may have the appearance of a patient in shock, with pallor, sweating, and peripheral cyanosis. Even though the patient may appear to be in shock, his blood pressure usually is in the hypertensive range, and he may even have marked hypertension, with the systolic blood pressure in excess of 200 mm Hg. Occasionally, patients in frank shock with a low blood pressure will demonstrate a rapid hypertensive response to the transfusion of only one to two units of blood.

Once the diagnosis of dissecting aneurysm is suspected, the patient should be placed in an intensive care unit and be carefully monitored. Cardiologists should be consulted, since the most common problem in differential diagnosis is to distinguish a dissecting aneurysm from acute myocardial infarction. If the diagnosis of acute myocardial infarction seems unlikely (electrocardiographic findings plus clinical picture) and the patient is hypertensive, it is usually wise to institute drug therapy to lower the blood pressure, control pain, and stabilize the patient's condition while confirming the diagnosis.

Laboratory findings

When the patient is admitted to the hospital, the laboratory findings are usually within normal limits unless the patient is actively bleeding, in which case the red blood cell count may be low. As time passes, the hematocrit tends to fall, probably as the result of sequestration of blood in the dissecting hematoma. There is usually a mild to moderate elevation of the white blood cell count to between 12,000 and 20,000.

Electrocardiogram

The electrocardiogram is helpful in that it usually shows no signs suggestive of myocardial infarction or of coronary insufficiency (subendocardial ischemia). There are usually signs of left ventricular hypertrophy (or left ventricular strain) related to the frequent association of hypertension.

Roentgenographic findings

The roentgenographic findings are the most important in confirming the diagnosis of dissecting aneurysm. A roentgenogram of the chest should be taken as soon as possible after admission because in most instances there will be widening of the mediastinal shadow. Obviously, it is very helpful to obtain previous chest roentgenograms for comparison because if recent significant widening of the mediastinum can be documented, the diagnosis has a much higher degree of certainty. However, lack of mediastinal widening does not rule out the diagnosis of dissecting aneurysm, since this sign can be absent in 40% to 50% of the cases. Classically, the mediastinum

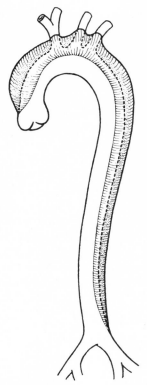

Fig. 13-3. Diagrammatic representation of usual path of dissecting hematoma (cross-hatched area) originating from an intimal tear in ascending aorta.

will bulge to the right with dissection of the ascending aorta and show widening on the left with involvement of the descending thoracic aorta.

When the dissection begins in the ascending aorta, it is usually to the right and posterior just above the level of the left coronary artery ostium (Fig. 13-3). As the hematoma advances into the arch, it passes posteriorly and superiorly. In the descending thoracic aorta and abdominal aorta, the dissection is most commonly posterior and to the left, resulting in a higher incidence of dissection into the left renal and left iliofemoral arteries than into the right.

Mediastinal widening is a highly suggestive but nondiagnostic sign of aortic dissection. Neoplastic or inflammatory processes involving the mediastinum can produce similar widening. Intramediastinal bleeding from a leaking saccular aneurysm of the thoracic or upper abdominal aorta can produce subadventitial dissecting hematomas. These hematomas, which do not involve the media of the aortic wall and therefore are not true dissecting aneurysms, can produce a false-positive diagnosis, even after arteriography. Calcium in the wall (intima) of the aorta, with obvious widening of the aortic shadow beyond the calcium of at least 4 to 5 mm, is highly suggestive but not conclusively diagnostic.

The chest roentgenograms can show pleural effusions, most commonly on the left, which are usually serous. A bloody pleural effusion does not necessarily mean that there is rupture or impending rupture of the aneurysm. The adventitia can weep red blood cells from the dissecting hematoma, producing a serosanguineous pleural effusion without actual rupture of the wall of the aorta. However, frankly bloody pleural fluid obviously means a leaking aneurysm.

The roentgenographic manifestations of dissecting aneurysm of the aorta on conventional films are: (1) a change in configuration of the mediastinum-thoracic aorta on successive films, (2) aortic wall thickening indicated by width of aortic shadow beyond intimal calcification, (3) localized hump on the aortic arch, and (4) mediastinal widening plus a pleural effusion. Since conventional chest roentgenograms are not diagnostic, aortograms should be performed promptly (ideally within 2 to 4 hours after the patient's admission) to either confirm or rule out the diagnosis. When the aortogram is made, the aorta should be visualized from just above the aortic valve to the abdominal aortic bifurcation (Wheat and Palmer, 1971). This complete visualization is necessary to delineate, if possible, the site of the intimal tear (most commonly ascending aorta), the status of the aortic valve, and the extent of

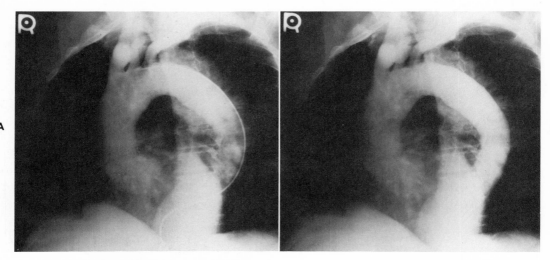

Fig. 13-4. A, Aortogram, left anterior oblique projection, in a patient with a dissecting aneurysm with intimal tear just distal to left subclavian artery. Catheter is against outer wall of the aorta; hematoma does not opacify with dye injection. **B,** Aortogram, left anterior oblique projection, illustrates compression of lumen of ascending aorta and 4+ aortic valve insufficiency.

Table 8. Drugs used in treating dissecting aneurysms of the aorta

Drug	Mechanism of action	Total effect
Reserpine	Depletes all catecholamines from all tissue stores; neurotransmitter (norepinephrine) release diminished after nerve stimulation	Decreases myocardial contractility; sedation, depression, bradycardia (reduces cardiac output); reduces peripheral resistance; stimulates gastric secretion
Trimethaphan (Arfonad)	Ganglionic blockade; direct relaxing effect on vascular smooth muscle; histamine release	Decreases myocardial contractility; lowers peripheral resistance; produces ileus, bladder distention, pupil dilatation
Guanethidine (Ismelin)	Selectively depletes catecholamines from postganglionic nerve terminals, particularly in the heart, gastrointestinal tract, blood vessels, but not central nervous system	Postural hypotension, diarrhea, bradycardia (reduces cardiac output); decreases peripheral resistance; no effect on central nervous system
Propranolol (Inderal)	Specifically blocks beta adrenergic stimulation at end-organ receptor (blood vessels, heart)	Bradycardia (reduces cardiac output); increases peripheral resistance; mild sedation; little hypotensive effect
Alpha-methyldopa (Aldomet)	Metabolized to alpha-methylnorepinephrine, a weak neurotransmitter and pressor agent, which replaces the more potent norepinephrine at nerve terminal; other unknown mechanisms	Sedation, little depression; reduces peripheral resistance; slight bradycardia
Thiazides (Diuril, Hydrodiuril)	Decreased tubular reabsorption of Cl^- and Na^+; some K^+ is lost; results in salt and/or extracellular fluid volume depletion, with possibly a direct cardiovascular effect	Decrease in blood pressure

the dissection, including the degree of involvement of major branches of the aorta, particularly of the carotid and renal arteries.

The definitive diagnosis of dissecting aneurysm requires that the aortogram show either the intimal tear and a false channel or some compression of the true aortic lumen by the dissecting hematoma (Fig. 13-4).

The aortographic findings in patients with dissecting aneurysms are:

1. Splitting of the contrast column
2. Distortion of the contrast column
3. Altered flow patterns in the aorta
   a. Failure of major vessels to fill (If there is renal calyceal filling without demonstration of blood flow to the kidney, or lack of filling of either renal artery in the absence of anuria, dissecting aneurysm is a strong possibility.)
   b. Flow reversal or stasis
4. Aortic valve insufficiency

After the diagnosis of acute dissecting aneurysm of the aorta is confirmed by definitive, competent aortography that delineates the site of the intimal tear and the extent of the dissecting hematoma, a rational approach to the use of the best treatment modalities available can be made.

Treatment

Intensive drug therapy refers to the use of drugs (Table 8) to decrease the cardiac impulse (dp/dt_{max}) and lower the systolic blood pressure as a method of treatment in the patient with an acute dissecting aneurysm (Wheat and Palmer, 1971). *Surgical therapy* refers to definitive surgery for the main dissecting process or its complications. Today, surgical therapy involves: (1) resection and graft replacement rather than fenestration procedures, (2) occasional repair and end-to-end anastomosis of the aorta, (3) resuspension or replacement of an insufficient aortic valve, and (4) local procedures to restore flow in major branches of the aorta (Wheat and Palmer, 1971; Wheat, 1973). The choice and use of the two main modes of therapy also must take into account the facilities and surgical expertise available.

*Treatment in a community hospital**

In this setting, the following treatment should be given as soon as the presumptive diagnosis of an acute dissecting aneurysm is made or suspected.

1. If the patient is hypertensive and in pain, institute appropriate drug therapy to reduce the blood pressure and control the pain. As soon as the patient's condition is stable and the pain relieved, usually within 1 to 2 hours, move him (along with any chest roentgenograms available) at once by ambulance to the nearest medical center where definitive angiographic and cardiovascular surgical expertise are available.

2. If the patient is not hypertensive but is in pain, institute drug therapy to decrease the blood pressure and cardiac impulse to the level necessary to relieve the pain, and carry out the transfer.

3. If the patient is not hypertensive and is also not in pain, then give either reserpine or propranolol or both IM, and transfer the patient immediately.

Treatment in a medical center†

Patients suspected of having acute dissecting aneurysms of the aorta should be placed in an intensive care unit, where they can be monitored carefully on a minute-to-minute basis. Other cardiovascular catastrophies, such as acute myocardial infarction or cerebrovascular hemorrhage, must be ruled out by appropriate studies and consultations.

It is mandatory that these patients be managed and followed on a cardiovascular surgical service. The surgeon must make

---

*Without 24-hour expertise available for definitive aortography and without an experienced cardiovascular surgical team available 24 hours a day (Wheat and Palmer, 1968).

†Definitive angiographic expertise and cardiovascular surgical expertise available 24 hours a day.

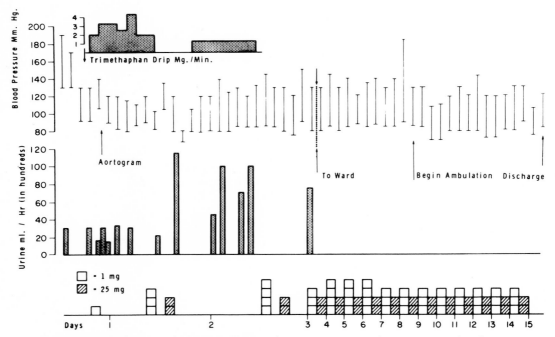

Fig. 13-5. Clinical course of patient with acute dissecting aneurysm of aorta managed with intensive drug therapy. Trimethaphan drip began soon after admission (arrow), with prompt blood pressure response. Open square, 1 mg reserpine; shaded square, 25 mg guanethidine.

the decision as to which type of therapy or combinations of therapy should be used. Probably all patients should be treated with drugs initially; but certain patients will need to be taken to surgery rather promptly, and the surgeon is the only one who can make the decision as to when it is appropriate to supplement drug therapy with definitive surgical intervention.

In the intensive care unit:

1. Monitor ECG, blood pressure, and central venous pressure, and insert Foley catheter to follow urinary output.

2. Reduce systolic blood pressure to 100 to 120 mm Hg (if appropriate). Give trimethaphan (Arfonad) (Fig. 13-5), 1 to 2 mg/ml as IV drip during the acute phase, and if necessary continue for 24 to 48 hours, with a flow rate to maintain the desired blood pressure. Keep the head of the bed elevated 30° to 45° to gain orthostatic effect of drugs.

3. Administer reserpine, 1 to 2 mg IM every 4 to 6 hours, or propranolol (Inderal), 1 mg IM every 4 to 6 hours. These drugs can be used in combination. For example, a small dose of reserpine, 0.25 mg twice daily, in combination with propranolol, 20 mg four times daily, can be given, with good control of hypertension and cardiac impulse but without the central nervous system side effects frequently seen with administration of larger doses of reserpine.

4. Give guanethidine (Ismelin), 25 to 50 mg twice daily by mouth. Continue to monitor ECG, blood pressure, pulses, and urine output. Examine stools for blood.

5. Take daily chest roentgenograms to check for progressive mediastinal widening and pleural fluid.

The management of a typical patient is outlined in chart form in Fig. 13-5. Usually the blood pressure response to trimeth-

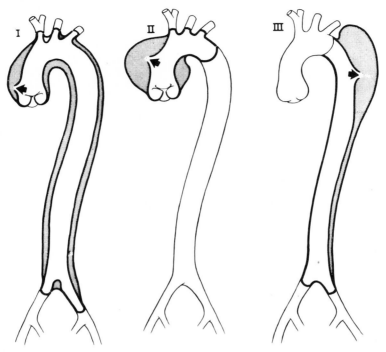

Fig. 13-6. Classification of dissecting aneurysms of the aorta, modified after DeBakey. Type I, dissecting hematoma involves ascending aorta and aortic arch and extends distally for varying distances. Type II, dissecting hematoma limited to ascending aorta. Type III, dissecting hematoma originates at or distal to left subclavian artery and extends distally for varying distances but does not involve aorta proximal to left subclavian artery.

aphan is rapid and can be profound if not carefully regulated. Renal complications usually can be eliminated by careful monitoring of the patient. As a rule, when the blood pressure is lowered, the chest or back pain or both are dramatically relieved.

Once the patient's blood pressure and pain are brought under control, indicating arrest of progress of the dissecting hematoma, and his condition stabilized, the diagnosis should be confirmed or ruled out by aortography (Anagnostopoulos and associates). If the aortogram does not clearly delineate the site of the intimal tear—the origin of the dissection—drug therapy should be continued.

If the site of the intimal tear is clearly identified, the type of dissecting aneurysm found will determine treatment.

Types I and II (Fig. 13-6). The intimal tear is in the ascending aorta or transverse arch, with the ascending aorta involved by dissecting hematoma. The key here is *involvement of the ascending aorta* by a dissecting hematoma with the threat of retrograde dissection and lethal pericardial tamponade (Wheat and Palmer, 1971; Wheat, 1973). There is good evidence from a number of centers that today this type of aneurysm, acute as well as chronic, can be corrected surgically, with a mortality of 12% to 25% (Wheat and Palmer, 1971; Wheat, 1973). Therefore, the patient with an acute type I or II dissecting aneurysm, who is otherwise a good surgical risk, should be taken to the operating room, and the appropriate corrective surgery should be performed as soon as the patient's condition can be stabilized with drug therapy and as soon as the diagnosis has been confirmed.

Type III. The intimal tear and dissecting hematoma are distal to the left subclavian artery. This type also includes dissections originating in the transverse aortic arch without involvement of the ascending aorta. All patients with dissecting aneurysms originating in the descending thoracic aorta should initially be given drug therapy. If the patient's condition stabilizes, if the patient is not in pain, and if there is no evidence of progress of the dissection, drug therapy should be continued into the chronic, long-term phase.

Surgery of the type III aneurysm is indicated as follows.

1. Progress of the dissecting process as shown by
   a. Significant increase in size of the dissecting hematoma while patient is receiving maximal intensive drug therapy
   b. Appearance of or changing murmurs over arterial branches of the aorta or the aortic valve area
   c. Signs of compromise or occlusion of a major branch of the aorta—deepening coma, stroke, painful cool extremity, marked decrease in or cessation of urinary output
2. Impending rupture of the dissecting hematoma as evidenced by
   a. Acute saccular aneurysm by angiocardiography
   b. Significant increase in size of the aneurysm within hours
   c. Blood in the pleural space or pericardium
   d. Lack of ability to control pain with intensive drug therapy
3. Inability to bring blood pressure or pain or both under control within 4 hours with intensive drug therapy

Summary of treatment
Indications for intensive drug therapy

1. Drug therapy is initial treatment of choice in all acute dissecting aneurysms
2. Site of intimal tear cannot be identified on aortogram
3. Site of origin in transverse arch of aorta without extension of dissecting hematoma into ascending aorta
4. Patients who are poor surgical risks in general

5. Stable chronic aneurysm, onset more than 14 days earlier
6. Community hospital that lacks facilities for definitive aortography and experienced cardiovascular surgical team
7. Failure of opacification of false channel
8. Type III aneurysm—intimal tear distal to left subclavian artery

Indications for definitive surgical therapy

1. Types I and II aneurysm—tear in ascending aorta or ascending aorta involved by dissecting hematoma
2. Aortic valve insufficiency secondary to dissecting aneurysm
3. Localized or impending rupture
4. Progress of dissecting hematoma
5. Compromise or occlusion of a major branch of aorta
6. Acute saccular aneurysm
7. Blood in pleural space or pericardium or both
8. Inability to relieve and control pain
9. Inability to bring blood pressure and cardiac impulse under control within 4 hours

Follow-up of acute phase

Drug therapy should be continued in those patients with dissecting aneurysms who have undergone definitive surgical correction. The basic underlying pathological process, cystic medial necrosis, is still present, and these patients are prone to have either a redissection or sustain a second dissection of the aorta. Therefore, the management and follow-up after the acute phase is the same whether drugs alone or drugs plus surgery have been used.

As the patient's clinical status stabilizes and administration of trimethaphan, if used, is discontinued, the patient can be transferred to routine floor care, where progressive ambulation and final regulation of drugs take place (Fig. 13-6). Orthostatic hypotension is frequently observed, particularly in patients taking guanethidine, and the drug dosage must be regulated to maintain the desired hemodynamic effects while permitting relatively normal activity. I prefer to discharge these patients with a systolic blood pressure no higher than 130 mm Hg (supine) and a minimal oral dosage of 0.5 mg reserpine or 60 mg propranolol per day.

During hospitalization the patients receiving reserpine are fed a bland ulcer diet with antacids between meals because of the gastric hypersecretion induced by reserpine. As the amount of reserpine is reduced to maintenance levels, the diet is liberalized, and most patients continue eating a regular bland diet.

Follow-up after discharge from hospital

Follow-up care consists of a first visit to the physician at 1 month and then visits at 3-month intervals. At each visit the patients are checked for pain, presence of peripheral pulses and murmurs, level of blood pressure, murmurs in the aortic valve area, particularly those of aortic valve insufficiency, prosthesis sounds if the aortic valve has been replaced, and the status of the chest roentgenograms. The chest roentgenograms are important for continued evaluation of the size of the aneurysm or the area of graft insertion or both or of aortic anastomosis.

Localized saccular aneurysms can develop in as many as 15% of patients with type III aneurysms in the chronic follow-up phase. When saccular aneurysms are suspected, they should be documented by aortograms and replaced with a prosthesis promptly.

It is worthwhile, if circumstances permit, to teach a member of the family to check and record the patient's blood pressure daily. The blood pressure check should be performed at the same time each day, with the patient supine and then standing. A daily record available for review at each clinic visit is helpful for continuous regulation of the blood pressure. I do not know of a single instance of a dissecting aneurysm followed continuously in this manner that has ruptured abruptly. In my experience, with one possible exception impending trouble in the follow-up period has always been evident, on the basis of (1)

signs and symptoms of progressive aortic valve insufficiency, (2) chest pain, or (3) visible enlargement of a saccular area of the aneurysm by chest roentgenogram. These indications have allowed sufficient time for appropriate elective surgical therapy.

Prognosis

In a series of patients with acute dissecting aneurysms of the aorta, unselected and treated with drug therapy alone, one should anticipate the development of localized saccular aneurysms in about 15% and progressive aortic valve insufficiency ultimately requiring aortic valve replacement in about 10% following discharge from the hospital. Those patients whose dissecting hematoma does not opacify at the time of initial aortography and who are (or should be) treated with drugs alone can be expected to do well without the development of saccular aneurysms (Wheat and Palmer, 1968).

In those patients with aneurysms involving the ascending aorta (types I and II) whose ascending aorta is either reanastomosed or replaced without aortic valve replacement, the results for 3 to 5 years appear to be good.

REFERENCES

Anagnostopoulos CE, Prabhakar MJS, Kittle CF: Aortic dissections and dissecting aneurysms, Am J Cardiol **30**:263, 1972.

Cooley DA, Bloodwell RD, Hallman GL, Jacobey JA: Aneurysms of the ascending aorta complicated by aortic valve incompetence; surgical treatment, J Cardiovasc Surg **8**:1, 1967.

DeBakey ME, Henly WS, Cooley DA, Morris GC Jr, Crawford ES, Beall AC Jr: Surgical management of dissecting aneurysms of the aorta, J Thorac Cardiovasc Surg **49**:130, 1965.

McFarland J, Willerson JT, Dinsmore RE, Austen WG, Buckley MJ, Sanders CA, DeSanctis RW: The medical treatment of dissecting aortic aneurysms, N Engl J Med **286**:115, 1972.

Najafi H, Dye WS, Javid H, Hunter JA, Goldin WS, Julian OC: Acute aortic regurgitation secondary to aortic resection, Ann Thorac Surg **14**:474, 1972.

Sorensen HR, Olsen H: Ruptured and dissecting aneurysms of the aorta; incidence and prospects of surgery, Acta Chir Scand **128:**644, 1964.

Webb WR, Ecker RR, Holland RH, Sugg WL: Aortic aneurysm with aortic insufficiency; repair without prosthesis, Am J Cardiol **26:**416, 1970.

Wheat MW Jr: Treatment of dissecting aneurysms of the aorta; current status, Prog Cardiovas Dis **16:**87, 1973.

Wheat MW Jr, Boruchow IB, Ramsey HW: Surgical treatment of aneurysms of the aortic root, Ann Thorac Surg **12:**593, 1971.

Wheat MW Jr, Harris PD, Malm JR, Kaiser G, Bowman FO Jr, Palmer RF: Acute dissecting aneurysms of the aorta, J Thorac Cardiovasc Surg **58:**344, 1969.

Wheat MW, Jr, Palmer RF: The management of dissecting aneurysms in the community hospital, Med Times **96:**221, 1968.

Wheat MW Jr, Palmer RF: Dissecting aneurysms of the aorta, Curr Probl Surg, July 1971, p 1.

14 / Acute cardiac tamponade

Acute cardiac tamponade is acute compression of the heart by fluid (usually blood) in the pericardium. When blood or fluid rapidly fills the pericardium, the pericardial sac cannot stretch rapidly enough and the intrapericardial pressure rises greatly. Because of the increased intrapericardial pressure, venous blood is unable to return to the right atrium and the right ventricle, and the central venous pressure rises.

The increased intrapericardial pressure also prevents the heart from expanding adequately during diastole. Therefore, less blood enters the heart, and the stroke volume, the blood pressure, and the cardiac output decrease. The heart rate increases to compensate for these changes. When the intrapericardial pressure reaches a level of approximately 15 cm water, there is a sudden further decrease in stroke volume, blood pressure, and cardiac output, and clinical signs of shock appear. If the intrapericardial pressure is not lowered (by removal of the blood or fluid), the patient will die. A volume of only 200 ml blood or fluid can be lethal.

Clinical aspects

The most common cause of acute cardiac tamponade is intrapericardial hemorrhage. This is usually due to rupture of a myocardial infarct (p. 142), penetrating wound of the heart, rupture of a coronary or aortic aneurysm or of the base of the aorta, perforation of the heart during cardiac catheterization, perforation by a transvenous catheter electrode (when the patient is receiving anticoagulants), rupture of a cardiac contusion, or rupture of the atrium. Less common causes of cardiac tamponade include tuberculosis or neoplasm of the pericardium, or bleeding from scurvy or thrombocytopenia. Rarely, cardiac tamponade occurs from a pericardial exudate, pus, or gas (due to a pressure pneumothorax or a gas-producing infection).

The three fundamental signs of acute cardiac tamponade are:

1. A falling arterial blood pressure. The blood pressure progressively falls until it is no longer measurable. When this occurs, clinical signs of shock, including anxiety, restlessness, pallor, cold moist skin, and finally unconsciousness, occur.

2. A rising venous pressure. The venous pressure may rise to 15 to 20 cm water. This is associated with marked engorgement of the neck veins. (However, the liver is not enlarged in acute tamponade.)

3. A small, quiet heart. The heart sounds are distant and muffled. Cardiac pulsations cannot be observed over the precordium.

In addition, pulsus paradoxus may be present. Abnormal pulsus paradoxus is an exaggeration of the normal inspiratory fall (less than 10 mm Hg) in systolic blood pressure. Kussmaul's sign (inspiratory distention of the neck veins) may also be present.

Differential diagnosis

Acute right-sided congestive heart failure can simulate cardiac tamponade because it can produce an acute enlargement of the cardiac shape with clear lung fields as revealed by x-ray examination. In addition, an increased central venous pressure and a decreased arterial blood pressure can be present. However, congestive heart failure rarely causes significant pulsus paradoxus.

A noncompressive hydropericardium may be associated with congestive heart failure in patients with rheumatic heart disease. Here again, pulsus paradoxus is rare, and auscultation reveals the murmurs of rheumatic heart disease rather than the distant heart sounds of pericardial tamponade.

X-ray examination

When acute cardiac tamponade occurs in the absence of prior pericardial effusion, x-ray examination may reveal normal findings because a pericardial effusion of less than 250 ml (which can be lethal) cannot be recognized on conventional x-ray films.

When acute cardiac tamponade occurs in a patient who has a pericardial effusion, the x-ray film may show a bulging, saclike, or globular cardiac shape, with a very acute angle between the right lower edge of the pericardium and the diaphragm. Although no shape in itself is diagnostic of pericardial effusion, this condition should be suspected if the cardiac shape increases rapidly and is associated with clear lung fields.

A pericardial scan will indicate effusion, but not necessarily tamponade.

Electrocardiogram

Total electrical alternans (of P, QRS, and T waves) is diagnostic of pericardial effusion or tamponade. However, this sign does not always appear.

A characteristic electrocardiographic sign of hemorrhage into the pericardium consists of the sudden development of tall, peaked T waves in the precordial leads. This may occur even if the T waves had previously been downward.

In addition, acute cardiac tamponade

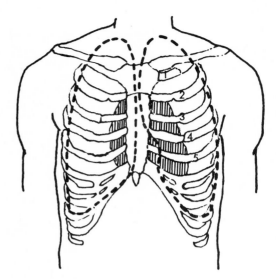

Fig. 14-1. Diagram of the chest showing how pleura (broken lines) does not cover left lower sternal and parasternal area ("triangle of safety" for pericardiocentesis).

due to cardiac rupture may produce sudden bradycardia and electromechanical dissociation (p. 12).

Emergency treatment

Perform a pericardiocentesis as soon as a diagnosis of acute pericardial tamponade has been made. Numerous sites of insertion of the aspirating needle have been used. The left lateral xiphoid site of insertion (between the xiphoid process and the left costal margin) is satisfactory because the pleura does not reach this area (Fig. 14-1) and the left internal mammary artery, which runs along the length of the sternum, lies laterally to the point of needle insertion.

The following equipment is needed.

5-ml and 50-ml syringes
No. 25 ⅝-inch and No. 20 and No. 18 3-inch needles (A 5-inch or 6-inch lumbar puncture needle may be necessary if the subxiphoid approach is used [Cobbs and associates]. Do *not* use a plastic-sheathed needle. A regular needle allows the diffusion of any stray electrical currents through the tissues surrounding the heart. A plastic-sheathed needle con-

centrates such currents at its tip and therefore increases the danger of accidental ventricular fibrillation.)

1% procaine solution
Antiseptic solution
Sterile gloves and towels
Sterile hemostat
Sterile three-way stopcock
Sterile rubber connecting tubing
Sterile length of insulated wire with an alli-
gator clamp on each end
Adequately grounded ECG
Defibrillator

The patient is placed in a comfortable
position, either sitting or supine. No sedatives are given prior to the pericardiocentesis. However, if the patient is apprehensive, diazepam (Valium)* can be given
IM.

The angle between the xiphoid process
and the left costal margin is palpated and
noted. The anterior chest wall is then
painted with the antiseptic solution, and
sterile towels are draped around the puncture site.

The 5-ml syringe is filled with the procaine solution, and a wheal is made at the
puncture site, using the No. 25 needle. The
No. 20 needle is then attached to the syringe and advanced inward and upward at
an angle of 45° to the abdominal wall.
When the needle is advanced approximately 1½ inches, it will reach the parietal
pericardium. (The operator will sense a
"give" as the pericardium is pierced.)

When local anesthesia has taken effect,
the No. 18 needle is attached to the three-
way stopcock and to the 50-ml syringe. The
short length of rubber tubing is attached
to the side arm of the stopcock so that if
blood or fluid is found in the pericardium,
it can be aspirated without disconnecting
the needle.

At the same time, one of the alligator
clamps is attached to the hub of the needle,
and the other alligator clamp is attached
to the V cable of the ECG. The No. 18

needle is advanced along the same tract as
the anesthetic needle. Negative pressure is
created by pulling on the syringe barrel.
Therefore, as soon as the needle enters the
pericardial sac, blood or fluid will enter
the syringe.

The ECG is turned on, and a continuous
V lead is taken while the needle is being
advanced. (The defibrillator is also
charged in case it has to be used.)

The ECG will continue to show the
usual pattern. However, if the needle
touches the epicardium of the heart, an
abnormal RS-T elevation will immediately
appear (Fig. 14-2). If this happens, the
needle should be withdrawn slightly.

When the pericardial sac has been entered, the hemostat is clamped to the
needle just where it penetrates the skin.
This will prevent the needle from advanc-
ing and penetrating the heart.

When the blood or fluid is removed, the
needle can be withdrawn. If there is a
large amount of fluid in the pericardial
sac, it may be convenient to substitute a
flexible catheter for the No. 18 needle.

When pericardiocentesis is done and
bloody pericardial fluid is found, it is important to determine if it is pericardial
fluid or intracardiac blood. If bloody pericardial fluid is present, it will show a lower
hematocrit value than a simultaneously determined venous hematocrit value. Similarly, bloody pericardial effusion fluid will
not clot. However, if the cardiac tamponade is due to rupture of the heart, the
pericardium may contain frank blood. (If
rupture of the heart is suspected, a large
quantity of the bloody fluid should be aspirated as quickly as possible. This will
result in clinical improvement, though
not always immediately.)

If the patient's condition is not critical,
indocyanine green dye can be injected
through the pericardiocentesis needle, and
its passage through the body can be recorded by means of a photoelectric densitometer attached to the pinna of the ear.

---

*This and other drugs are described in Part three.

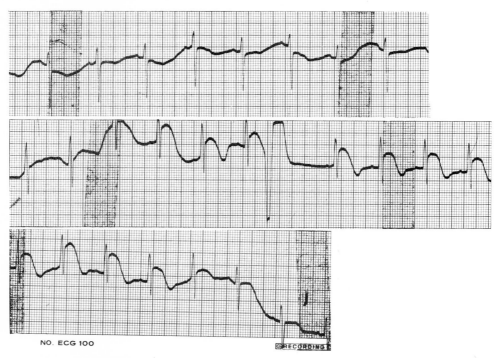

NO. ECG 100   RECORDING

Fig. 14-2. Electrocardiographic monitoring of pericardiocentesis. Upper strip and first two complexes of the middle strip recorded as needle entered pericardial sac. Needle was touching the epicardium as remainder of complexes of second strip were recorded. Notice the RS-T elevations that developed. Artifact in center of second strip occurred when the patient took a deep breath. Lower strip shows disappearance of RS-T elevation when the needle was withdrawn slightly.

If the needle tip is in the pericardium, the densitometer will not show any pickup of dye (Stone and Martin).

If shock persists when the blood or fluid is removed, the patient can be given IV fluids (Chapter 3). Oxygen can be given by nasal catheter. Oxygen under positive pressure must *not* be used, because it will increase the intrapericardial pressure and aggravate the cardiac tamponade.

Even though the venous pressure is high, phlebotomy or diuretics are contraindicated because the high venous pressure is required to counterbalance the high intrapericardial pressure and maintain adequate filling of the heart.

If acute cardiac tamponade reappears, surgical pericardiotomy or pericardiectomy may be necessary.

REFERENCES

Arbeit SR, Parker B, Rubin IL: Controlling the electrocution hazard in the hospital, JAMA **220:** 1581, 1972.

Beck CS: Two cardiac compression triads, JAMA **104:**714, 1935.

Beck CS: Acute and chronic compression of the heart, Am Heart J **14:**515, 1937.

Bishop LH Jr, Estes EH Jr, McIntosh HD: Electrocardiogram as a safeguard in pericardiocentesis, JAMA **162:**264, 1956.

Cobbs BW Jr, Hatcher CR Jr, Robinson PH: Cardiac rupture; three operations with two long-term survivals, JAMA **223:**532, 1973.

Cortes FM, editor: The pericardium and its disorders, Springfield, 1971, Charles C Thomas, Publisher.

Hancock EW: Subacute effusive-constrictive pericarditis, Circulation **43:**183, 1971.

London RE, London SB: The electrocardiographic sign of acute hemopericardium, Circulation **25:** 780, 1962.

Spodick DH: Differential diagnosis af acute pericarditis, Prog Cardiovasc Dis 14:192, 1971.

Stone JR, Martin RH: Bloody pericardial fluid or intracardiac blood? A method for quick and ac-curate differentiation, Ann Intern Med 77:592, 1972.

Usher BW, Popp RL: Electrical alternans; mechanism in pericardial effusion, Am Heart J 83: 459, 1972.

Part two

Apparatus used for cardiac emergencies

15 / Modes of cardiac pacing

Myocardial cells are excitable and can be stimulated by very small electrical currents of approximately 1.2 mA, 2 V, for a duration of 1 to 2 msec (pulse duration). Because small batteries that can duplicate these currents are now available, artificial cardiac pacemakers can be used to stimulate either the ventricles or the atria at any desired rate.

The term *electrical threshold* describes the smallest amount of electrical current, or of voltage, needed to produce consistent cardiac contractions when the pacemaker spike occurs at a time in ventricular diastole when the heart is no longer refractory and when the pulse duration is constant (1 to 2 msec). The electrical threshold varies with the duration of the pulse and also with the type of metal used for the electrodes.

Since 1960, when a totally implanted pacemaker was developed, the pacemaker has become the preferred method for the treatment of symptomatic complete AV block. It has also been used to treat symptomatic bradyarrhythmias from other causes. It can also be used to treat refractory tachyarrhythmias (Chapter 17).

A cardiac pacemaker basically consists of an electrode or electrodes in contact with either the endocardial or epicardial surface of the heart, connected to a pacing unit that contains a *pulse generator* and a battery or batteries. More complicated pacemakers contain an amplifier to magnify currents sensed from the atrium or ventricle.

There are two basic ways (modes) of either temporary or long-term cardiac pacing: fixed rate pacing and demand, or standby, pacing.

FIXED RATE CARDIAC PACING

In the usual form of fixed rate cardiac pacing, an electrode catheter is passed transvenously into the right ventricle.

A fixed rate pacemaker emits an electrical pulse at a fixed rate. The rate of an *external* fixed rate pacemaker can be adjusted by turning a dial on the control panel. Fixed rate pacemakers are also available for implantation for long-term use.

Each stimulus from the pacemaker is recorded on the ECG by a pacemaker spike (artifact), which may show one of two patterns.

1. Sharp, narrow spikes may appear (Fig. 15-1). The spikes may be upward or downward, depending on the leads in which they appear. The amplitude of the spikes also varies, depending on the lead being recorded. However, in any one lead the direction and amplitude of the spikes should be constant.

2. Large biphasic spikes, with a slow return of the deflection to the base line may also appear (Fig. 15-1). These biphasic spikes should not be confused with the RS-T patterns of either pericarditis or myocardial infarction. Also, if acute myocardial infarction occurs in a patient with a pacemaker, the ECG will usually *not* show a characteristic abnormal Q wave and the RS-T deviations, because the pacemaker ECG usually shows a left bundle branch block type of pattern, which masks

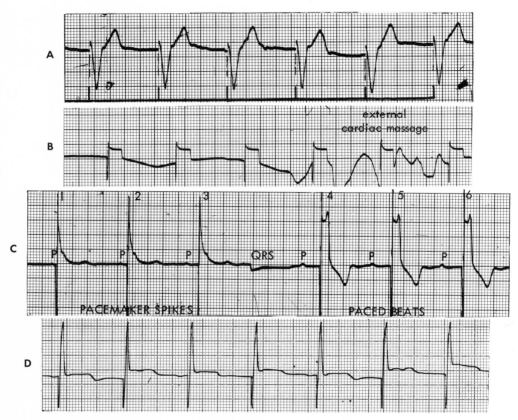

Fig. 15-1. Pacemaker spikes. **A** to **D** from different patients. **A,** Pacemaker functioning at a fixed rate; monitor lead. Each vertical pacemaker spike is followed by a QRS complex and a T wave. It is difficult to determine if P waves (which would indicate atrial activity) are present. **B,** Biphasic pacemaker spikes in a patient with cardiac arrest due to asystole; lead II. Spikes show an elevated end-deflection, suggestive of an RS-T segment. Distortion at the end of the strip is due to external cardiac compression. **C,** Biphasic pacemaker spikes; lead II. Patient had an Adams-Stokes syndrome (complete AV block with periods of ventricular standstill) and was being temporarily paced with an external battery-operated pacemaker. P waves occur regularly, but only one spontaneous QRS complex is present. In beats 1, 2, and 3, pacemaker spikes are present; but because of pacemaker malfunction, they are not followed by QRS complexes and T waves. After spike 3, the milliamperage of the pacemaker was increased. Beats 4, 5, and 6 show the pacemaker spikes followed by paced QRS complexes and T waves. The spikes in this patient also have a biphasic shape and return slowly to the base line. This is suggestive of an RS-T segment but is solely due to the pacemaker. **D,** Biphasic pacemaker spikes recorded in a monitor lead. ECG shows only the pacemaker spikes because the amplitude of the pacemaker spikes was so large that the standardization of the monitor was decreased greatly. As a result, the patient's QRS complexes and T waves were not visible.

myocardial infarction. However, nonspecific changes in the ECG may occur. In such patients, the diagnosis of acute myocardial infarction must be made on the basis of clinical findings and enzyme changes unless the pacemaker can be turned off temporarily.

In addition, when a catheter electrode has been implanted for a long time, it may cause focal injury to the endocardium and T wave changes, which may persist for a long time, even after the catheter electrode has been removed.

When a spike occurs at a time when the heart is not refractory, it will be followed by a QRS and T wave. When a spike occurs when the heart is refractory (approximately from the beginning of the QRS to slightly before the end of the T wave), it will be superimposed on the QRS or T and will not result in an additional heartbeat.

When a fixed rate pacemaker is functioning in a patient with complete AV block and when the pacing rate is set faster than the patient's ventricular rate, the ECG will show regular pacemaker spikes, followed by QRS complexes and T waves. However, P waves or other electrocardiographic signs of atrial activity, such as AV junctional P waves, AV junctional premature beats, atrial flutter, or atrial fibrillation, may also be present. In addition, if ventricular premature contractions or escape beats occur, they will also be recorded on the ECG (see Fig. 17-1).

The patient's own ventricles may begin beating spontaneously while the fixed rate pacemaker is functioning. When this occurs, the ventricular rate will become very irregular. Spontaneous ventricular beats may occur when the heart is not refractory from the pacemaker-induced beats, and pacemaker-induced beats will occur when the heart is not refractory from the spontaneous beats. Because of these characteristics, the term *competitive pacing* is used to describe fixed-rate pacing. This irregular ventricular rate may cause palpitations.

Another complication of fixed rate pacing is the development of the so-called pacemaker syndrome, due to variations in blood pressure because atrial and ventricular systoles are not synchronous. The patient may experience odd sensations.

There is still another danger from fixed rate pacemakers. Theoretically, when the pacemaker spike occurs during the so-called vulnerable period (namely, just before or on the apex or nadir of the T wave), it may cause ventricular premature beats, ventricular tachycardia, or ventricular fibrillation. This is particularly possible when hypoxia, myocardial injury, myocardial infarction, hypokalemia, other electrolyte disturbances, acidosis or alkalosis, or digitalis toxicity is present.

Another problem may develop when a patient with acute myocardial infarction has a fixed rate pacemaker and the tip of the catheter electrode lies against the endocardium of an infarcted area of the heart. The infarcted heart muscle is excessively irritable throughout the entire cardiac cycle, and the repeated pacemaker pulses of the fixed rate pacemaker may irritate the heart and produce ventricular tachycardia or ventricular fibrillation. Therefore, in acute myocardial infarction, a demand type of pacemaker should be used.

Increased vulnerability of the ventricles to ventricular fibrillation can also be produced by the administration of sympathomimetic amines such as isoproterenol (Isuprel). If the patient has been receiving isoproterenol, administration of the drug should be stopped before the pacing starts.

Usually, fixed rate pacing is used to stimulate the right ventricle. However, the right atrium can also be paced, or a catheter electrode can be inserted into the coronary sinus (see below).

Fig. 15-1 shows the effect of a fixed rate pacemaker on the ECG.

Right atrial pacing

Right atrial pacing is usually a form of fixed rate pacing.

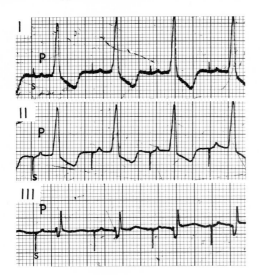

Fig. 15-2. Right atrial pacing. A temporary transvenous catheter electrode had been placed in right atrium. Notice pacemaker spike before each P wave. P waves show normal shapes, indicating that stimulus is spreading through atria in a normal way.

A catheter electrode can be passed into the cavity of the right atrium, placed in contact with the right atrial wall, and connected to a fixed rate pacemaker. Each pacemaker pulse will stimulate the right atrium. The stimulus will spread to the AV junction and into the ventricles if AV conduction is normal (Fig. 15-2).

One of the problems of right atrial pacing is that it is very difficult to keep the tip of the catheter electrode in contact with the endocardium of the right atrium, even when a special catheter electrode with a J-shaped tip is used.

Temporary right atrial pacing has been used to overdrive tachyarrhythmias (Chapter 16). Right atrial pacing is also used for bifocal demand pacing (see below).

Coronary sinus pacing

Coronary sinus pacing is also usually a form of fixed rate pacing.

Occasionally, when transvenous cardiac pacing is done, the tip of the catheter electrode may enter the coronary sinus and

pace from there, instead of pacing from the right ventricular cavity.

Coronary sinus pacing can be recognized in several ways.

1. The pacemaker spikes are usually immediately followed by P waves, QRS complexes, and T waves, rather than by just the QRS and T (Fig. 15-3).

Since the coronary sinus may lie above or below the AV junction, P waves may appear with a so-called left atrial pattern—downward P in leads I and V_6 or with downward P waves in leads II, III, and aV_F (and an upward P in lead aV_R).

2. When x-ray films of the heart are taken in the posteroanterior view, the tip of the catheter electrode in the coronary sinus resembles the posteroanterior view of the tip when it is placed in the apex of the right ventricle. However, in the lateral view, the tip of the catheter electrode in the coronary sinus characteristically lies posteriorly rather than anteriorly (see Figs. 16-9 and 16-10).

When the tip of the catheter electrode is wedged tightly into the coronary sinus, it may actually pass into the cavity of the left ventricle through a venous communication between the coronary sinus and the left ventricular cavity, or it can enter the great cardiac vein and reach the epicardial surface of the left ventricle this way. In either case, the paced QRS complex will show a right bundle branch block pattern (Fig. 15-4) rather than the usual left bundle branch block pattern (Fig. 15-5).

Under fluoroscopic control, it is possible to direct the catheter tip into the coronary sinus deliberately. The entrance of the coronary sinus is located on the posterior wall of the right atrium, just above the inlet of the inferior vena cava. The catheter electrode used for insertion into the coronary sinus should have an angle of approximately 110° in its last 7 cm. The catheter electrode is inserted into the right atrium and is advanced through the tri-

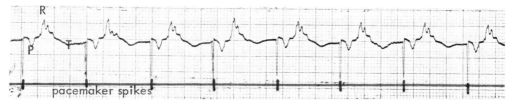

Fig. 15-3. Coronary sinus pacing; monitor lead. Pacemaker spikes are immediately followed by downward P waves, QRS complexes, and T waves. Shape of P waves in monitor leads cannot be used to indicate whether site of stimulus formation is sinus node, coronary sinus, or AV junction.

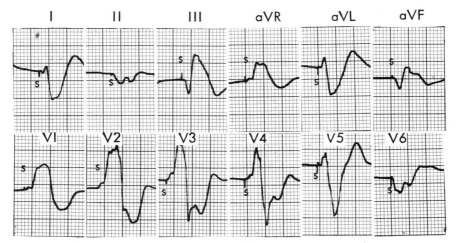

Fig. 15-4. Right bundle branch block pattern in a pacemaker ECG (tall, notched R waves in leads V_1 and V_2). This was produced when tip of catheter electrode was wedged into coronary sinus. Location of catheter electrode tip was confirmed by x-ray examination. A pacemaker spike (s) appears before each QRS complex.

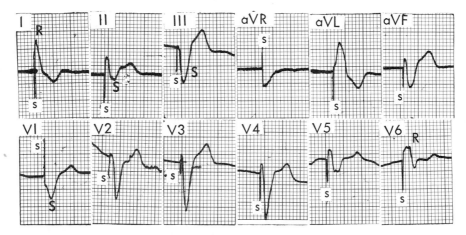

Fig. 15-5. Left bundle branch block pattern produced by transvenous catheter electrode in right ventricular cavity. Standard leads show marked left axis deviation (R_1, S_2, S_3), indicating that tip of catheter electrode is in apex of right ventricle. R, R wave; S, S wave; s, pacemaker spike.

cuspid valve toward the inferior vena cava. It can then be withdrawn slightly and its tip rotated to point in a posterior and medial direction. It then easily enters the coronary sinus. To perform this procedure, Gorlin finds it preferable to place the patient in a left lateral position.

DEMAND, OR STANDBY, CARDIAC PACING

Demand, or standby, cardiac pacing can be accomplished by either a QRS inhibited pacemaker or a QRS synchronous pacemaker. Atrial synchronous pacing and bifocal pacing are specialized forms of demand pacing.

QRS inhibited and QRS synchronous pacing

QRS inhibited pacemakers are also called *R wave inhibited* or *ventricular inhibited* pacemakers.

QRS inhibited pacemakers emit pulses only when the spontaneous ventricular stimuli (which are represented by the R wave, or the QRS complex of the ECG) do not occur. For example, if the pacemaker rate (escape rate) is set at 70 per min, the interval between each pacemaker pulse (when spontaneous ventricular activity is absent) will be 0.86 sec (860 msec).

The QRS inhibited pacemaker does not emit pulses when the patient's heart rate is faster than the escape rate of the pacemaker. This occurs because each time the pacemaker senses an R wave, it blocks the formation of a pacemaker pulse. Therefore, a QRS inhibited pacemaker will show pacemaker spikes only when the spontaneous heart rate is slower than the escape rate of the pacemaker (Fig. 15-6). The spikes appear before each QRS complex.

The QRS inhibited pacemaker also has a *refractory period*—for example, 0.40 sec (400 msec)—which begins when the pacemaker emits a pulse or when it senses an R wave. During this refractory period, the pacemaker can neither stimulate the ventricles nor sense another R wave. However, if spontaneous ventricular beats or

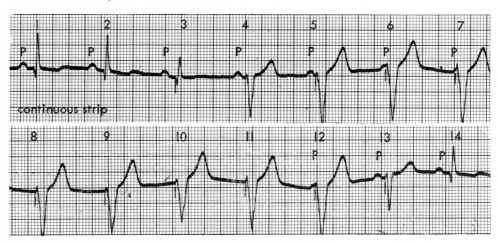

Fig. 15-6. QRS inhibited pacing; lead II. Beats 1 and 2 show regular sinus rhythm. In beat 3, ventricular rate has slowed slightly so that a pacemaker spike appears at approximately same time as regular stimulus spreads through ventricles from AV node. Result is a fusion beat. In beats 4 through 12, pacemaker is functioning because patient's spontaneous heart rate has slowed below escape rate of pacemaker (in this case, 70 per min). Then patient's spontaneous ventricular rate becomes more rapid, so that beat 13 is a fusion beat, and beat 14 again shows regular sinus rhythm. P waves merge into QRS complexes in beats 4 through 7, and then reemerge in beats 12 and 13.

ventricular premature contractions occur during the refractory period of the pacemaker, they will not be inhibited and will appear in the ECG (see Fig. 17-1). The refractory period is followed by an *alert period*, during which the pacemaker can sense an R wave. If it does not sense an R wave at the end of the alert period, it will emit another pulse, for example, 0.86 sec after the last pulse. However, if it senses an R wave during the alert period, it will be recycled into another refractory period and into another alert period.

The escape rate and the refractory period vary with different makes of QRS inhibited pacemakers.

When a QRS inhibited pacemaker is used, the catheter tip not only stimulates the heart muscle, but it also serves as a *sensing* electrode for the patient's R waves. The electrical threshold for the sensing is approximately 2 mV. Therefore, to make certain that the electrode tip is consistently sensing the R waves, the amplitude of the QRS complex of a right ventricular unipolar lead should be at least 6 mV. If this does not occur, the pacemaker will not be inhibited by the R waves and will not be able to function as a demand pacemaker.

The effects of a QRS inhibited pacemaker on the cardiac rhythm are shown in Fig. 15-6.

QRS synchronous pacemakers are also called *QRS blocking, QRS triggered, ventricular blocking, ventricular triggered, R wave blocking,* or *R wave triggered* pacemakers.

A QRS synchronous pacemaker emits electrical pulses at a fixed rate, just as occurs in a fixed rate pacemaker. However, it is also synchronized with the patient's own ventricular activity (which is simultaneous with the QRS complex of the patient's ECG). When the catheter electrode tip senses the spontaneous spread of a stimulus through the patient's right ventricle, it emits a pulse, which is recorded on the ECG as a spike superimposed on the patient's QRS complex (Fig. 15-7). (This spike does not appear in all leads.) However, this pacemaker spike is blocked because the heart is refractory during systole. Therefore, the QRS synchronous pacemaker is in a *standby* state as long as spontaneous ventricular activity is present. When the patient's heart rate slows below the escape rate of the pacemaker, the spikes will appear before each pacemaker QRS complex (Fig. 15-7).

Like the QRS inhibited pacemaker, the QRS synchronous pacemaker also has a long *refractory period* (p. 202). The purpose of the refractory period is to limit

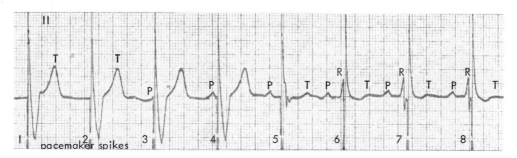

Fig. 15-7. QRS synchronous pacing; lead II. In beats 1 through 4 patient's spontaneous ventricular rate has slowed below escape rate of QRS synchronous pacemaker, which has started to form stimuli at a regular rate of 70 per min. In the meantime, patient's spontaneous heart rate is increasing (notice P waves emerging) so that beats 5 through 8 are spontaneous regular sinus beats with pacemaker spikes occurring within QRS complexes. Notice how shapes of QRS and T of beats 5 through 8 are different from their shapes in beats 1 through 4.

the maximum rate at which the pacemaker will respond to QRS complexes. Otherwise, it could respond to very high ventricular rates. The long refractory period also prevents the pacemaker from sensing and responding to very tall T waves. Therefore, the refractory period is set (preset) between 0.4 and 0.5 sec. This will give a maximum rate of 120 to 150 beats per min. (If the refractory period is 0.4 sec [400 msec], only 2½ pulses can be formed in each sec, 5 pulses in each 2 sec, 150 pulses per min.)

The refractory period is followed by an *alert period,* during which the pacemaker can sense R waves. If the pacemaker does not sense an R wave at the end of the alert period, it will begin to function as a fixed rate pacemaker and will emit another pulse. The interval between these pacemaker pulses is preset by the manufacturer. For example, if it is preset at 0.86 sec, the escape rate of this pacemaker is 70 beats per min. If the QRS synchronous pacemaker senses an R wave during the alert period, it will emit a pulse that will appear as a spike on the R wave, and the refractory period will start again.

Both the QRS inhibited pacemakers and the QRS synchronous pacemakers have the same effects on the peripheral pulse because neither competes with stimuli that arise spontaneously in the heart. For this reason, both these pacemakers are called *demand, standby,* or *noncompetitive pacemakers.* In addition, both these pacemakers allow the paced ventricular rate to vary. However, they ordinarily do not suppress ventricular premature contractions or atrial or ventricular tachycardia. (The treatment of paroxysmal tachyarrhythmias by means of pacemakers is described in Chapter 16.)

When a patient has either a QRS inhibited or QRS synchronous pacemaker and his spontaneous rate is faster than the escape rate of the pacemaker, he will be free from symptoms. If his spontaneous heart rate suddenly slows, the pacemaker will shift to an automatic fixed rate of approximately 70 beats per min. However, the patient may respond to this sudden decrease in heart rate with symptoms of dizziness, faintness, or even momentary unconsciousness *(pacemaker syncope).* This is not serious, but the patient should be told that these symptoms may occur.

The effects of a QRS synchronous pacemaker on the cardiac rhythm are shown in Fig. 15-7.

Atrial synchronous pacing

Atrial synchronous pacing is a form of demand pacing.

In an atrial synchronous pacemaker, the spread of the stimulus through the atria is sensed by an electrode that is in contact with the epicardium of the left atrium. After a delay of 0.12 sec and a latent period of 0.04 sec (which approximates the normal P-R interval of 0.16 sec), the pacemaker emits a pulse that is sent to another electrode in contact with the epicardium of the left ventricle. This is recorded by a sharp spike immediately before the QRS complex (Fig. 15-8). In this way, atrial and ventricular contractions are synchronized and resemble a normally conducted impulse.

If the P-R interval is less than 0.16 sec, the pacemaker spike will occur within or even after the QRS complex, when spontaneous beats are present.

If no signal from the atrial sensor is received within a certain time, usually 1 sec after a previous pulse, another pulse is sent, and the atrial synchronous pacemaker becomes a fixed rate pacemaker at a rate of approximately 60 beats per min (Fig. 15-8, complexes 6, 7, and 8).

The atrial synchronous pacemaker has a long refractory period like the QRS synchronous pacemaker. This prevents it from responding to too rapid atrial stimuli.

Two models of atrial synchronous pacemakers are manufactured. One has a maxi-

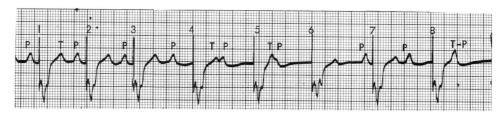

Fig. 15-8. Atrial synchronous pacing; lead II. In beats 1 through 3, sinus P waves are present. These P waves are sensed by left atrial electrode, so that 0.16 sec later (actually 0.18 sec in this patient), pacemaker emits a pulse that stimulates ventricles and produces wide, aberrant QRS complexes followed by T waves. After these three beats, heart rate slows below escape rate of atrial synchronous pacemaker. Therefore, in beats 4 through 8, pacemaker automatically beats at a preset rate of 65 per min. Notice that in these beats there is no constant P-R interval.

mum pacing rate of 125 beats per min. The other, for use in children, has a maximum pacing rate of 150 beats per min.

Rapid spontaneous atrial stimuli will *not* be inhibited by the atrial synchronous pacemaker. These spontaneous atrial beats can pass through the AV node and cause the ventricles to beat rapidly. When this happens, an irregular heart rate occurs, due partly to paced beats and partly to spontaneous beats.

If the heart rate suddenly increases beyond the maximum rate of the atrial pacemaker in a patient with complete AV block, the atrial synchronous pacemaker will become refractory to every other stimulus from the atrium, and the heart rate may suddenly become slow, producing dizziness and other symptoms. This is not serious, but the patient should be told that this may happen. It is very difficult to detect pacemaker failure with an atrial synchronous pacemaker because there are so many clinical conditions that can produce a very irregular ventricular rate when the pacemaker is functioning.

An atrial synchronous pacemaker has to be implanted in a special way. The pulse generator is implanted subcutaneously, like all implanted pacemakers. However, one electrode (the sensing electrode) must be sutured to the base of the left atrial appendage. Two other electrodes (the stimulating electrodes) must be implanted at the base of the left ventricle. This requires open thoracotomy. In spite of the direct contact of the electrodes with the heart, failure of pacing does occur.

The effects of an atrial synchronous pacemaker on the cardiac rhythm are shown in Fig. 15-8.

Bifocal demand pacing

A new type of pacemaker system, called a *bifocal AV sequential demand pacemaker* that stimulates sequential atrial and ventricular systole has recently been developed. This pacemaker unit consists of two pulse generators in a single package: a conventional QRS inhibited pacemaker and a QRS inhibited atrial demand pacemaker. Each has a separate escape rate. In this way, the unit may be dormant, or it may stimulate the atria or both the atria and the ventricles.

Two endocardial catheter electrodes are needed. They are inserted transvenously. One is inserted into the right atrial cavity. It has a special J-shaped end to maintain close contact with the atrial endocardium. The second catheter electrode is inserted into the right ventricular cavity.

The ventricular electrode serves as a sensing device to pick up the QRS complexes. It is also able to stimulate the ventricles when required. The atrial electrode stimulates only the atria. It has no sensing function. Therefore, the signal detected by the ventricular electrode is responsible for both atrial and ventricular pacing.

The atrial and the ventricular pulse generators have different escape intervals. The escape interval of the atrial pulse generator is shorter than that of the ventricular pulse generator. The atrial pulse generator has an escape interval of 0.6 sec, the ventricular pulse generator an escape interval of 0.84 sec. Therefore, the difference of 0.24 sec between these two escape intervals describes the AV sequential interval of the pacemaker.

The pulse generators work in the following way. If a patient has sinus bradycardia and normal AV conduction and the sensing electrode in the right ventricular cavity does not detect a QRS complex within 0.6 sec (600 msec, equivalent to an atrial rate of 100 per min; the atrial escape interval), a pulse is delivered to the atria. Therefore, a stimulus spreads through the atria, through the AV node, and into the ventricles. When this happens, a pacemaker spike will appear immediately before the P wave.

The ventricular escape interval is set at 0.84 sec (840 msec, equivalent to a ventricular rate of 72 per min). Therefore, if the atrial impulse is conducted normally through the AV node in less than 0.24 sec, the ventricular pacemaker is inhibited. However, if first-degree AV block is present and the P-R interval is longer than 0.24 sec, the ventricular pulse generator will stimulate the ventricles 0.24 sec after the atrial pulse. When this happens, a pacemaker spike will also be present before the QRS complex.

Theoretically, bifocal demand pacing should be particularly effective for patients with intermittent AV block. However, experience with this type of pacemaker is still limited.

COMPLICATIONS OF CARDIAC PACING

Cardiac pacing is not always innocuous. There are two types of complications that can occur: complications related to improper functioning of the pacemaker (Chapters 16 and 17) and complications related to the insertion or presence of the pacemaker system in the body. For example, infection may occur at any point in the pacemaker system, with a resultant bacteremia. It most commonly occurs at the skin site of the temporary catheter electrode. Prophylactic antibiotic therapy is usually not helpful.

The complications of percutaneous subclavian vein insertion of the catheter electrode are discussed on p. 212.

When a long-term pacemaker is implanted under the skin, the implanted pacemaker may be mobile in its pocket. This is not serious. However, if the subcutaneous pocket of the pacemaker is so large that the pacemaker can twist, breakage of the electrode wires is possible.

Pacemaker extrusion may occur due to acute or chronic infection and necrosis of the overlying skin. When an implanted pacemaker erodes through the skin, it can be treated in several ways: the area can be kept covered with sterile gauze, even for months, until the pacemaker begins to fail; the pacemaker can be removed and another one implanted, with aseptic technic, on the other side of the body; the infected wound can be irrigated with antibiotics.

Excessive fibrosis of the myocardium at the site of the electrode tip may occur. This may impede or block the spread of the pacemaker pulse to the myocardium.

Other mechanical complications include fracture of the electrode wires and loosening of the connections of the catheter to the pacemaker.

Perforation of the thin right ventricular wall of the myocardium has occurred in as many as 5% of patients with a transvenous pacemaker. It is a serious complication. It usually occurs in the first few weeks after implantation and is more common when a small-caliber electrode (2-mm diameter) is used. If the catheter electrode is inserted when the patient's heart is dilated, perforation may occur when cardiac compensation is restored, and the heart size shrinks.

Signs of perforation of the myocardium by the tip of the catheter electrode include loss of pacing, with recurrence of the patient's symptoms, and stimulation of the adjacent phrenic nerve, with signs of contractions of the diaphragm or contractions of the intercostal or abdominal muscles. (However, stimulation of the diaphragm can occur in the absence of perforation.) A pericardial friction rub may appear. Hemopericardium rarely occurs, unless the patient is receiving anticoagulants. X-ray examination may or may not show the tip of the catheter outside the right ventricle.

Characteristic electrocardiographic signs may appear.

1. A marked change (more than 90°) in the electrical axis of the pacemaker

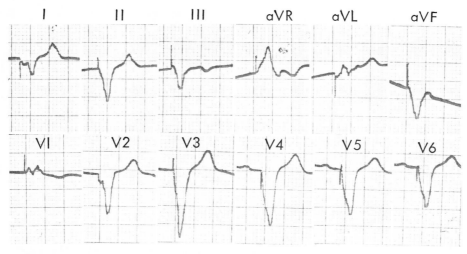

Fig. 15-9. Right bundle branch block (rsR' in lead VI) with unusual left axis deviation in the standard leads. This pattern has been described as a sign of perforation of the right ventricle by the catheter electrode tip. However, it may also occur when the catheter electrode tip remains in the right ventricle.

spike, as measured in the frontal plane. (This is done in the extremity leads in the same way that the electrical axis of the QRS is measured.)

2. A marked change in the QRS complexes of the paced ECG. For example, when the electrode tip is in the right ventricular cavity, the 12-lead ECG usually shows a pattern similar to left bundle branch block (Fig. 15-5), rarely a right bundle branch block type of pattern. After perforation, the electrode tip lies on the free epicardial wall of the heart, and the precordial leads may change and show a right bundle branch block type of pattern (Fig. 15-9). Treatment consists in withdrawing the catheter tip from the pericardial sac and repositioning it in the right ventricular cavity, under fluoroscopy.

REFERENCES

Baird CL Jr, editor: Cardiac pacing, Symposium, Med College of Virginia Quart 7:127, 1971.

Barold SS: Clinical significance of pacemaker refractory periods, Am J Cardiol 28:237, 1971.

Bauman DJ, Lamb KC, Tsagaris TJ: Unusual QRS wave forms associated with permanent pacemakers, Chest 64:480, 1973.

Bilitch M, Cosby RS, Cafferky EA: Ventricular fibrillation and competitive pacing, N Engl J Med 276:598, 1967.

Castellanos A: Technical problems with pacemakers, Letter, N Engl J Med 284:1385, 1971.

Castellanos A Jr, Lemberg L: Electrophysiology of pacing and cardioversion, New York, 1969, Appleton-Century-Crofts.

Castillo CA, Berkovits BV, et al: Bifocal demand pacing, Chest 59:360, 1971.

Center S, Berger RA, Tarjan P: The diagnosis of acute myocardial infarction in patients with permanent pacemakers, Arch Intern Med 127:932, 1971.

Chatterjee K, et al: Electrocardiographic changes subsequent to artificial ventricular depolarization, Br Heart J 31:770, 1969.

Chatterjee K, et al: T-wave changes after artificial pacing, Lancet 1:759, 1969.

Escher DJW: Types of pacemakers and their complications, Circulation 47:1119, 1973.

Furman S, Escher DJW: Principles and techniques of cardiac pacing, New York, 1970, Harper & Row, Publishers.

Furman S, Reicher-Reiss H, Escher DJW: Atrioventricular sequential pacing and pacemakers, Chest 63:783, 1973.

Gorlin R: Coronary blood flow. In Warren JV, editor: Methods in medical research, vol 7, Chicago, 1958, Year Book Medical Publishers, Inc.

Langendorf R, Pick A: Artificial pacing of the human heart; its contribution to the understanding of the arrhythmias, Am J Cardiol **28:** 516, 1971.

Lown B, Kosowsky BD: Artificial cardiac pacemakers, N Engl J Med **283:**907, 1971.

Meltzer LE, Kitchell Jr, editors: Current concepts of cardiac pacing and cardioversion, Philadelphia, 1971, The Charles Press.

Parker DP, Kaplan MA: Demonstration of the supranormal period in the intact human heart as a result of pacemaker failure, Chest **59:**461, 1971.

Parsonnet V: Types of pacemakers, Letter, JAMA **207:**367, 1969.

Rubenfire M, et al: Clinical evaluation of myocardial perforation as a complication of permanent transvenous pacemakers, Chest **63:**185, 1973.

Siddons E, Sowton E: Cardiac pacemakers, Springfield, Ill, 1967, Charles C Thomas, Publisher.

Singer E, Gooch AS, Morse D: Exercise-induced arrhythmias in patients with pacemakers, JAMA **224:**1515, 1973.

Wanatabe Y, Dreifus LS: Newer concepts in the genesis of cardiac arrhythmias, Am Heart J **76:** 114, 1968.

Whalen RE, Starmer CF: Electric shock hazards in clinical cardiology, Mod Concepts Cardiovasc Dis **36:**7, 1967.

Whalen RE, Starmer CF, McIntosh HD: Electrical hazards associated with cardiac pacemaking, Ann NY Acad Sci **111:**922, 1964.

16 / Temporary cardiac pacing

There are two types of cardiac pacing: temporary and long-term. Temporary cardiac pacing can be accomplished in two ways: by temporary external cardiac pacing and by temporary percutaneous or transvenous cardiac pacing.

TEMPORARY EXTERNAL CARDIAC PACING

It has been found that heart muscle can be stimulated when 25 to 150 V are applied to the closed chest wall for a duration of 2 to 3 msec. External pacemakers capable of doing this are available. The voltage and the rate of discharge of the pacemaker can be adjusted manually. The usual rate of pacing is 75 beats per min.

Small flat disc electrodes are applied to the patient's closed chest. The negative electrode is placed just outside the cardiac apex at the point used to record lead V_5 or V_6. The positive electrode is placed just to the left of the sternum at the point used to record lead V_2 to V_4. The electrodes should be at least 3 inches apart. Occasionally, it may be necessary to place electrodes in different positions on the anterior chest and the left axilla to get adequate pacing.

The skin should be shaved, if necessary, and gently cleansed with an alcohol swab to remove surface oil and dead skin. A suitable electrode paste is gently rubbed into the skin at the site of the electrodes. To prevent irritation, the rubbing should not be too vigorous. Also, the electrode paste should not extend beyond the surface of the electrodes. If this occurs and the two paste areas touch each other, the two electrodes will short-circuit and the current will be prevented from penetrating to the heart.

The electrodes are held firmly in place with a perforated rubber chest strap or with adhesive tape. The paste should be renewed as it dries, every 2 to 3 hours. The electrode paste has a corrosive action on the electrodes. Therefore, they should be cleaned with scouring powder after use. If long-term monitoring is being done, the disc electrodes should be moved to a new skin site every time the electrode paste is renewed, to prevent skin irritation.

Each pacemaker pulse will be associated with a large pacemaker deflection, which should not be confused with the patient's ECG.

External cardiac pacing can also be done with needle electrodes and a lower voltage for the pacing. This will prevent the local muscle contractions that occur when disc electrodes are used. Conventional hypodermic needles that have been sterilized are used. Although any size of needle is satisfactory, a needle with a thin gauge and a 1-inch length is recommended. The needles are inserted in the same areas as the disc electrodes, to a depth of $1/2$ inch. The exposed $1/2$ inch is secured to the skin with adhesive tape. Plastic hub needles or needles that have been siliconized should not be used, because they will not conduct the current properly. The needles are attached to the patient cable of the pacemaker with Luer-Lok adapters.

The temporary external cardiac pacemaker can also be used to stimulate the exposed heart, during open-heart surgery, for example. In such a case, one wire (electrode) is attached to the myocardium and connected to the negative pole of the pacemaker. It can remain in the myocardium even when the chest is closed. The peripheral end is then brought out through the chest wall. A second wire is attached subcutaneously and connected to the positive pole of the pacemaker. When direct pacing of the myocardium is done this way, not more than 15 V are needed.

Adequate pacing occurs only when each paced beat is associated with a palpable pulse.

External cardiac pacing is usually not effective in a patient with acute myocardial infarction who develops asystole, because such a severely damaged heart usually does not respond.

Battery-operated pacemakers for external cardiac pacing are available. Pacemakers for external cardiac pacing, powered by alternating current are also available. These must be grounded very carefully to prevent accidental ventricular fibrillation.

Temporary transthoracic cardiac pacing

In an emergency, a transthoracic needle and cannula can be passed transthoracically (between the fourth or fifth left intercostal space or in the subxiphoid area) into the ventricle. A special curved pacing stylus (available from Electro-Catheter Corp) can then be passed into the ventricle and attached to an external battery-operated pacemaker.

TEMPORARY TRANSVENOUS CARDIAC PACING

The heart can also be temporarily paced by inserting a catheter electrode through a vein, either percutaneously or transvenously through a cutdown, and guiding it into the cavity of the right atrium or right ventricle, with electrocardiographic monitoring. The catheter electrode is then connected to an external battery-operated pacemaker.

Small external battery-operated pacemakers for temporary use are available. Some of the pacemakers are the fixed rate or demand type. Others can be adjusted to provide either fixed rate or demand temporary pacing.

Sites for venipuncture
Subclavian venipuncture

The best way to insert a transvenous catheter into the heart at the bedside is by way of the subclavian vein. However, this should be done only by one who is thoroughly familiar with the anatomy of the area and with the technic, and who is aware of possible complications. Before using this technic, one must know the anatomical relationships of the subclavian vein to the clavicle, the subclavian artery, and the pleura. The subclavian vein lies posterior to the clavicle and to the pectoralis and subclavian muscles. It lies above the first rib and is anterior to the subclavian artery and to the pleural cavity (Fig. 16-1).

The subclavian vein can be entered from either above or below the clavicle.

Supraclavicular subclavian venipuncture (Yoffa). The needle is inserted at the point where the lateral (posterior) margin of the sternomastoid muscle meets the upper border of the clavicle (Fig. 16-2). This point can be identified by having the patient tense the sternomastoid muscle by raising his head against the resistance of the operator's hand on the forehead. The sternomastoid muscle can always be felt even if it is difficult to see. This point is marked on the skin, and a local anesthetic is injected at this point. Then a 14-gauge 2¼- or 2½-inch Bardic needle with a plastic outer shield is connected to a 5-ml syringe. The needle is then directed inferiorly toward the center of the chest at an angle of 45° to the sagit-

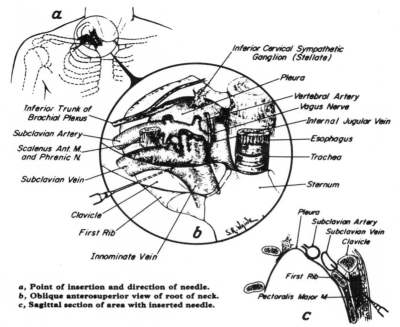

a, Point of insertion and direction of needle.
b, Oblique anterosuperior view of root of neck.
c, Sagittal section of area with inserted needle.

Fig. 16-1. Technic for infraclavicular subclavian venipuncture. Patient lies flat on his or her back, with head facing forward. Needle is inserted immediately below clavicle at junction of its middle and medial thirds, **A** and **B**. Needle is directed backward, inward, and slightly upward to a point where the subclavian, internal jugular, and innominate veins join, **C**. Negative pressure is applied through syringe attached to needle until a free flow of venous blood occurs. Syringe is then disengaged, and a sterile plastic cannula is passed through needle into vein. (From Davidson JT, Ben-Hur N, Nathen H: Lancet **2:**1139, 1963.)

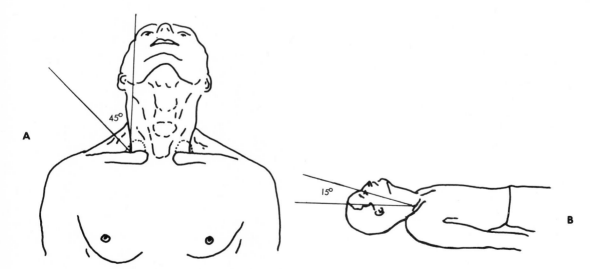

Fig. 16-2. Technic for supraclavicular subclavian venipuncture (technic after Yoffa). **A,** Posteroanterior view. **B,** Lateral view.

tal plane (which divides the body into a right and a left half) and posteriorly (backward) at an angle of 15° to the coronal plane (which divides the body into an anterior and a posterior half) (Fig. 16-2).

As the needle is advanced, negative pressure is applied to the syringe until a free flow of venous blood is aspirated. The needle enters the vein with a slight "give." The syringe and needle are removed, and the catheter electrode is passed through the plastic cannula into the heart, with electrocardiographic monitoring (see below).

The patient must be lying flat or be in Trendelenburg's position to prevent venous air embolism, which may occur when the syringe and needle are removed and when the catheter electrode is being passed through the open vein.

Infraclavicular venipuncture (Davidson, Ben-Hur, Nathen). The patient lies on his back, looking forward. The same preparation and the same type of needle as for supraclavicular venipuncture are used.

The needle is inserted about 1 cm below the clavicle at the junction of its middle and medial thirds. (At this point the clavicle crosses the first rib and begins to diverge from it.) The needle is directed backward, inward, and slightly upward toward the upper border of the substernal notch. The needle should be kept at an angle of 10° to 15° to the chest wall (Fig. 16-1). Negative pressure is applied to the syringe until the free flow of venous blood is aspirated. The syringe and needle are removed, and the catheter electrode is inserted through the plastic cannula into the heart, just as in supraclavicular subclavian venipuncture.

To avoid possible injury to the thoracic duct, which enters the junction of the left jugular and subclavian veins, the right subclavian vein, rather than the left, should be cannulated.

Percutaneous insertion of a catheter electrode through the subclavian vein can be accomplished in about 80% of patients.

About 10% will require fluoroscopic guidance as well as electrocardiographic monitoring. (Fluoroscopic guidance alone should not be used, because there is an increased incidence of ventricular arrhythmias developing during the procedure.) In about 10% of patients, the jugular, the femoral, or even the brachial vein will have to be used.

Complications of subclavian venipuncture. Passing a catheter electrode percutaneously through a subclavian vein can result in hematoma, sepsis, thrombophlebitis, partial pneumothorax, injury to the thoracic duct or the brachial plexus, air embolism, partial pneumothorax, accidental puncture of the subclavian artery, perforation of the right ventricle (p. 206), and other complications (p. 36). No specific treatment is needed for the pneumothorax. If the subclavian artery is punctured, local compression beneath the clavicle for 5 min will stop the bleeding.

Late displacement of the catheter electrode occurs in one third or more of patients.

Brachial venipuncture

A catheter electrode can be inserted by way of the brachial (or jugular or femoral) vein if the operator is concerned about possible complications from subclavian vein insertion. However, when the brachial vein is used, displacement of the catheter electrode tip quickly occurs when the patient moves his arm.

To insert a catheter electrode by way of the brachial vein, the patient's arm is elevated, and the basilic or median antecubital vein in the antecubital fossa is identified. The cephalic vein should *not* be used because it makes an acute angle when it pierces the fascia in the deltopectoral triangle to reach the axillary and subclavian veins.

A blood pressure cuff is placed around the arm and is inflated to the level of the diastolic pressure to make the vein more prominent. The vein is punctured with a

Bardic 14-gauge needle with a plastic outer sheath, attached to a syringe. When the vein is entered, the needle and syringe are removed, leaving the sheath in the vein. The catheter electrode is then inserted into the vein and advanced toward the heart, with electrocardiographic monitoring (see below).

Just before the tip of the catheter electrode is positioned in the right ventricle, the patient's arm should be brought back to the side of the chest and immobilized because movement of the arm can easily displace the catheter electrode tip.

Other sites for venipuncture

The *internal jugular vein* can also be entered percutaneously (Jernigan and associates).

The *femoral vein* can also be entered percutaneously. It lies just medial to the femoral artery in the femoral triangle. Puncture is therefore made just medial to the point where the femoral artery pulse is felt.

When the femoral vein is used to insert a temporary catheter electrode, there is increased danger of thrombophlebitis. Therefore, temporary femoral vein pacing should not exceed 10 to 14 days, whereas temporary pacing through the subclavian, brachial, or jugular vein can continue for 3 weeks or more.

Catheter electrodes

Two types of catheter electrodes can be used for temporary transvenous cardiac pacing: (1) floating or semi-floating catheter electrodes and (2) fixed-position catheter electrodes.

Floating or *semi-floating catheter electrodes* do not have a rigidly fixed position in the right ventricular cavity. *Fixed-position catheter electrodes* are rigid and will maintain any position into which they are placed in the heart cavity. However, they can perforate the right ventricular wall very easily.

Unipolar or bipolar stimulation of the heart

Unipolar or bipolar catheter electrodes can be used to stimulate the heart. Physiologically, both are equally effective.

In a *unipolar* system, the *cathode* is in contact with the heart, and the *anode* is placed elsewhere. If a temporary pacemaker is used, the anode can be attached to the skin by means of an ordinary metal electrocardiographic electrode with conductive paste between it and the skin, or the anode may be connected to a wire that is attached to the skin by means of a braided stainless steel suture.

In a unipolar system, if the anode is placed in contact with the heart, much larger currents are needed to stimulate the heart muscle.

A *bipolar* catheter electrode has a *dipole,* anode and cathode, close to each other and in contact with the heart muscle. The potentials at the two poles may be similar. If this occurs, they will tend to cancel each other out, and the resultant current flow may not be large enough to stimulate the underlying heart muscle. This can be corrected by a slight change in the position of the bipolar electrode tip within the right ventricle.

A bipolar catheter electrode has one advantage over a unipolar catheter electrode. If one wire of a bipolar catheter electrode breaks or does not function, the electrode can be converted into a unipolar system by connecting the functioning lead wire to the *negative* pole of the pacemaker (and grounding the *positive* pole of the pacemaker to the skin or subcutaneous tissue).

A unipolar catheter electrode is more sensitive than a bipolar catheter electrode to stimuli, such as the QRS complexes, that arise in the heart. However, the unipolar catheter electrode is also much more sensitive to external electrical interference.

Preston has recently pointed out that every documented case of pacemaker-induced ventricular fibrillation in humans has been associated with a bipolar catheter electrode system. He therefore suggests that when temporary transvenous pacing is done, particularly in a patient with acute myocardial infarction, a unipolar catheter electrode should be used.

Characteristics of intracardiac electrocardiograms
Technic and equipment

The location of the catheter tip in the heart is monitored by means of unipolar lead ECGs taken from the cavity of the heart. This is done in the following way.

Metal electrocardiographic electrodes are attached to the patient's arms and legs. The electrocardiograph is set to take a V lead, and the free proximal end of the catheter electrode is attached to the V cable of the electrocardiograph by means of an insulated wire with an alligator clip at each end.

These unipolar lead ECGs should be taken with a battery-operated electrocardiograph or with a properly grounded high-impedance electrocardiograph to prevent accidental leakage of alternating current from the electrical outlet into the patient's heart, which can cause ventricular fibrillation.

Until the equipment is tested, no one can assume that an electrocardiograph operating on alternating current, or that any other electrically operated hospital equipment, such as electrically controlled hospital beds, suction equipment, and foot switches, does not leak alternating current. Therefore a defibrillator and resuscitative equipment should be immediately available whenever intracardiac ECGs are taken or whenever a catheter electrode is passed. Even when a battery-operated electrocardiograph is used, the physician should be careful not to touch any electrical equipment while handling the exposed wires of the catheter electrode.

If 50- or 60-cycle (Hz) alternating cur-

rent interference artifacts are noted on the ECG, the procedure should be stopped at once.

Characteristics

In the right atrium, the P wave is usually downward near the entrance of the superior vena cava and upward near the entrance of the inferior vena cava. Elsewhere in the right atrium, the P wave is large and biphasic (Fig. 16-3). It is usually larger than the QRS complex.

If the catheter tip produces pressure on the atrial wall, an elevation of the P-Ta segment may occur, which resembles the pattern of myocardial injury (Fig. 16-3, C). This is similar to the elevated RS-T segment that occurs when the electrode tip presses on the right ventricular cavity wall. The elevated P-Ta segment disappears when the position of the electrode is shifted.

When the electrode tip is in the right subclavian vein, the ECG resembles lead aV_R. When it is in the left subclavian vein, the ECG resembles lead aV_L.

When the electrode tip is in the coronary sinus, the intracardiac ECG may show downward P waves in leads II, III, and aV_F, or a so-called left atrial pattern (downward P waves in leads I and V_6).

If the electrode tip is pushed deeply into the coronary sinus, it may enter the left ventricular cavity because the coronary sinus communicates with the left ventricular cavity. When this happens the intracardiac ventricular ECG will show a QS (instead of an rS) and a downward T wave.

When atrial arrhythmias are present, the intra-atrial P waves will not show these characteristic shapes. For example, if atrial tachycardia is present, biphasic P waves at a fast rate will be present. A similar pattern will be present in atrial flutter, but the atrial rate will be 300 per min or faster. If atrial fibrillation is present, the biphasic atrial waves will show varying shapes with a rate faster than 300 per min

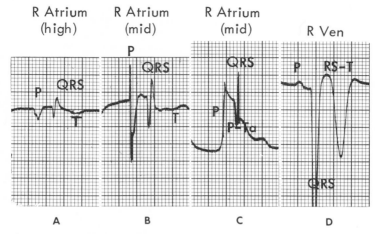

Fig. 16-3. Intracardiac unipolar lead ECGs. **C,** Atrial current of injury when catheter electrode tip is pressed against endocardium of right atrium.

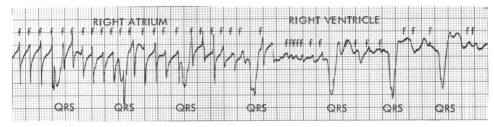

Fig. 16-4. Intracardiac unipolar lead ECG in a patient with atrial fibrillation. Fibrillatory *(f)* waves are large and biphasic in right atrium, but become small in right ventricle.

(Fig. 16-4). If AV junctional rhythm is present, the intra-atrial P waves will resemble normal P waves. However, the shape of the P wave in the superior vena cava will be upward instead of downward; and when a right ventricular cavity lead is taken, P will be downward instead of upward. In addition, P waves may be seen interrupting the QRS complexes. If either complete AV block or the Wenckebach or Mobitz type of incomplete AV block is present, P waves not followed by QRS complexes will appear (Fig. 16-5).

When the tip of the catheter electrode passes the tricuspid valve and enters the right ventricular cavity, the unipolar intracardiac ECG changes markedly. An rS

ventricular pattern with a very deep S and deep T wave appears, and it is usually necessary to decrease the standardization to one half or one fourth. The P wave is small and upward and may be difficult to see when the standardization is decreased (Fig. 16-3).

When the catheter tip produces pressure on the endocardial wall of the right ventricle, an elevated RS-T segment will develop, due to a current of injury (Fig. 16-6). This indicates that the catheter tip has good contact with the right ventricular endocardium. The tip should be kept in this location.

When the catheter tip enters the right ventricular cavity, it may produce a few

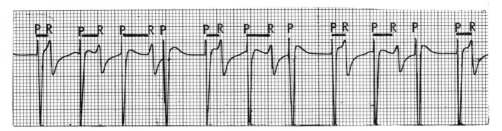

Fig. 16-5. Right atrial unipolar lead ECG in a patient with Wenckebach type of AV block. P-R intervals progressively prolong until a P wave is not followed by a QRS complex.

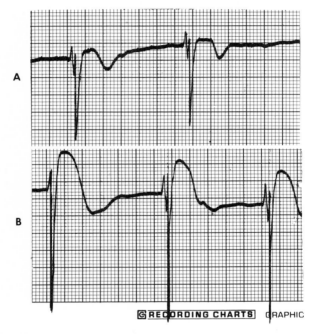

Fig. 16-6. Endocardial current of injury. **A,** Right ventricular cavity lead. **B,** RS-T elevation occurs when tip of catheter electrode is pressed against endocardium.

ventricular premature contractions. However, ventricular fibrillation is always a possibility.

If the tip of the catheter electrode moves into the pulmonary artery, the QRS voltage will decrease.

If right or left bundle branch block is present, the QRS will be wide and will show an aberrant shape.

When the tip of the catheter electrode is in the right ventricular cavity, the con-

ventional 12-lead ECG will show a left bundle branch block pattern (because the right ventricle is stimulated before the left ventricle).

Fig. 15-5 shows a typical 12-lead ECG of such a patient. The precordial leads show widened QRS complexes with deep S waves in leads V_1 to V_4 and a tall R wave in lead V_6, typical of left bundle branch block. Pacemaker spikes appear before each QRS complex.

The standard leads show marked left axis deviation (R_1, S_2, S_3). This indicates that the tip of the catheter electrode is in the apex of the right ventricle. If the standard leads show moderate left axis deviation (R_1, R_2, S_3) or a normal electrical axis (R_1, R_2, R_3), the tip of the catheter electrode is in the mid–outflow tract of the right ventricle. If right axis deviation is present (S_1, R_2, R_3), the tip of the catheter electrode is in the outflow tract of the right ventricle. However, these rules are not absolute.

The directions of the pacemaker spikes cannot be used to determine the location of the electrode tip. However, if displacement of the electrode tip occurs, the electrical axis of the pacemaker spikes (calculated in the same way that the electrical axis of QRS is calculated) may shift 90% or more.

Rarely, pacing with a catheter electrode in the right ventricular cavity will be associated with a 12-lead ECG showing a right bundle branch block pattern. This can occur if the tip of the catheter electrode touches the upper portion of the ventricular septum. A right bundle branch block pattern can also occur if the tip of the catheter electrode is wedged into the coronary sinus and in this way enters the left ventricular cavity. (The catheter may also pass from the coronary sinus through the great vein to the epicardium of the left ventricle.) A right bundle branch block pattern may also develop if the tip of the catheter electrode perforates the wall of the right ventricle (pp. 200 and 207).

Testing the catheter electrode

After a catheter electrode has been placed within the heart, the pacemaker must be tested. If a fixed rate pacemaker is used, the electrical threshold of the catheter electrode tip is tested. If a demand pacemaker is used, the ability of the electrode tip to sense R waves must be tested, in addition to the electrical threshold.

The peripheral wires of the catheter electrode are connected to an external battery-operated pacemaker whose milliamperage can be varied by the physician. The patient is connected to a battery-operated or adequately grounded electrocardiograph, which is set to take any of the standard leads.

Testing the electrical threshold

The amperage of the pacemaker is slowly lowered until the paced QRS complexes and T waves just disappear, leaving only the pacemaker spikes and electrocardiographic signs of the patient's spontaneous heart activity. Then the amperage is slowly raised until pacing is reestablished. This point is the *electrical threshold* (Fig. 16-7). Since the pacemaker may not consistently stimulate the heart muscle at this amperage, its amperage should be raised to two to four times this threshold level.

The term *hysteresis* describes the difference between the amplitude at which pacing becomes ineffective when the pacemaker current is reduced and the amperage at which pacing again becomes effective when the pulse generator current is increased. A satisfactory low hysteresis value is 20% or less the amperage needed for effective pacing. For example, if 2.0 mA are needed for pacing, the hysteresis value should be 0.4 mA or less. (One should also remember that mA readings may not be accurate because of the small space intervals on the pacemaker dial.)

If the hysteresis value is high in a newly implanted catheter electrode, the catheter should be repositioned. If the hysteresis value becomes high in a catheter electrode that has been implanted for a long time, it suggests that there is an intermittent break in the leads, or a short-circuit.

Ordinarily, a newly implanted catheter electrode should show an electrical threshold of less than 2.0 mA. If pacing does not occur at this amperage, the catheter electrode should be repositioned. If the cath-

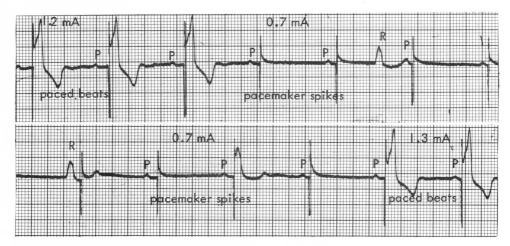

Fig. 16-7. Testing electrical threshold of a transvenous pacemaker; lead II, continuous strip. When a current of 1.2 mA is used, pacing occurs. When current is decreased to 0.7 mA, effective pacing stops. Regular pacemaker spikes continue but are not followed by paced QRS complexes and T waves. R waves indicate spontaneous QRS complexes of this patient. When current was raised to 1.3 mA, effective pacing again returned. The hysteresis value is high (p. 217).

eter electrode has been in place 3 months or longer, the electrical threshold will be higher, but it should not exceed 4.0 mA.

The electrical threshold can vary greatly under normal and abnormal conditions. During sleep or after a heavy meal, it rises. Exercise is associated with a decreased threshold. All antiarrhythmic drugs increase the electrical threshold slightly. Hypokalemia and hyperkalemia are also associated with an increased threshold.

Malfunction of an implanted pacemaker may occur in the first 12 weeks after implantation because the electrical threshold may rise even ten times the initial level at the time of implantation. After this period, the threshold gradually falls.

Corticosteroids lower the electrical threshold. Sowton has used prednisone in a daily oral dose of 40 mg for 3 to 4 days to reestablish pacing if the electrical threshold becomes high shortly after a catheter electrode is implanted. (When pacing failure associated with a high threshold occurs more than 2 or 3 months after a catheter electrode is inserted, corticosteroids should not be given; instead, the catheter electrode should be repositioned or replaced.)

When a bipolar catheter electrode is used, the potentials recorded by each of the electrodes in the right ventricular cavity may be similar. When this occurs, they tend to cancel each other, and the resultant current flow may not be large enough to stimulate the underlying heart muscle. If this is suspected, the bipolar catheter electrode tip should be repositioned, or the catheter electrode should be converted for unipolar use.

The pacemaker rate depends on the clinical needs of the patient. If a fixed rate pacemaker is used on a patient with uncomplicated AV block, a rate of 70 beats per min is satisfactory. Some cardiologists have paced the heart rate of their older patients at 90 to 100 per min. However, the higher the pacing rate, the greater the oxygen needs of the heart. Therefore, the pacing rate should be kept as low as possible.

Testing the sensing of demand pacemakers

If a demand pacemaker is used, the *sensing* of the catheter electrode, in addition to the electrical threshold, must also be tested to determine if the catheter tip is able to sense electrical stimuli (R waves) from the endocardium of the right ventricle, which allows it to act in a demand or standby mode.

A QRS inhibited or a QRS synchronous pacemaker has an electrical sensing threshold of approximatey 2 to 3 mV. Therefore, the amplitude of the QRS complex of a unipolar or bipolar lead from the right ventricular cavity should be at least 1 to 2 mV greater than the sensing threshold, to make certain that it is strong enough to trigger the pacemaker. (The sensing thresholds of different makes of implantable pacemakers vary. The manufacturer's brochures should be consulted for these data.)

When a bipolar catheter electrode is used, the signal from the electrode at the catheter tip and the signal from the electrode proximal to the tip should be checked individually by taking a unipolar lead ECG from each of these locations. This is done as follows.

Metal electrodes are placed on the pa-

tient to take a conventional ECG. The electrocardiograph is set to take a V lead. The end of the catheter wire (that leads to the distal electrode at the catheter tip) is connected by means of an insulated wire with an alligator clip on each end to the V cable of the electrocardiograph. A unipolar lead is then taken (at one-fourth standardization). Another unipolar lead is taken in a similar way from the end of the catheter wire that leads to the proximal electrode in the heart (Fig. 16-8).

The voltage of the QRS complex (multiplied by 4) of each of these unipolar leads indicates whether each electrode has adequate contact with the endocardium.

Next, the electrocardiograph is set at lead I. The wire from the distal electrode is connected to the LA cable. The wire from the proximal electrode is connected to the RA cable, and lead I is taken (Fig. 16-8).

If the QRS (multiplied by 4) of this synthetic lead I has a small amplitude (less than 1 or 2 mV more than the sensing threshold of the pacemaker), the electrode tip should be repositioned; or, if one of the unipolar lead ECGs from the cavity of the heart shows adequate voltage, the catheter can be converted to unipolar use.

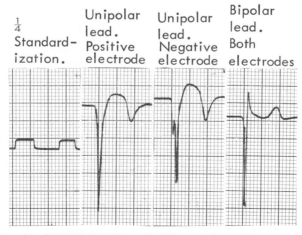

Fig. 16-8. Testing a bipolar catheter electrode. Electrocardiograph is set at one-fourth standardization because endocardial deflections are so large.

If a *unipolar* catheter electrode is used, the amplitude of the endocardial QRS complex should be checked by taking a V lead with the distal end of the catheter electrode attached to the V cable of the electrocardiograph, as described above.

The voltage of S is measured and multiplied by 4. Here again, to obtain adequate sensing, the sum should be at least 1 to 2 mV larger than the sensing threshold of the pacemaker. If massive myocardial infarction occurs, the endocardial QRS voltage may decrease greatly. This may prevent a demand pacemaker from functioning. (Some demand pacemakers may also not sense ventricular premature contractions, particularly if a bipolar catheter electrode is used.)

Testing temporary battery-powered pacemakers

If pacing stops and the ECG does not show spikes, the following can be done.

1. Inspect the electrode wires. One or both wires may be disconnected or short-circuited, may have poor contact, or may be broken.

If a *unipolar* catheter is used, the electrode that serves as an anode on the skin may be loose, or the electrode paste underneath it may have dried. If an anode suture wire is used, it may have extruded or broken.

2. If this does not reveal the source of the trouble and if a *bipolar* catheter electrode is used, check each of the catheter electrode wires in the following way. Connect the patient to take a conventional ECG. Set the electrocardiograph for a V lead (at one-half or one-fourth standardization). Connect the negative wire of the catheter electrode to the V cable (using an insulated wire with an alligator clip on each end), and take a V lead. If this electrode wire is intact, a regular unipolar lead ECG from the right ventricular cavity will be recorded. If the wire is broken, no ECG will be recorded. Alternating current inter-ference may indicate a partial break in the wire.

Next, test the positive wire of the catheter electrode in the same way.

Next, connect one wire of the catheter electrode to the RA cable of the electrocardiograph, the other wire to the LA cable, and take a synthetic lead I. Recording of an ECG indicates that the electrode wires are intact.

If there is a break in one of the catheter electrode wires and if the catheter electrode is bipolar, the problem can be corrected by converting the bipolar catheter electrode for use as a unipolar unit. This can be done simply by connecting the intact wire (or both wires) of the catheter electrode to the negative pole of the pacemaker and connecting the positive pole of the pacemaker to the skin.

If there is no detectable break in the catheter electrode wires, examine the pacemaker to make certain that the on-off switch is functioning. If the switch is satisfactory, replace the pacemaker battery.

If the pacemaker still does not function, replace it.

If pacing stops, but the ECG continues to show spikes, it may be due to the following.

1. The pacemaker battery may be depleted so much that it cannot pace even though it still has enough current to form pacemaker spikes.

2. The electrical threshold may have become too high. This can be determined quickly by increasing the amperage of the pacemaker. If pacing begins again with a higher amperage, measure the threshold and reset the amperage at three times the threshold, unless the measured threshold is too high. In this case, reposition the catheter electrode to obtain a low threshold.

3. The catheter electrode tip may have moved away from the endocardium. This often can be confirmed by taking an x-ray film of the chest.

Also notice if the pacemaker spikes show

a constant amplitude in any one lead, and a constant rate. Battery failure may be associated with changes in the amplitudes of successive spikes (this is *not* true for monitor leads) or changes in the rate of pacing or with both.

Usually, the pacing rate slows with battery failure. Rarely, the pacemaker spike rate becomes faster than its set rate. This may indicate the possibility of a *runaway pacemaker*. When this occurs, the pacing rate may reach or exceed 300 per min. Disconnect such a pacemaker immediately to prevent hypotension, congestive heart failure, ventricular fibrillation, and death.

If demand pacing stops, but the pacemaker continues to function at a fixed rate, it is due, in most cases, to an abnormally high electrical threshold. (Paradoxically, sensing may reappear when the pacemaker amperage is decreased rather than increased.)

Check the electrical threshold (p. 217). If the threshold is satisfactory, check the amplitudes of the intracardiac unipolar ECGs (p. 219), to determine if the sensing is adequate.

If the unipolar leads show low voltage, reposition the catheter electrode.

If a bipolar catheter electrode is used and the unipolar leads show high voltage, convert the catheter electrode for unipolar use (p. 213).

If pacing stops with a demand pacemaker but the pacemaker continues to show regularly recurring spikes, it indicates not only that the pacemaker is not pacing, but that it is also not sensing the R waves, because it would be inhibited if it were sensing. This type of problem is usually due to displacement of the catheter tip away from the endocardium. This often can be confirmed by an x-ray film of the chest. Reposition the catheter tip.

Care of patient after insertion of temporary transvenous catheter electrode

Anticoagulants are not given to the patient for either temporary or permanent catheter electrode placement. Prophylactic antibiotic therapy may or may not be helpful in preventing infection at the site of insertion of the catheter electrode.

The patient should be connected to a cardiac monitor for at least several hours after the catheter electrode has been inserted. If premature beats or signs of unstable pacing are present, the monitoring should be continued until the rhythm becomes stable.

A 12-lead ECG and a long rhythm strip should be taken immediately after the catheter electrode has been inserted. Pacemaker spikes should appear regularly if fixed rate pacing is being done. If the patient has a demand pacemaker and the spontaneous heart rate is faster than the escape rate of the pacemaker, the ECG will not show any pacemaker spikes until the heart slows or until the pacemaker is momentarily converted to fixed rate pacing, if possible.

Posteroanterior and lateral x-ray films of the chest should also be taken to make certain that the tip of the catheter electrode is in place. In the posteroanterior view, the electrode tip should be close to the left border of the heart. In the lateral view, the electrode tip should lie anteriorly (Fig. 16-9). If it is in the coronary sinus, it will lie posteriorly in the lateral view (Fig. 16-10).

The patient is allowed to walk immediately after the catheter electrode has been placed.

Removal of catheter electrodes

When it is no longer necessary to continue temporary transvenous pacing, the catheter electrode can be removed at the bedside simply by withdrawing it. If bleeding from the vein occurs, it is controlled by simple pressure. If the catheter electrode had been implanted into the subclavian vein by means of a cutdown, the incision will have to be reopened to remove the retention sutures.

If a temporary catheter electrode is removed after a long-term transvenous cath-

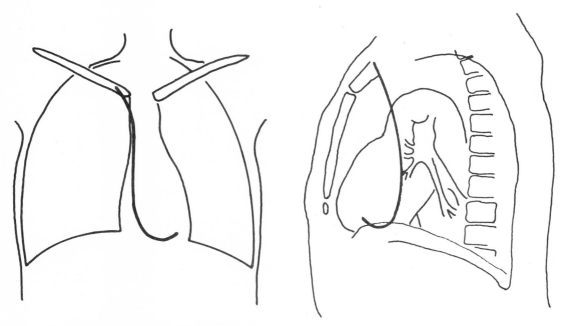

Fig. 16-9. Posteroanterior *(left)* and lateral *(right)* x-ray views of a catheter electrode in right ventricular cavity.

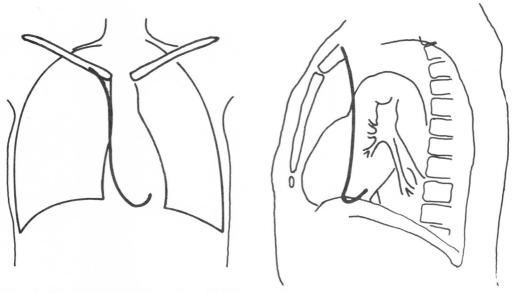

Fig. 16-10. Posteroanterior *(left)* and lateral *(right)* x-ray views of a catheter electrode whose tip is in the coronary sinus.

eter electrode has been introduced, postero-anterior and lateral x-ray films of the heart should be taken to make certain that the location of the long-term catheter electrode has not been disturbed.

When a long-term catheter electrode is introduced, the temporary catheter electrode is left in place for several days. Occasionally the two catheter electrodes may become entangled. This can be prevented by using the left side for the temporary catheter electrode and the right side for the permanent catheter electrode, or vice versa.

INDICATIONS FOR TEMPORARY CARDIAC PACING

The indications for temporary cardiac pacing are discussed in the chapters on the bradyarrhythmias, the tachyarrhythmias, and acute myocardial infarction. I believe that there has been a tendency to use pacemaker therapy too enthusiastically. One must always remember that cardiac pacing is not innocuous and that it can cause serious tachyarrhythmias, particularly in patients with acute myocardial infarction.

Indications for temporary ventricular pacing

The following is a brief resumé of the indications for temporary ventricular pacing.

1. Bradyarrhythmias associated with acute myocardial infarction, particularly complete AV block and anterior infarction, or complete AV block and inferior infarction when a complication, such as severe congestive heart failure, cardiogenic shock, or syncope is present (also see p. 147)
2. AV block following cardiac surgery
3. Symptomatic bradyarrhythmias associated with drug toxicity, or electrolyte disturbances, such as hyperkalemia, not responding to drug therapy
4. Tachyarrhythmias (see below)
5. Preparatory to inserting a long-term pacemaker, to determine if pacing is helpful

Indications for temporary right atrial (or coronary sinus) pacing

When AV conduction is normal, temporary right atrial (or coronary sinus) pacing has been used in patients with the following conditions.

1. Symptomatic bradyarrhythmias
2. Tachyarrhythmias (see below)
3. Prevention of bradyarrhythmias during selective coronary arteriography

It has also been used during stress testing (using rapid atrial pacing) to determine the presence of coronary artery disease.

Pacemaker "overdriving" of tachyarrhythmias

Electrical pacing (overdriving, overriding) of the heart for tachyarrhythmias has been used in patients with the following conditions.

1. Tachyarrhythmias due to digitalis toxicity (DC shock would be dangerous)
2. Tachyarrhythmias occurring in acute myocardial infarction, when drug therapy or DC shock is not effective
3. Tachyarrhythmias occurring after cardiac surgery
4. Tachyarrhythmias that do not respond to the usual cardiac-depressant drugs
5. Tachyarrhythmias associated with bradyarrhythmias (bradycardia-tachycardia syndrome) so that cardiac-depressant drugs are contraindicated
6. Allergy to cardiac-depressant drugs

Even if the cardiac pacing is not completely successful in terminating a tachyarrhythmia, it can be used in combination with cardiac-depressant drugs, which otherwise might be contraindicated because of the possibility of slowing the heart rate too much. (This can occur, for example, in patients with complete AV block complicated by tachyarrhythmias or with other bradycardia-tachycardia syndromes; see Chapter 9.)

Right atrial (or coronary sinus) pacing or right ventricular pacing can be used for both supraventricular and ventricular tachyarrhythmias (when AV conduction is normal). However, right ventricular pacing is preferable because a catheter electrode in the right ventricle has less tendency to be displaced than one in the right atrium or coronary sinus. Right atrial (or coronary sinus) pacing can be used for a supraventricular tachyarrhythmia when AV block is present but cannot be used for a ventricular tachyarrhythmia when AV block is present.

Fixed rate pacemakers are needed for either atrial or ventricular pacing.

When right atrial pacing is done, the pacemaker should be capable of delivering 400 or more pulses per min. Atrial pacing up to 1,200 pulses per min has been used. These rapid rates require the use of special pacemakers. The amperage needed can vary from 0.5 to 15 mA.

Supraventricular tachyarrhythmias, with the exception of atrial fibrillation, can be terminated by atrial (or ventricular) pacing for a brief period of seconds or minutes in one of three ways.

1. A single stimulus or two successive stimuli in quick succession
2. Repetitive stimulation at a rate slower than the tachyarrhythmic rate
3. Repetitive stimulation at a rate faster than the tachyarrhythmic rate

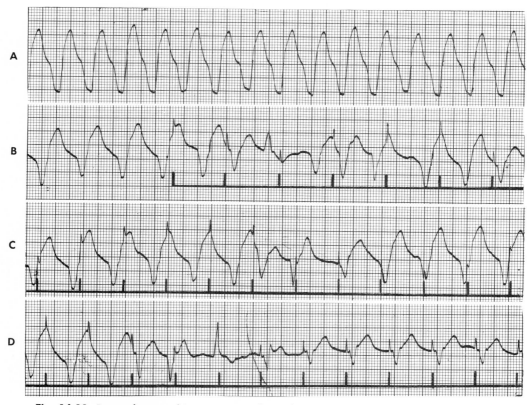

Fig. 16-11. Pacemaker overdriving a ventricular tachycardia; lead II. **A,** Ventricular tachycardia with a rate of approximately 160 per min. The patient was in cardiogenic shock and had not responded to lidocaine or to other cardiac-depressant drugs. **B,** Transvenous battery-operated pacemaker catheter electrode was inserted into right ventricle. At first, rate of pacing was approximately 80 per min. This was not effective. However, pacing became effective, **C** and **D,** when the pacemaker rate was increased to 100 per min.

When repetitive atrial pacing is done at a rate faster than the supraventricular tachyarrhythmia rate, one of three results may occur.

1. Sinus rhythm may result.
2. Atrial fibrillation may develop. When this happens, the ventricular rate can be slowed with digitalis.
3. The ventricular rate may decrease without conversion of the tachyarrhythmia.

The stimulation must be interrupted every few minutes to determine if sinus rhythm or atrial fibrillation has developed. Atrial fibrillation is usually transient (lasting seconds to hours) and is followed by sinus rhythm. If it persists, the ventricular rate can be slowed with digitalis.

Atrial pacing with a high overdriving rate can be dangerous because it can precipitate angina, hypotension, or congestive heart failure.

When right ventricular pacing is done, the pacing rate should be faster than the patient's usual heart rate. It is not always necessary to increase the pacing rate above that of the tachyarrhythmia.

Fig. 16-11 shows the effect of a ventricular pacemaker overdriving a ventricular tachycardia when lidocaine was ineffective.

REFERENCES

Baird CL: Transvenous pacing; a bedside technique, Br Heart J **33**:191, 1971.

Bing OHL, et al: Pacemaker placement by electrocardiographic monitoring, N Engl J Med **287**:651, 1972.

Cheng TO: Coronary sinus pacing masquerading as interventricular septal perforation by transvenous catheter, Am J Cardiol **26**:547, 1970.

Davidson, JT, Ben-Hur N, Nathen H: Subclavian venipuncture, Lancet **2**:1139, 1963.

Elder RL, Furman S: Electric razor interference with cardiac pacemakers, Questions and Answers, JAMA **222**:1658, 1972.

Evans GL, Glasser SP: Intracavitary electrocardiography as a guide to pacemaker positioning, JAMA **216**:483, 1971.

Jernigan WR, Gardner WC, et al: Use of the internal jugular vein for placement of central venous catheter, Surg Gynecol Obstet **130**:520, 1970.

Jernigan WR, Gardner WC, et al: The internal jugular vein for access to the central venous system, JAMA **218**:97, 1971.

Johnson CL, Jazarchick J, Lynn HB: Subclavian venipuncture; preventable complications, Mayo Clin Proc **45**:719, 1970.

Killip T, Kimball JTJr: Percutaneous techniques for introducing flexible electrodes for intracardiac pacing, Ann N Y Acad Sci **167**:597, 1969.

Kimball JT, Killip T: A simple bedside method for transvenous intracardiac pacing, Am Heart J **70**:35, 1965.

Meister SG, et al: An improved method for temporary transvenous pacing without fluoroscopy, Circulation **46**(Suppl 2):191, 1972.

Preston TA: Anodal stimulation as a cause of pacemaker-induced ventricular fibrillation, Am Heart J **86**:366, 1973.

Preston TA: Electrocardiographic diagnosis of pacemaker catheter displacement, Am Heart J **85**:445, 1973.

Rutenberg HL, Soloff LA: Simulation of "left atrial rhythm" by right atrial pacing, Am J Cardiol **26**:427, 1970.

Samet P, Bernstein WH, Korn M: Methodology of cardiac pacing, part 1, Geriatrics **25**:87, 1970.

Sowton E: Discussion. In Meltzer LE, Kitchell JR, editors: Current concepts of cardiac pacing and cardioversion, Philadelphia, 1971, The Charles Press.

Yoffa D: Supraclavicular subclavian venipuncture and catheterization, Lancet **2**:614, 1965.

17 / Long-term transvenous cardiac pacing

When a patient has a chronic cardiac condition that responds to temporary cardiac pacing, a long-term transvenous pacemaker can be implanted. This consists of a small sealed battery-operated pulse generator, implanted subcutaneously, and a catheter electrode passed into the right ventricle.

TYPES OF IMPLANTED PACEMAKERS

There are 5 different types of implanted pacemakers (pulse generators) and approximately 30 different models available for long-term cardiac pacing.

Fixed rate pacemakers
Demand pacemakers
  QRS inhibited pacemakers
  QRS synchronous pacemakers
  Atrial synchronous pacemakers
  Bifocal demand pacemakers (p. 205)

The usual energy source for an implanted pacemaker is the zinc-mercuric oxide primary battery cell. Most implanted pacemakers contain four to six such cells in series. These batteries provide a stable output of about 8 V for approximately 80% to 90% of the life of the battery. The voltage then decays rapidly in a period of several weeks and is accompanied by changes in the pacemaker rate and amplitude of the pacemaker spikes.

The pacemaker is implanted subcutaneously, usually in the right or left pectoral region, and is connected to the peripheral ends of the catheter electrode. The various types and makes of implanted pacemakers can be recognized by x-ray examination of the chest. The technic of implanting a pacemaker is described in Furman and Escher's excellent textbook. Some manufacturers recommend the use of bipolar or unipolar catheter electrodes with their implanted pacemakers. These recommendations should be followed.

Implanted fixed rate pacemakers

The electrical characteristics of fixed rate pacemakers have been described in Chapter 15.

The fixed rate pacemaker emits an electrical pulse at a fixed rate, usually 60 to 70 beats per min. The rate may be preset by the manufacturer. In some models, such as the Medtronic fixed rate pacemaker, model 5910, the rate can be adjusted even after the pacemaker has been implanted by passing a sterile Keith triangular needle through the skin into a self-sealing silicone-rubber nipple in the center of the pacemaker.

The methods of testing the function of implanted fixed rate pacemakers are described below.

Implanted QRS inhibited pacemakers

The electrical characteristics of QRS inhibited pacemakers have been described in Chapter 15.

The refractory period and the escape period of various implanted QRS inhibited pacemakers vary. In addition, these pacemakers vary in their response to external alternating current interference, to radio-frequency stimulation, and to battery depletion. As the batteries fail, some of the pacemakers may become slower, some faster. The manufacturers' instruction booklets should be consulted for details.

The rate of some of the Medtronic implanted QRS inhibited pacemakers can be varied, as was described for implanted fixed rate pacemakers. The rate of the General Electric QRS inhibited pacemakers can also be varied through inductive coupling by placing a radio frequency coil connected to a control box, on the skin overlying the pacemaker.

The Cordis Company now makes implantable (Omnicor) fixed rate, QRS inhibited, QRS synchronous, and atrial synchronous pacemakers whose current output and fixed rate pacing can be changed whenever desired without penetration of the skin and without removal of the pacemaker. This is done by placing an external portable battery-operated programmer on the skin overlying the implanted Omnicor pacemaker. The programmer emits a pulse that can be recognized only by the implanted pacemaker.

Methods of testing implanted QRS inhibited pacemakers are described below.

Implanted QRS synchronous and atrial synchronous pacemakers

The electrical characteristics of these pacemakers have been described in Chapter 16.

METHODS OF ELECTRODE PLACEMENT

There are two methods of placing the pacemaker electrodes in contact with the heart for long-term pacing: epicardial and transvenous.

In *epicardial pacing,* the pacing electrodes are sewn to the epicardium. The pacemaker is then implanted in the subcutaneous tissue of the chest wall, usually over the right or left pectoral muscles. However, this method requires thoracotomy, with the patient under general anesthesia, and may be associated with a mortality of 5% to 20%, as well as with serious postoperative complications, including post-

operative myocardial infarction, in elderly patients with cardiac disease.

In *transvenous pacing,* a catheter electrode is passed transvenously through a cutdown on a cephalic vein, the external jugular vein, or the subclavian vein, and is guided with the ECG and fluoroscope (using image intensification, if possible) into the right ventricular cavity until it comes into contact with the endocardium. The catheter is then wedged into the trabeculae near the apex of the right ventricle. After the catheter electrode is placed, its position should be checked with posteroanterior and lateral x-ray views of the chest, as has been described for the insertion of temporary transvenous catheter electrodes (see Fig. 16-9).

Before the skin overlying the pacemaker is sutured, the patient should cough and turn on the operating room table, to confirm that stable pacing is present.

Recently, Mansour and associates have described a new sutureless screw-in epicardial electrode that can be implanted by way of a transxiphoid approach under general or local anesthesia. In this way, epicardial pacing is achieved without the dangers of open thoracotomy. Experience with this technique is still limited.

Catheter electrodes that are used for long-term implantation in right ventricular cavity have a flared or special tip that can be wedged into the trabeculae of the right ventricle.

When a long-term transvenous pacemaker is installed in a patient who has a temporary catheter electrode, the temporary catheter electrode should be kept in place for 2 to 3 days. When it is withdrawn, the long-term catheter electrode should be rechecked by x-ray films to make certain that its position has not been disturbed.

The removal of a chronically implanted catheter electrode may be difficult and dangerous because the catheter may become attached to the endocardium or to the tricuspid valve. If this occurs, the gentle steady application of pulley traction, using a weight of 250 gm (½ pound), may be helpful.

TESTING IMPLANTED PACEMAKERS

The causes of malfunction of implanted pacemakers are similar to those of temporary pacemakers. However, because the pulse generator and the catheter electrode of the implanted pacemaker are not accessible, it is more difficult to find the exact cause of the malfunction.

With all implanted pacemakers, it is important to know the name of the manufacturer, the model of the pacemaker, the date of insertion, the pacing site within the heart, and the preset rate of the pacemaker. With QRS inhibited and synchronous pacemakers, it is also necessary to know the refractory period of the pacemaker, in addition to its escape rate. It is also important to know the underlying cardiac rhythm of the patient before the pacemaker was inserted. If this information is lacking, the make and model of the pacemaker can usually be recognized by its configuration in an x-ray film of the chest.

A patient with an implanted pacemaker should be examined at regular intervals after 1 month, and then at intervals of 4 to 6 months for the first year, then every 2 months for the next 6 months, and monthly thereafter. This is the best way to detect battery failure.

There are many sensitive electronic methods to detect pacemaker function, such as using an oscilloscope to evaluate the shape, amplitude, duration, polarity, and firing rate of the implanted pacemaker. A recent method determines pacemaker rate via the telephone. The pacemaker pulse is transformed into a sound tone, which is transmitted over the telephone to a central receiving station. There it is converted back into an electronic signal and fed into a rate counter. However, the conventional ECG is very valuable for detecting pacemaker function and failure (see below).

Malfunction of implanted pacemakers may occur for several reasons.

1. The catheter electrode wires may break. This can be determined by taking posteroanterior and lateral x-ray films of the heart.

2. The catheter tip may shift in the right ventricular cavity. This may stop the pacing; or if a demand pacemaker has been inserted, the pacemaker may revert to fixed rate pacing.

3. The electrical threshold may have increased, so that pacing stops or becomes intermittent. This can be determined only by exposing the catheter electrode wires surgically.

4. A demand pacemaker may lose its sensing ability (p. 219).

5. Perforation of the right ventricular wall may occur (p. 206).

6. Battery failure may occur. There are several ways of determining this. Battery failure in an implanted pacemaker is usually associated with slowing of the pacemaker rate and a decrease in the spike amplitude. However, in some implanted pacemakers, battery failure may be associated with an increased rate. (The manufacturers' instruction booklets should be consulted.) Battery failure in a QRS inhibited or synchronous pacemaker is associated at the beginning with loss of demand pacing and a reversion of the pacemaker to fixed rate pacing only. Battery failure in an atrial synchronous pacemaker is associated with a change in pacemaker rate or loss of ability to function synchronously or both.

If the rate of a fixed rate pacemaker (or the escape rate of a demand pacemaker) changes more than 10%, the implanted pacemaker should be promptly replaced. It has been calculated that an atrial synchronous pacemaker will last about 1½ years; the others will last about 2 years. The demand type of implanted pacemakers may last longer than fixed rate pacemakers because their battery drain is less. However, the heat of the body may accelerate battery failure even when the batteries are not used.

Using the electrocardiogram to test pacemaker function

When an ECG is taken of a patient with a cardiac pacemaker, the ECG should show the pacemaker spikes if a fixed rate pacemaker is used. However, when a demand pacemaker is used, the pacemaker spikes will not appear when the patient's spontaneous heart rate is faster than the escape rate of the pacemaker, for reasons already discussed.

The ECG can also be used to determine the location of the tip of the catheter electrode in the right ventricular cavity. Because the catheter electrode is in the right ventricular cavity, each pacing pulse stimulates the right ventricle first, producing a left bundle branch block pattern (wide QS in lead V_1 and a wide, tall R in lead aV_L or V_6; see Fig. 15-5). The location of the tip of the catheter electrode in the right ventricle can be determined by the electrical axis of the standard leads, as described in Chapter 16 for temporary transvenous pacemakers.

The ECGs of patients with pacemakers will also show, in addition to the pacemaker spikes and the paced beats, atrial arrhythmias and abnormal ventricular rhythms. The atrial arrhythmias include sinus rhythm, SA block, AV block, AV dissociation, atrial flutter or atrial fibrillation, AV junctional rhythm, unidirectional AV block (retrograde spread of the stimulus from the paced ventricles through the AV node to the atria when forward conduction from the atria to the ventricles through the AV node is blocked), and signs of concealed conduction through the AV node. The abnormal ventricular rhythms include parasystole, fusion beats, AV junctional or ventricular premature contractions (Fig. 17-1). However, the discussion of these phenomena is outside the scope of this book.

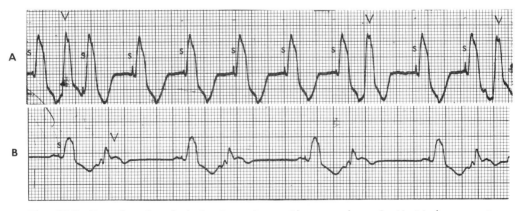

Fig. 17-1. Examples of arrhythmias in patients with pacemakers. **A,** Ventricular premature contractions *(V)* occurring in a patient with a ventricular demand (QRS inhibited) pacemaker. First ventricular premature contraction occurs during refractory period of pacemaker and is not sensed. Therefore, it does not interfere with the pacemaker rate. Second ventricular premature contraction *(V)* is sensed, causing the next pacemaker beat to occur after the preset escape interval; *s,* pacemaker spike. **B,** Ventricular premature contractions *(V)* occurring in a patient with a ventricular demand (QRS inhibited) pacemaker. The pacemaker was set to beat at a rate of approximately 58 per min. (The interval between pacemaker spikes is therefore 1.02 sec.) The ventricular premature contractions occur during alert period of pacemaker. Therefore, they reset pacemaker so that next spike occurs 1.02 sec after beginning of ventricular premature contraction.

*Electrocardiographic signs of
malfunction of fixed rate pacemakers*

Malfunction of a fixed rate pacemaker can cause cessation of pacing, intermittent pacing, or a change in pacing rate.

The following electrocardiographic signs of pacemaker malfunction may occur.

1. The pacemaker may stop forming pulses, and the pacemaker spike may disappear for one or more beats (Fig. 17-2, *D*).

A fixed rate pacemaker always shows regularly occurring spikes. The spikes have no relation to the spontaneous rhythm of the patient's heart and may be superimposed on spontaneously occurring P waves or on spontaneously occurring QRS complexes and T waves (Fig. 17-2, *D*). However, a QRS and T should appear after each pacemaker spike that does not occur in the refractory period after a spontaneous heartbeat (approximately the interval from the beginning of the QRS to just before the end of the T).

If pacemaker spikes are not visible, the pacemaker can also be checked as follows. Take an inexpensive AM battery-powered transistor radio, tuned between stations, with the volume turned up. Place the radio over the pacemaker, and rotate it until clicks are heard on the radio. These are the audible pacemaker pulses. Count the number of clicks for 2 minutes, then divide by 2 to obtain an accurate pacemaker rate.

2. The pacemaker rate may be faster or slower than the preset rate of the pacemaker, or the rate may vary from spike to spike.

The pacemaker spike rate can be measured in several ways.

Method A

Count the number of 0.04-sec time intervals between two successive spikes. Divide the constant 1,500 by this number. The result is the rate per minute.

Example: In Fig. 17-3 there are nineteen 0.04-sec time intervals between two successive spikes (or between R-R or P-P intervals). Therefore, the pacing rate is: 1,500/19 = 79 beats per min.

Method B

Measure the interval in hundredths of a second between two successive spikes (or between two R-R or P-P intervals). Divide the constant 60 by this value. The result is the rate per minute.

Example: In Fig. 17-3 the interval between two successive spikes is 0.76 sec (nineteen 0.04-sec intervals). Therefore, the pacing rate is 60/0.76 = 79 beats per min.

Each 0.04 sec time interval = 40 msec. Each 0.2 sec time interval = 200 msec.

Method C

Electrocardiographic paper has a vertical mark or dot at the top of the paper, occurring every 3 sec (Fig. 17-3). Therefore, the number of pacemaker spikes (or P or R waves) that occur within a 6-sec interval multiplied by 10 gives the rate per minute. (If the first and last spike or wave are both simultaneous with the first and last vertical marks, count only one of the spikes or waves.)

Example: In Fig. 17-3 there are nine pacemaker spikes in a 6-sec time interval. However, the first and last QRS complexes occur simultaneously with the 3-sec time marks. Therefore, the pacing rate is: 9 − 1 × 10 = 80 beats per min.

The pacemaker rate should be checked further in the following way.

Count the interval between two successive spikes in any lead. Repeat this in two different leads. All these values should not differ by more than one half of a 0.04-sec time interval.

Example: The time interval between successive spikes in three separate leads is: 22, 21½, and 22 0.04-sec time intervals. This is satisfactory. (However, one should remember that variations in paper speed of the electrocardiograph may also cause apparent variations in pacemaker escape intervals.)

In addition, the patient can be taught to count his pulse for a full minute daily and to report when his heart rate consistently varies more than 2 beats per min. (This method can be used only when there are no spontaneous beats.)

3. The pacemaker may not stimulate the ventricles during a nonrefractory period. Therefore, the pacemaker spike will not be followed by a QRS complex and T wave at a time when the ventricles should

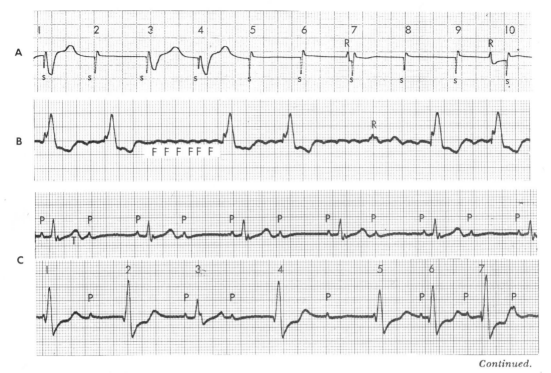

Fig. 17-2. Examples of pacemaker malfunction. **A** to **G** are from different patients. **A,** Malfunction of a fixed rate pacemaker; monitor lead. Beats 1, 3, and 4 show the pacemaker spikes (s) and normally paced QRS complexes and T waves. The remaining beats show only pacemaker spikes. R represents the patient's slow spontaneous QRS complexes. R waves show low voltage because standardization of monitor had been greatly decreased. **B,** Malfunction of a QRS inhibited pacemaker. Pacemaker was set to pace at a rate of 75 per min. However, rate of pacing is variable. In addition, pacemaker does not pace when heart rate spontaneously slows. R represents a spontaneous QRS complex. F, atrial flutter. **C,** Malfunction of a QRS inhibited pacemaker in a patient with a Mobitz type II AV block; monitor lead. Upper strip merely shows a 2:1 AV block with a slow ventricular rate of approximately 40 per min. A QRS inhibited pacemaker had been inserted several hours previously, but it was no longer pacing. Lower strip was taken a few seconds later. Pacemaker beats appear (1, 2, 4, 5, 6, 7), but pacemaker is beating irregularly and does not pace when heart rate slows. **D,** Malfunction of a QRS inhibited pacemaker; lead II. Pacemaker had been implanted 2 days before ECG was taken. P, R, and T represent patient's spontaneous sinus rhythm, which had reappeared. Pacemaker had reverted to fixed rate pacing but shows malfunction because pacemaker spikes appear only irregularly. In addition, first pacemaker spike occurs simultaneously with apex of preceding T wave (R on T phenomenon). However, this did not precipitate ventricular premature contractions or ventricular tachycardia in this patient. Pacemaker was removed, and a new pacemaker was inserted shortly after this ECG was taken. **E,** Malfunction of a QRS inhibited pacemaker in a patient with complete AV block. Pacemaker had been implanted 3 days earlier. Pacemaker is now firing in fixed rate mode, but it is malfunctioning. This is indicated by loss of a pacemaker spike after fourth beat. P, patient's spontaneous P waves. **F,** Malfunction of a QRS synchronous pacemaker in a patient with complete AV block. Beats 1 and 2 are normally paced, but the remaining pacemaker spikes are not followed by QRS complexes and T waves. R represents QRS complexes of patient's slow idioventricular rhythm. **G,** Malfunction of a pacemaker that had been inserted into coronary sinus; monitor lead. Pacemaker spikes occur regularly, but only occasionally stimulate the heart and produce paced beats (beats 2, 3, and 4). P, R, and T show patient's spontaneous sinus rhythm, which had reappeared. J, AV junctional P waves produced by pacemaker.

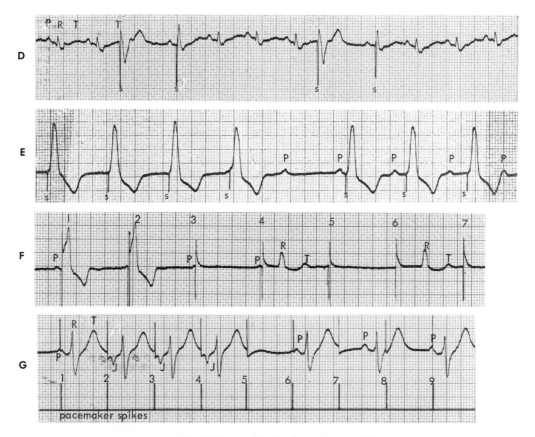

Fig. 17-2, cont'd. For legend see p. 231.

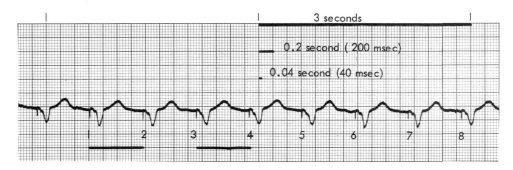

Fig. 17-3. Measurement of pacemaker rate. ECG shows a fixed rate pacemaker.

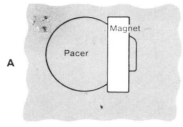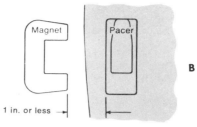

Fig. 17-4. Use of external magnet test to determine function of a ventricular demand (QRS inhibited or QRS synchronous) pacemaker. **A,** Front view of magnet overlying skin of implanted pacemaker. **B,** Side view. (Courtesy the Cordis Corp.)

be responsive (from just before the end of the T wave to the next QRS complex) (Fig. 17-1, *A*).

A fixed rate pacemaker may appear to be defective because pacing occurs only sporadically. This may be due to inadequate amperage of the pacemaker. Therefore, pacing occurs only when the pacemaker pulse is simultaneous with the *supernormal phase of recovery* of the ventricular muscle, at the end of the T wave (just before the U wave). This is corrected by increasing the milliamperage.

Testing an implanted QRS inhibited pacemaker

Demand pacemakers (QRS inhibited and synchronous) are more complex than fixed rate pacemakers and must be tested for their ability to *pace* at a fixed rate when the patient's heart slows and for their ability to *sense* R waves. This can be done by two special tests: the external magnet test and the external pacemaker test.

External magnet test. The external magnet test determines the demand pacemaker's ability to *pace* at a fixed rate. When a suitable magnet is applied externally over an implanted demand pacemaker (either a QRS inhibited or QRS synchronous pacemaker), a magnetically controlled reed switch will close, and the pacemaker will revert automatically to fixed rate pacing (Figs. 17-3 and 17-4).

The magnet should be placed 1 inch or less from the implanted pacemaker (it can be placed over the patient's clothing), and a standard lead ECG is taken. When the pacemaker spikes occur at a time when the heart is not refractory, paced QRS complexes and T waves will appear. When the pacemaker spikes occur during the refractory period of the heart, paced QRS complexes and T waves will not appear. As soon as the magnet is withdrawn, the reed switch opens and the pacemaker returns to its standby state.

The fixed rate of the pacemaker produced by the magnet may be slightly different from the pacemaker's spontaneous rate. This information is found in the manufacturers' instruction booklets.

When the magnet has been applied and the pacemaker is functioning at a fixed rate, a pacemaker spike may occur during the vulnerable period of the heart (at or near the apex or nadir of the T wave) (Fig. 17-2, *D*).

When this occurs, there is a possibility that ventricular tachycardia or ventricular fibrillation may develop. Therefore, the magnet test should be done only in a hospital setting where defibrillation equipment, supplies, and personnel are available. The patient's heart can also be slowed below the escape rate of the QRS inhibited pacemaker by means of carotid sinus pressure or by IV injection of a cholinergic drug, such as edrophonium chloride (Tensilon). However, this can produce

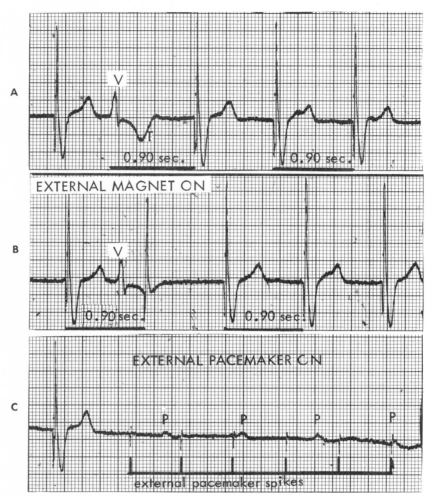

Fig. 17-5. Implanted QRS inhibited pacemaker. **A,** Normal functioning of pacemaker. It had been set at a rate of approximately 66 per min (with an interval between spikes of 0.90 sec). *V,* a ventricular premature contraction that occurs outside refractory period of pacemaker. Therefore, it is sensed by pacemaker, which recycles and fires again after 0.90 sec. **B,** Effect of external magnet test. Pacemaker reverts to a fixed rate pacing mode. *V,* ventricular premature contraction, but now it is not sensed by pacemaker. Therefore, interval between pacemaker beats remains 0.90 sec. **C,** Effect of an external battery-operated pacemaker applied to skin over implanted pacemaker. It completely inhibits QRS inhibited pacemaker. This patient had complete AV block. Ventricles did not respond when pacemaker activity stopped, so that only P waves appeared.

a dangerous bradyarrhythmia or cardiac arrest if the pacemaker is not able to function at a fixed rate. Conversely, if a patient has intermittent AV block and if the QRS inhibited pacemaker is pacing at a fixed rate, the patient can be exercised in an attempt to inhibit the pacemaker to determine if it can temporarily stop functioning.

External pacemaker test. The external pacemaker test determines the *sensing* ability of a demand pacemaker. This is im-

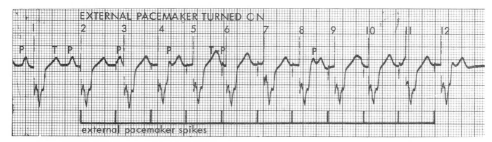

Fig. 17-6. Effect of a battery-operated pacemaker applied to skin over atrial synchronous pacemaker; lead II. Same patient as in Fig. 15-8. Pacemaker had been pacing at a rate of approximately 80 per min (beats 1 and 2). External pacemaker was then set to pace at a rate of approximately 115 per min. Therefore, atrial synchronous pacemaker rate increased similarly.

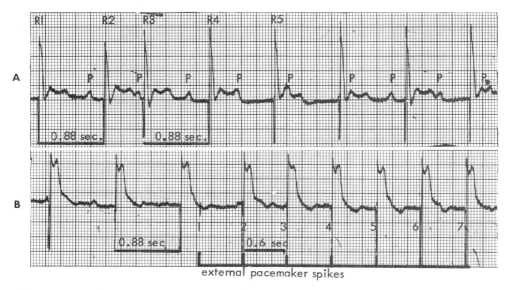

external pacemaker spikes

Fig. 17-7. Implanted QRS synchronous pacemaker in a patient with almost complete AV block. **A,** Normal functioning of pacemaker. Rate had been set at approximately 70 per min (0.88-sec interval between spikes). An occasional P wave is able to penetrate AV node and stimulate ventricles when they are not refractory. This causes an irregular ventricular rate (R_3). **B,** Effect of an external battery-operated pacemaker applied to skin over implanted pacemaker. External pacemaker was set to beat at a rate of 100 per min (0.6-sec interval between pacemaker spikes). This causes implanted QRS synchronous pacemaker rate to increase.

portant because the sensing circuits often fail before the pacing circuits fail.

When an external pacemaker is applied over an implanted QRS inhibited pacemaker at a rate slightly faster than the implanted pacemaker (overdriving), a normally functioning QRS inhibited pacemaker will stop pacing (Fig. 17-5, *C*). A normally functioning atrial or QRS synchronous pacemaker, on the other hand, will begin to pace faster (Figs. 17-6 and 17-7).

The test is done as follows. Two additional electrodes (preferably suction cup electrodes), which are attached to an external fixed rate pacemaker whose rate can

A

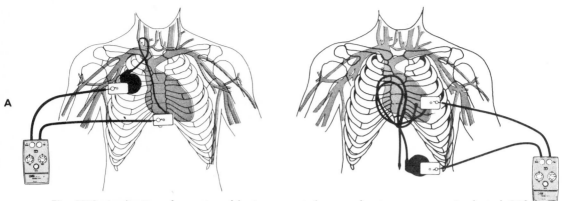

B

Fig. 17-8. Application of an external battery-operated pacemaker to suppress an implanted QRS inhibited pacemaker or to stimulate an implanted QRS synchronous pacemaker. **A,** Implanted pacemaker with unipolar lead electrode in heart. **B,** Implanted pacemaker with epicardial leads. (Courtesy the Cordis Corp.)

be varied, are connected in the following locations. When an implanted demand pacemaker with a *unipolar* electrode is within the heart, one cup electrode is placed on the skin overlying the implanted pacemaker. The other cup electrode is placed on the skin overlying the apex of the heart (the general area of the catheter electrode tip) (Fig. 17-8, *A*). If epicardial leads have been used, one electrode cup is placed on the skin overlying the epicardial leads; the other electrode is placed on the skin over the implanted pacemaker (Fig. 17-8, *B*). When an implanted demand pacemaker with a *bipolar* electrode is within the heart, the cup electrodes of the external pacemaker are applied closely together over the apex of the heart.

The external fixed rate pacemaker is activated with an amperage of 4 mA or higher. The external rate is set faster than the patient's heart rate. It may be necessary to vary the rate of the external pacemaker so that the induced pacemaker spikes fall outside the patient's QRS complexes and T waves (the refractory period of the heart). A standard lead ECG is simultaneously recorded.

If the implanted QRS inhibited pace-

maker is sensing adequately, it will stop pacing as long as the external pacemaker is activated. Regularly recurring spikes from the external pacemaker will appear in the ECG, but there will not be any spikes from the implanted pacemaker (Fig. 17-5).

As soon as the external pacemaker is turned off, the patient's implanted pacemaker should begin to pace again.

The patient may or may not show spontaneous heart activity during the period when the external pacemaker is activated. Therefore, the test should be done for only 2 to 3 sec. In addition, the test should be done only in a hospital setting in case the implanted pacemaker does not start to pace again when the external pacemaker is turned off.

Electrocardiographic signs of malfunction of QRS inhibited pacemakers

It is more difficult to identify malfunction of demand (QRS inhibited or synchronous) pacemakers than fixed rate pacemakers because it is necessary to know the refractory periods of the demand pacemakers in addition to their preset escape rates. This information is not always available.

In addition, the measured escape rates and the refractory periods of demand pacemakers may be different from the values given by the manufacturers.

The following electrocardiographic changes may occur.

1. The QRS inhibited pacemaker may be unable to initiate pacing when the heart slows. Therefore, one or more pacemaker spikes will not appear when the escape interval has been exceeded or when the magnet test is done (Fig. 17-2, *B, C,* and *E*).

2. The escape rate may become either faster or slower than the preset escape rate, or the rate may vary from spike to spike.

3. When the external pacemaker test is done, the implanted QRS inhibited pacemaker may not stop pacing.

4. A pacemaker spike may occur when the heart is not refractory, but it may not be followed by a QRS complex and T wave.

The following electrocardiographic signs can be used only when the refractory period and the escape period of the pacemaker are known.

5. The QRS inhibited pacemaker may be recycled by a spontaneous QRS complex or a ventricular premature contraction that occurs during the refractory period of the pacemaker. Therefore, the interval from this QRS to the next spike will equal the escape interval of the pacemaker.

6. A spontaneous QRS complex or a ventricular premature contraction, which occurs during the alert period of the pacemaker, may not recycle the pacemaker. Therefore, the interval from this QRS to the next spike will be shorter than the normal escape interval of the pacemaker.

Some QRS inhibited pacemakers may sense and be recycled from different portions of the QRS complex in different beats. This causes slight differences in the intervals between pacemaker spikes. This should not be considered a sign of malfunction. In addition, when the heart slows

and the QRS inhibited pacemaker begins fixed rate pacing, the fixed rate pacing may not start for 1 sec, for example, even though the rate of fixed pacing is faster (with an interval between paced beats of 0.84 sec, for example). This difference, which is known as *rate hysteresis,* is not a sign of pacemaker malfunction.

Testing an implanted QRS synchronous pacemaker

It is necessary to know the refractory period of a QRS synchronous pacemaker, in addition to its preset escape rate, just as for a QRS inhibited pacemaker. However, this information is not always available. In addition, the measured escape rate and the refractory period of the pacemaker may be different from the values given by the manufacturer.

The external magnet test response of a QRS synchronous pacemaker is similar to the response of a QRS inhibited pacemaker (p. 234).

The external pacemaker test response of a QRS synchronous (or atrial synchronous) pacemaker is different from that of a QRS inhibited pacemaker because the synchronous pacemaker responds to the external pacemaker by a change in pacing rate. therefore, when the external pacemaker is set at a rate faster than the patient's rate, the QRS (or atrial) synchronous pacemaker will respond with the similar faster rate of pacing (Fig. 17-8).

Electrocardiographic signs of malfunction of QRS synchronous pacemakers

A QRS synchronous pacemaker shows electrocardiographic signs of pacemaker malfunction similar to those of a QRS inhibited pacemaker (see above). In addition, the following changes may appear. Each spontaneous QRS complex may not be associated with a pacemaker spike superimposed on it. However, one should remember that the pacemaker spikes of a

QRS synchronous pacemaker do not appear in all leads. In addition, the characteristic spike superimposed on the QRS will not appear when the pacemaker is functioning at a fixed rate.

Testing an implanted atrial synchronous pacemaker

Current models of atrial synchronous pacemakers respond like QRS synchronous pacemakers to an external magnet and to an external pacemaker. The external magnet test causes the pacemaker to revert to fixed rate pacing. The external pacemaker, when set at a rate faster than the patient's heart rate, will induce the same faster rate of pacing in the atrial synchronous pacemaker (Fig. 17-6).

Electrocardiographic signs of malfunction of atrial synchronous pacemakers

The following electrocardiographic signs may occur.

1. P waves may be present, but they may not be regularly followed by pacemaker spikes after 0.16 sec.

2. Pacemaker spikes may be present, but they may not be followed by QRS complexes and T waves.

3. The pacemaker does not act as a fixed rate pacemaker when the atrial rate falls below the preset rate of the pacemaker, usually 60 beats per min, or when a magnet is applied. Therefore, the pacemaker spikes do not appear.

4. The pacemaker does not block atrial stimuli when the atrial rate exceeds the preset maximum pacemaker rate of 125 per min (or 150 in junior models).

5. Occasionally, when the pacemaker does not sense P waves, it may respond to ventricular depolarization. When this happens, the mechanical contraction of the ventricles stimulates the pacemaker, and a pacemaker spike, superimposed on the RS-T segment or T wave, occurs. Such a pacemaker spike is ineffectual because it occurs when the heart is refractory. This is not necessarily abnormal.

INDICATIONS FOR LONG-TERM CARDIAC PACING

One should remember that an implanted pacemaker is not a permanent pacemaker and will require surgical replacement approximately every 2 years.

The following is a brief resumé of some of the indications for long-term ventricular pacing.

1. Complete AV block with:
   a. One proved attack of syncope. A long-term pacemaker can be inserted into such a patient without a trial of temporary pacing.
   b. Congestive heart failure.
   c. Angina that does not respond to the usual antianginal drugs.
   d. Symptoms of cerebrovascular insufficiency, such as dizziness or lightheadedness, or failing memory of recent events.
   e. Progressive azotemia.
   Patients in groups *b* to *e* should receive a trial of temporary cardiac pacing to determine if the pacing is associated with clinical improvement.
2. Bradycardia-tachycardia syndrome (Chapter 8).
3. Carotid sinus syncope that does not respond to drug therapy.
4. Recurrent refractory ventricular tachycardia. Long-term pacing (ventricular or right atrial) has been used to control recurrent ventricular tachycardia that has not responded to drug therapy. The effective rate of pacing should be the lowest that effectively suppresses the tachycardia. Johnson and associates found that a pacing rate between 70 and 100 per min was satisfactory.

Long-term pacing with an atrial *synchronous* pacemaker can be used in the following groups of patients.

1. Young patients with *symptomatic* complete AV block
2. Postsurgical patients with AV block

CHOICE OF AN IMPLANTED PACEMAKER

Implanted *fixed rate pacemakers* have the simplest electrical circuitry and the lowest battery drain and are less affected by extraneous electrical interference than implanted demand pacemakers. However, it is not possible for the patient to increase his heart rate, except with premature ventricular contractions, when an increased rate may be temporarily necessary, as during exercise or fever (unless a fixed rate pacemaker with variable rate control is used). In addition, the pacemaker spikes can occur near the peak of the T waves (the vulnerable period of the ventricles) (R on T phenomenon), and ventricular fibrillation may be precipitated (p. 199).

An implanted fixed rate pacemaker can be used in patients with chronic complete AV block. However, it should not be used if the patient shows changing degrees of AV block or has persistent ventricular premature contractions.

Many cardiologists believe that a demand type of pacemaker (QRS inhibited or QRS synchronous) should be used in all patients.

Implanted *demand pacemakers* can, of course, be used in patients with chronic complete AV block. They are also valuable in patients with intermittent AV block or drug-induced AV block, in patients with complete AV block and persistent ventricular premature contractions, or in patients with bradyarrhythmias alternating with tachyarrhythmias (Chapter 7).

The atrial synchronous pacemakers are capable of stimulating the ventricles up to 125 (or 150) beats per min. This rapid rate can precipitate congestive heart failure or angina in an elderly patient. Therefore, the atrial pacemakers have been used chiefly in young patients with congenital AV block or in patients with postsurgical AV block.

EFFECTS OF ELECTRICAL INTERFERENCE ON CARDIAC PACEMAKERS

Fixed rate pacemakers are usually very resistant to external electrical interference because they do not have sensing circuits. However, patients with fixed rate pacemak-

ers should not receive diathermy treatments in the area of the implanted pacemaker, because the inductive heating produced by the diathermy treatment can stop the pacemaker from functioning.

A similar effect occurs if electrocautery treatment is used near the pacemaker. Electrocautery should not be used within 6 inches of an implanted pacemaker or lead. If a transurethral prostatectomy is done with electrocautery, the ground plate of the electrocautery should be placed under the buttocks, not in the chest area.

The patient should be monitored with repeated blood pressure recordings in addition to the ECG, because the cauterizing current interferes with the recording of the ECG.

Fixed rate pacemakers are not usually affected by radiation produced by electrical particle accelerators (see below).

Demand pacemakers can show several types of responses to external electrical interference. A QRS inhibited pacemaker can revert to fixed rate pacing or may stop pacing if the electrical interference is very strong. A QRS (or atrial) synchronous pacemaker may respond to electrical interference with its maximal rate of pacing, or it may revert to fixed rate pacing, or it may stop pacing.

Demand pacemakers may or may not be affected by external electrical interference from numerous sources, including household appliances, hair dryers, television sets, radios, electric shavers, electric blankets, microwave ovens (when the patient is less than 1 foot away from the oven), gasoline engine ignition systems, spark coils, power tools, electric garage door openers, computer tape erase heads, golf carts, 50- and 60-cycle (Hz) leakage currents, fluorescent lamps, electric motors, radio or television transmitters; x-ray, diathermy, and electrocautery apparatus; and cardiac telemetry transmitters.

Preflight screening of airplane passengers with an electromagnetic weapons detector does not affect fixed rate or demand pacemakers.

SAFETY RECOMMENDATIONS FOR PACEMAKER PATIENTS IN THE HOSPITAL

Patients with pacemakers and patients with or without pacemakers who have exteriorized wires from the heart are subject to electrical shock hazards in many ways, particularly in a hospital. Therefore, many hospitals have devised safety regulations to prevent electrical shock.

Patients with *completely implanted fixed rate pacemakers* can be treated in a normal way, with the exception of diathermy or electrocautery treatment, as noted above.

Patients with *completely implanted demand pacemakers* can also be treated in a normal way, with some exceptions. The patient with an implanted demand pacemaker can use an electric shaver for the usual cosmetic reasons. However, he must not use an electric shaver to shave the skin over the implanted pacemaker. The patient can use the bedside call button and can be placed in an electric bed. The precautions noted above for diathermy and electrocautery treatments also apply. When radiation therapy is given, cobalt radiation is preferable to radiation produced by electrical particle accelerators. The accelerators produce large alternating current magnetic fields or intense radiation that may interfere with the function of a demand pacemaker. If the patient must be treated with an electric particle accelerator, the ECG must be monitored continually during the treatment. Electrical stimulation procedures are also not recommended for a patient with a demand pacemaker.

Patients with *exteriorized wires, with or without pacemakers,* are particularly vulnerable to electrical shock. The following precautions are required. The patient must be in a nonelectric bed. Only adequately grounded cardiac monitors and electrocardiographs may be attached to the patient. Exteriorized conductors must be insulated

with flexible plastic tubing or should be of the insulated wire type. They should be taped to the skin. Uninsulated pacemaker terminals must be covered with *electrical tape.* No bare wire must ever touch the skin directly. (*Medical* adhesive tape is not a satisfactory insulator.) Conductive leads should be labeled to show the site of insertion; for example, atrium, ventricle, ground. Rubber gloves must be worn when exteriorized conductors are handled. Every person who handles an exteriorized wire or wires must avoid contact with any electrically operated devices, including lights, monitors, foot switches, inhalation therapy equipment, x-ray equipment, and communication and entertainment equipment (radios and television sets). When these precautions are followed, the patient may use any equipment, including the bedside call-bell normally found in the hospital room. However, he may use only battery-operated radios and hospital-approved television sets. The patient may use an electric razor if the charge nurse determines that its wires are properly insulated.

When a patient with exteriorized wires is transferred to another unit, the charge nurse of the original unit must inform the charge nurse of the new unit that the patient has exteriorized wires and that precautions must be continued. When a patient with exteriorized wires is transferred to another room, a member of the engineering department of the hospital must check the new room to make certain that all equipment, monitors, and so on are properly grounded *before* the patient is transferred.

For patients with *external pacemakers* all the precautions described for patients with exteriorized wires should be followed. In addition, a patient with an external demand pacemaker should remain at least 10 feet away from a television set, electrical calculating machine, or diathermy equipment that is in operation.

USE OF CARDIAC MONITORS IN PACEMAKER PATIENTS

When a patient with a pacemaker is connected to a cardiac monitor and the heart either stops or slows but the pacemaker spikes continue, the monitor may continue to respond to the pacemaker spikes, which it confuses for the QRS complexes of the patient. If this happens, the monitor will not sound an alarm. This can be avoided by placing the electrodes of the cardiac monitor over areas of the chest that will give a much larger QRS complex than the pacemaker spike. The monitor can then be set to respond only to the large QRS complexes and not to the pacemaker spikes.

CARDIOVERSION IN PACEMAKER PATIENTS

DC shock may be needed in a patient with a pacemaker if a tachyarrhythmia or ventricular fibrillation occurs. If the patient is attached to a battery-operated external pacemaker, it should be disconnected just before the patient receives the shock, to prevent damage to the pacemaker. DC shock ordinarily will not damage an implanted pacemaker.

REFERENCES

Barold SS, Gaidula JJ: Failure of demand pacemaker from low-voltage bipolar ventricular electrograms, JAMA **215**:923, 1971.

Barold SS, Gaidula JJ: Pacemaker refractory periods, Letter, N Engl J Med **284**:220, 1971.

Barold SS, Gaidula JJ: Selected electrocardiographic manifestations of cardiac pacing, Cardiol Digest, July 1972, p 16.

Barold SS, Linhart JW: Recent advances in the treatment of ectopic tachycardias by electrical pacing, Am J Cardiol **25**:698, 1970.

Beller BM, Kotler MN, Collens R: The use of ventricular pacing for suppression of ectopic ventricular activity, Am J Cardiol **25**:467, 1970.

Berstein V, Rotem CE, Peretz DI: Permanent pacemakers; 8 year follow-up study; incidence and management of congestive cardiac failure and perforations, Ann Intern Med **74**:361, 1971.

Castellanos A Jr, Hendrix L: The manufacturer and the physician; the brave new world of in-tracardiac pacing, Editorial, Chest **61**:409, 1972.

Castellanos A, Lemberg L, et al: Atrial synchronous pacemaker arrhythmias revisited, Am Heart J **76**:199, 1968.

Cohen HE, Kahn M, Donoso E: Treatment of supraventricular tachycardia with catheter and permanent pacemakers, Am J Cardiol **20**:735, 1967.

Davis RH, Knoebel SB, Fisch C: Pacemaker-induced arrhythmias, Cardiovasc Clin **2**:163, 1970.

Escher DJW, Furman S: Modern methods of follow up of the patient with an implanted cardiac pacemaker, Am J Cardiol **28**:359, 1971.

Fein RL: Transurethral electrocautery procedures in patients with cardiac pacemakers, JAMA **202**:101, 1967.

Friesen WG: Atrial pacing to control heart rate and rhythm in acute cardiac conditions, Can Med Assoc J **104**:900, 1971.

Furman S: Bifocal pacemakers, Communication, Chest **62**:237, 1972.

Furman S: The cardiac pacemaker and the manufacturer's responsibility, Editorial, Chest **61**:411, 1972.

Furman S, Escher DJW: Principles and techniques of cardiac pacing, New York, 1970, Harper & Row, Publishers.

Geha AS, Anderson RA: Permanent transvenous demand pacing of the heart, J Thorac Cardiovasc Surg **60**:63, 1970.

Goswami M, et al: Perforation of the heart by flexible transvenous pacemaker, JAMA **216**:1340, 1971.

Heiman D, Helwig J Jr: Suppression of ventricular arrhythmias by transvenous intracardiac pacing, JAMA **195**:1150, 1966.

Hollingsworth JH, Muller WH, Beckwith JR, McGuire LB: Patient selection for permanent cardiac pacing, Ann Intern Med **70**:263, 1969.

Huang T-Y, Baba N: Cardiac pathology of transvenous pacemakers, Am Heart J **83**:469, 1972.

James PM Jr, Bevis A, Myers RT: Experiences with central venous and pulmonary artery pressure in a series of 3,500 patients, South Med J **65**:1299, 1972.

Johnson RA, et al: Chronic overdrive pacing in the control of refractory ventricular arrhythmias, Circulation **46**(Suppl 2):109, 1972.

Kaltman AJ: Indications for temporary pacemaker insertion in acute myocardial infarction, Am Heart J **81**:837, 1971.

Kastor J, DeSanctis R, et al: Transvenous atrial pacing in the treatment of refractory ventricular irritability, Ann Intern Med **66**:939, 1967.

Keshishian JM, et al: The behavior of triggered unipolar pacemakers in active magnetic fields, J Thorac Cardiovasc Surg **64**:772, 1972.

Kosowsky BD: Barr I: Complications and malfunctions of electrical cardiac pacemakers, Prog Cardiovasc Dis **14**:501, 1972.

Langendorf R, Pick A: Artificial pacing of the human heart; its contribution to the understanding of the arrhythmias, Am J Cardiol **28**:516, 1971.

Mansour KA, Dorney ER, Tyras EH, Hatcher CR Jr: Cardiac pacemakers; comparing epicardial and pervenous pacing, Geriatrics **28**:151, 1973.

Margolis J: Complete heart block; procrastination suggested in using pacemaker, Letter, JAMA **212**:1524, 1970.

Massumi RA: An unusual complication of the transvenous pacemaker catheter, Am Heart J **81**:259, 1971.

Massumi RA, et al: Apparent malfunction of demand pacemaker caused by nonpropagated (concealed) ventricular extrasystoles, Chest **61**:426, 1972.

Meibom J, Andersen JD: Inhibition of demand pacemaker by leakage current from electrocardiographic recorder, Br Heart J **33**:326, 1971.

Misra KP, Korn M, Ghahramani AR, Samet P: Auscultatory findings in patients with cardiac pacemakers, Ann Intern Med **74**:245, 1971.

Moss AJ, Rivers RJ, et al: Transvenous left atrial pacing for the control of recurrent ventricular fibrillation, N Engl J Med **278**:1968.

Parsonnet V, Giedwoyn JOL: Pacemaker failure following external defibrillation, Letters, Circulation **45**:1144, 1972.

Patton RD, et al: Pacemakers for digitalis associated bradyarrhythmia, Chest **57**:194, 1970.

Rosenberg AS, Furman S, Escher DJW, Lister J: Emergency cardiac pacing in hyperkalemia, Arch Intern Med **126**:658, 1970.

Rubin IL, Arbeit SR, Gross H: The electrocardiographic recognition of pacemaker function and failure, Ann Intern Med **71**:603, 1971.

Schwartz IS, Pervez N: Bacterial endocarditis associated with a permanent transvenous cardiac pacemaker, JAMA **218**:736, 1971.

Smyth NP, Bacos JM, Keller JW: Experimental and clinical use of a variable parameter cardiac pacemaker, Dis Chest **53**:93, 1968.

Somerndike JM, Ostermiller WE Jr, et al: Sleeping threshold change causes failure of artificial cardiac pacing, Letter, JAMA **215**:980, 1971.

Sowton E: Discussion. In Meltzer LE, Kitchell JR, editors: Current concepts of cardiac pacing and cardioversion, Philadelphia, 1971, The Charles Press.

Tulgan H: Electrocardiographic misrepresentation of impending pacemaker failure, Ann Intern Med **72**:251, 1970.

Waisser E, Kuo C-S, Kabins SA: Septic pulmonary embolism arising from a permanent transvenous cardiac pacemaker, Chest **61**:503, 1971.

Walter WH: Radiographic identification of commonly used pulse generators—1970, JAMA **215**:1974, 1971.

Watson CC, Goldberg MJ: Evaluation of pacing for heart block in myocardial infarction, Br Heart J **33**:120, 1971.

Youman CR, et al: Electroshock therapy and cardiac pacemakers, Am J Surg **118**:931, 1969.

Zipes DP, et al: Treatment of ventricular arrhythmias by permanent atrial pacemaker and cardiac sympathectomy, Ann Intern Med **68**:591, 1968.

Zucker IR, Parsonnet V, Gilbert L: A method of permanent transvenous implantation of an atrial electrode, Am Heart J **85**:195, 1973.

18 / Defibrillation and cardioversion

DEFIBRILLATION

It has been known for many years that if an electric current passes through the body, it may induce ventricular fibrillation. In addition, many investigators have shown the reliability and effectiveness of electric shock (countershock) to the exposed heart in abolishing ventricular fibrillation. Beck used it successfully in a patient in 1947. Subsequently, Zoll developed an AC defibrillator for applying an external electric shock across the closed chest of patients to terminate ventricular fibrillation. He also predicted that this method might be useful in terminating other tachyarrhythmias. Zoll's external defibrillator used 60-cycle alternating current, 150 to 450 V, with a duration of 0.15 sec, applied with large paddle electrodes to the closed chest.

The DC defibrillator

In 1962 Lown and associates described a new electronic defibrillator, which employed a DC discharge. The basic component of the DC defibrillator is a large capacitor. A capacitor is a condensor, a device for storing electrical energy, and discharging it when needed, through appropriate electronic circuitry. It consists of two conductive plates separated by an insulator (dielectric). Each of the plates has an opposite charge: one positive one negative. This sets up a considerable stress throughout the dielectric. This stress represents stored energy.

The maximum number of electrons that can be stored in a capacitor depends on its capacity, which in turn depends on the area of the plates, the space between the plates, and the material used for the dielectric between them. The two plates of the capacitor are charged by a battery or by some other suitable power supply. The capacitor is capable of accumulating an electrical charge within a period of several seconds. It can then release the electrical charge in an interval of milliseconds, to provide energy to defibrillate the heart or stop a tachyarrhythmia. The basic unit of capacity of the capacitor is the farad. The capacity is described in microfarads (millionths of a farad).

The energy delivered by a DC defibrillator is usually measured in watt-seconds (ws) or joules. A joule is the energy supplied when a power of 1 watt is applied for 1 sec. Since power in watts is equal to volts × amperes, energy in watt-seconds equals the product of volts × amperes × time in seconds.

Actually, the output of what is called a DC defibrillator is not direct current, because the current intensity changes with time. However, it is essentially unidirectional in contrast to alternating current, which flows equally in both directions. The exact wave form produced by a DC defibrillator is determined by the circuitry used in the discharge pathway of the capacitor and varies with different manufacturers. Lown's original instrument employed an underdamped DC discharge of 2.5 msec duration. Other apparatus show slow rising, trapezoidal, triangular, rectiangular, and various ramp-shaped wave forms.

The energy of a DC defibrillator can be described in terms of the charge that is built up or, more accurately, in terms of the energy that is dissipated when the shock (countershock) is delivered to the patient. The stored energy level is recorded on a meter that is calibrated from 0 to 400 ws. The pulse width, usually 2.5 to 3 msec, is determined by electronic circuitry and cannot be varied by the operator.

The DC defibrillator is able to be recharged in approximately 7 sec after discharge, when the patient can be given another shock at the same or at a different energy level. The DC shock should not be given until the meter reads the amount of energy desired by the operator. As a safety device, the DC defibrillator has a built-in load resistor that automatically dissipates any charge remaining on the capacitors in a few seconds when the power is turned off.

It has been found that DC shock produces less myocardial injury and less frequent atrial and ventricular arrhythmias than an AC apparatus. In addition, the DC apparatus can be charged with batteries, and small portable models for use in ambulances and first aid stations are now available.

Technic of defibrillation

The patient becomes unconscious within a few seconds after ventricular fibrillation occurs. Therefore, it is not necessary to use any anesthetic agent. However, the DC shock must always be given in a room where pacemakers and cardiopulmonary resuscitative apparatus and medications are instantly available.

Two large, well-insulated circular metal paddles are applied to the chest. Conductive electrocardiographic paste is applied to the surfaces of the paddles.

The paddles can be applied to the chest in several ways.

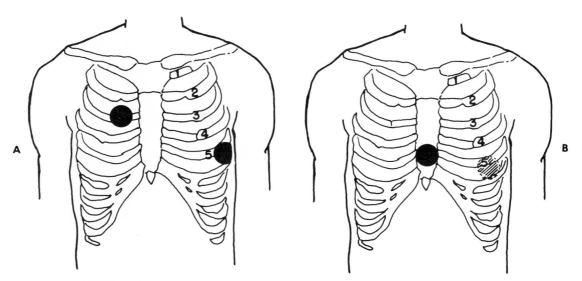

Fig. 18-1. Locations of paddles for defibrillation or cardioversion with DC shock. **A,** One paddle is placed to the right of sternum over second and third interspaces. Other paddle is placed on left anterior axillary line, just below level of apex of the heart, so that electric current passes through the heart. **B,** Anteroposterior locations of paddles. One paddle is placed over sternum at level of apex of the heart. Second paddle is placed under left interscapular area.

1. One defibrillator paddle is applied to the anterior chest wall, slightly to the right of the sternum, over the second and third interspaces. The second paddle is placed on the left anterior axillary line, just below the apex of the heart, so that the electric current passes through the heart (Fig. 18-1, *A*).

2. One defibrillator paddle is placed over the sternum at the level of the apex of the heart. The second paddle is placed under the left infrascapular area (Fig. 18-1, *B*). It should not be placed on the spinal column, because it is difficult to get good skin contact over this region. A towel can be folded and placed under this posterior paddle to keep it in good contact with the skin.

3. If the patient is connected to a bedside monitor and has chest electrodes applied, one of the defibrillator paddles should be applied at the suprasternal notch. The other paddle is placed on the left anterior axillary line in such a position that a line drawn between them will pass through the apex of the heart.

4. The DC defibrillator can also be directly applied to the exposed surface of the heart, as during open heart surgery, using special curved electrodes.

The defibrillator paddles should be pressed firmly against the chest surface. If this is not done, the electrodes may cause skin burns or dissipation of the DC shock or both.

The skin between the two electrode sites must be wiped dry before the DC shock is applied. If this is not done, the current will flow across the skin instead of through the heart and will make the DC shock ineffective. In addition, the electrodes must not touch each other. Also, there should not be any electrode paste between the electrodes. If the two paste areas touch, the current will short-circuit and will not penetrate to the heart.

If the apparatus has a hand or foot switch, one person can operate the DC de-

fibrillator. Otherwise, an additional person is needed to turn the current on.

To avoid receiving the current, the operator must hold only the electrode handles and must not touch the patient or the metallic surface of the paddles during the discharge All other personnel must avoid contact with the patient or the bed during the DC shock.

A cardiac monitor or electrocardiograph should be momentarily disconnected during the DC shock. A portable battery-operated pacemaker should also be momentarily disconnected during the DC shock. However, the DC shock will usually not injure an implanted pacemaker.

To prevent an explosion or fire, oxygen should be turned off during the DC shock.

To terminate ventricular fibrillation, an energy level of 400 ws is needed. If this is not successful, it is necessary to wait several seconds until the capacitators are fully recharged. Usually not more than three DC shocks will be needed. However, I have seen patients who required a total of nine or more DC shocks to stop ventricular fibrillation. A possible cause of failure of DC shock in ventricular fibrillation is faulty apparatus. Therefore, a different DC defibrillator should be tried if three DC shocks have not been effective.

Cardiopulmonary resuscitation should be used in conjunction with the electrical defibrillation (Chapter 2).

Defibrillation should be done as soon as possible after the diagnosis is made because it has been shown that the chance of recovery is excellent up to 1 min. However, if the ventricular fibrillation has been present 2 or more min, only about one third of patients can be resuscitated.

After the defibrillator has been used, the paddles should be carefully cleaned. Other wise a metallic oxide will form and interfere with the current flow. If the metal surfaces of the paddles become corroded, they can be cleaned with an abrasive cleaner, even with sandpaper. The paddles can be cold sterilized, if necessary.

CARDIOVERSION
The DC cardioverter

It has been long known that the heart is not uniformly susceptible to ventricular fibrillation during the cardiac cycle. The heart is particularly vulnerable in late systole at a time coinciding with a limited period of 30 msec just preceding the apex of the T wave of the ECG.

When ventricular fibrillation is treated with DC shock, the shock can be *unsynchronized;* that is, it can be given at any time in the cardiac cycle. However, if DC shock is used to terminate a paroxysmal tachycardia and if it is given during the vulnerable period of the cardiac cycle, the patient may develop ventricular fibrillation as a complication of the shock. Therefore, it is important to deliver the shock outside this vulnerable period.

In order to do this, Lown developed an electronic synchronizer in association with his DC defibrillator. He called this instrument a cardioverter, and the technic of terminating tachyarrhythmias this way, *cardioversion,* or *synchronized* DC shock. In this way, the DC shock is triggered by the R wave of the ECG. Actually, the synchronized DC shock occurs not with the peak of the R wave, but after a very slight delay of approximately 20 to 30 msec. (When the heart rate is faster than 100 per min, the synchronous signal may not always appear with each R wave, but with every other R wave.)

Theoretically, the timing of the synchronized shock can be varied, and it can be discharged at any preselected point in the cardiac cycle. Practically, this is not necessary, and the timing of the synchronization is preset in the cardioverter.

In order to deliver a synchronized DC shock, the cardioverter must be connected to an oscilloscope that records the patient's ECG. A lead, such as lead I or II, which shows a tall R wave, should be selected.

Regular metal electrocardiographic electrodes are then connected to the patient's right arm, left arm, left leg, and right leg (as a ground). The oscilloscope is then connected to the cardioverter.

When the synchronizer is connected to the cardioverter, one must make certain that the time delay circuit is triggered by the R wave because it can also be triggered by a large T wave if the sensitivity of the control is set too high. The apparatus is not able to distinguish R waves from any other wave form, and the discharge follows the highest wave in the cardiac cycle. Usually, this is an R wave. However, there are many conditions in which an rS pattern is present and the r wave is smaller than the succeeding T wave. If the countershock is triggered by a tall T wave, ventricular fibrillation may occur.

In addition, the sensitivity control should be checked before the DC shock is delivered, to make certain that it is not firing in response to a T wave. For example, in the BD Electrodyne DC pulse defibrillator, the sensitivity control is turned clockwise until the synchronizer button blinks with each heartbeat. This establishes the "threshold point." The control is then turned about one-fourth turn further to get the proper setting. However, if the sensitivity control is advanced too far, a double blink will occur. This indicates that the synchronizer is picking up a T wave in addition to the R wave.

Technic of cardioversion
Preparation

The general rules described for defibrillation also apply. The patient should not receive either fluids or solid food for at least 8 hours before elective cardioversion. This will prevent regurgitation and aspiration into the lungs during the cardioversion anesthesia. An anesthetist should be present because if complications occur, it may be necessary to intubate the patient and start artificial respiration.

A 12-lead ECG should be taken. The patient is then connected to the oscilloscope of the cardioverter. The synchronous discharge of the cardioverter is then tested and adjusted so that the discharge signal occurs simultaneously with the R wave of the patient's ECG.

When energies of 50 ws or less are needed, particularly in terminating atrial flutter, anesthesia may not be needed. Instead, the patient can be given premedication with 100 mg meperidine (Demerol) and 100 mg secobarbital (Seconal), both given IM. However, an analgesic should be given IV if higher energies are needed. This can be provided in several ways.

The anesthetist should give the patient 100% oxygen for 5 min before the anesthesia is given. The purpose of the oxygen is to avoid respiratory depression, which can produce serious postconversion arrhythmias. In addition, heavy sedation with meperidine, prochlorperazine (Compazine), or similar drugs prior to the anesthesia should be avoided.

Diazepam (Valium), 5 mg, can then be given IV every 5 min for a total dose of 10 to 20 mg. Each 5 mg should be injected in a period of at least 1 min. The diazepam should not be mixed with any other drugs or solutions. Diazepam may cause laryngospasm. Ventricular premature contractions and ventricular tachycardia have also been reported as side effects of IV administration of diazepam.

A short-acting barbiturate, such as thiopental (Pentothal), can be given in a concentration of 1%, for a dose of 150 to 400 mg. Sodium methohexital (Brevital) can also be given IV, up to a total of 30 to 50 mg. The purpose of these drugs is to produce transient amnesia rather than anesthesia.

It is not necessary to give atropine prior to the DC shock, although some cardiologists give it to prevent the marked slowing of the heart that often occurs immediately after the DC shock.

It is also not necessary to use smooth-muscle relaxants prior to the DC shock (although I know of one patient who developed a fracture of the spine because of excessive muscle contractions during the DC shock). A muscle relaxant, such as succinylcholine, can cause prolonged muscle paralysis and apnea when given to a patient who has received quinidine.

It is preferable to stop administration of digitalis before synchronized DC shock is given. If the patient has been taking a quickly excreted preparation, such as digoxin or lanatoside C (Cedilanid), it can be stopped 1 to 2 days prior to the DC shock. If a preparation that is slowly excreted, such as digitoxin or digitalis leaf, has been taken, it should be stopped 5 days or longer before the DC shock. If the patient's condition is critical, this may not be possible. In such a case, the DC shock should be started with a low discharge of even 5 ws. The energy can then be raised to 25, 50, 100, 200, 300, and even 400 ws, if necessary.

If digitalis toxicity is present and one uses a low charge, minor complications, such as ventricular premature contractions, may develop, rather than dangerous or lethal ventricular tachycardia or ventricular fibrillation. If ventricular premature contractions appear, they can be treated with an IV bolus of 75 mg lidocaine.

Propranolol (Inderal) should *not* be used prior to the synchronized DC shock, because it may cause cardiac standstill after the shock.

Serum electrolyte concentrations, particularly the serum potassium concentration, should be normal before synchronized DC shock is given.

Technic

The cardioverter is charged to 25 ws. The paddles are coated with a conductive electrocardiographic paste and applied to the chest as for terminating ventricular fibrillation (p. 244). If a countershock of 25 ws is not adequate, 50 ws is then given. If this is also not adequate, further energies of 100, 200, 300, and 400 ws are given.

After each DC shock, the ECG should be observed to see if sinus rhythm has returned. It may take a few seconds after a DC shock for the base line of the ECG to stabilize.

When the DC shock is given, a vertical spike will appear on the oscilloscope screen, and the energy level of the cardioverter will temporarily fall to zero. A second shock can be given in approximately 7 sec, when the capacitators have recharged fully.

If the patient's clinical situation is desperate, an unsynchronized DC shock can be given. If ventricular fibrillation develops, this usually can be terminated by a second DC shock.

The patient will respond to the DC shock with a twitching of the chest muscles, jerking of the arms, and occasionally with an audible sigh. The patient is usually awake within 1 to 5 min. The patient may notice a mild ache of his chest muscles, and an area of erythema may develop where the paddle edges touched the skin.

A 12-lead ECG should be taken as soon possible after the DC shock. The patient should be monitored for at least 8 hours after the DC shock, to detect the late development of postshock arrhythmias. Vital signs, including blood pressure should be checked every 15 min for 1 hour.

Indications for cardioversion

1. Atrial flutter. Synchronized DC shock, even with a very small energy discharge (as low as 1 to 5 ws) is very effective in abolishing atrial flutter. However, I and many other cardiologists still prefer to treat atrial flutter initially with drugs (Chapter 6).

2. Ventricular tachycardia. When the patient is critically ill and when congestive heart failure, hypotension, or cardiogenic shock is present and drug therapy has been ineffective, synchronized DC shock should be used.

When the patient is critically ill or in cardiogenic shock, there may not be time to adequately synchronize the DC shock. In such a patient, an unsynchronized DC shock of 400 ws can be given (Fig. 18-2). If ventricular fibrillation occurs, another unsynchronized DC shock will restore sinus rhythm.

3. Paroxysmal atrial tachycardia that does not respond to medical treatment.

4. Paroxysmal atrial tachycardia associated with Wolff-Parkinson-White syndrome. Drug treatment is preferable to synchronized DC shock because the patient usually has innumerable attacks of tachycardia (Chapter 8). However, if severe congestive heart failure or cardiogenic shock is present, synchronized DC shock should be used.

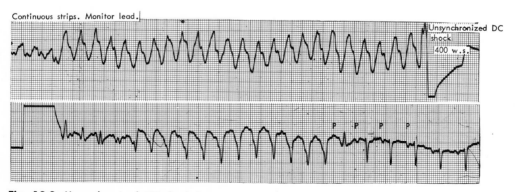

Fig. 18-2. Unsynchronized DC shock in a patient with ventricular tachycardia. Patient was unconscious. Notice that ventricular tachyarrhythmia continued for 7 sec after DC shock, before sinus rhythm returned (end of lower row).

5. Atrial fibrillation (paroxysmal or chronic) should be first treated with drugs (Chapter 6). However, synchronous DC shock can be used in the following conditions.

   a. When the rapid ventricular rate does not respond to medical treatment.
   b. When severe congestive heart failure persists in spite of adequate digitalization.
   c. When hyperthyroidism is the cause of the atrial fibrillation and the atrial fibrillation persists after the hyperthyroidism has been controlled.
   d. When atrial fibrillation persists for 2 to 3 months after cardiac surgery for rheumatic heart disease. (When mitral insufficiency is present with a giant left atrium, it may take 2 to 3 months for the left atrium to shrink after cardiac surgery. If DC shock is given before the left atrium shrinks adequately, the atrial fibrillation usually recurs.)
   e. When the atrial fibrillation is acute or has been present less than 1 year. (The atrial fibrillation tends to recur in patients who have had it longer than 1 year.)

Technic of cardioversion for atrial fibrillation

Quinidine is given in a dose of 0.3 to 0.4 gm orally every 6 hours starting 1 to 2 days prior to the cardioversion. In an emergency, it can be started as soon as the DC shock is given. There are several reasons for using quinidine this way. First, the oral doses of quinidine may cause sinus rhythm to reappear without the DC shock. Second, the atrial fibrillation will usually reappear unless the quinidine therapy is continued indefinitely. Therefore, if the patient shows intolerance to quinidine, such as cinchonism, gastrointestinal symptoms, or other symptoms (see Quinidine in Part three), or if the patient has developed thrombocytopenia prior to administration of the quinidine, DC shock should not be given.

It is preferable to stop administration of

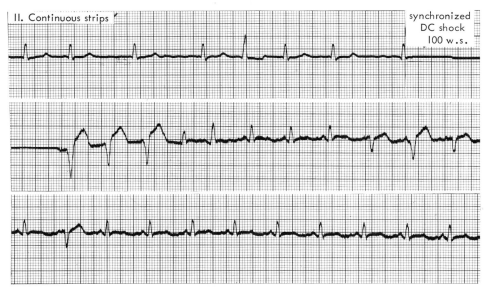

Fig. 18-3. Cardioversion for atrial fibrillation; lead II. A few ventricular premature contractions occurred after DC shock (second row) but quickly disappeared without medication.

digitalis before synchronized DC shock is given (see Technic of Cardioversion.)

Anticoagulants are not given routinely when atrial fibrillation is treated with DC shock. However, they should be used if: (1) the patient gives a history of pulmonary or systemic emboli, (2) the atrial fibrillation has been present for 3 months or longer, or (3) the patient has rheumatic heart disease with mitral insufficiency or mitral stenosis. Anticoagulants should be started 10 days to 2 weeks prior to the DC shock and should be continued for at least 1 week afterward.

One should remember that thrombosis of the left or right atrial appendage occurs chiefly in rheumatic heart disease due to myocarditis, rather than to the atrial fibrillation, and that thrombosis and embolism occur much less commonly when atrial fibrillation is associated with conditions other than rheumatic heart disease.

The initial discharge should be 50 ws. If this is not effective, higher energy discharges should be used (see Technic of Cardioversion, above).

Contraindications to cardioversion

1. Chronic atrial fibrillation, particularly if rheumatic heart disease with mitral stenosis or mitral insufficiency has been present for several years. The atrial fibrillation usually returns shortly after the DC shock, even when quinidine therapy is continued.

2. Atrial fibrillation or atrial flutter with a slow ventricular rate of approximately 60 per min.

3. Atrial fibrillation or atrial flutter, with complete AV block.

4. Atrial fibrillation, when the patient is sensitive to quinidine, because the atrial fibrillation will reappear unless the quinidine is given continually for an indefinite time.

5. When hypokalemia is present. This should be corrected before the DC shock is given.

6. When digitalis toxicity is present (Chapter 8).

7. When atrial fibrillation is present and the patient is scheduled for cardiac surgery, and for 2 to 3 months after cardiac surgery (see above).

8. When the patient has repeated attacks of paroxysmal tachycardia, unless severe congestive heart failure or cardiogenic shock is present.

9. When atrial fibrillation is associated with acute hyperthyroidism. The hyperthyroidism should be treated first (see above).

10. If two previous attempts at cardioversion have failed.

Complications of cardioversion
Supraventricular arrhythmias

For 1 to 2 sec after DC shock (synchronized or unsynchronized) the patient's muscular contractions may interfere with the recording of the ECG. Theoretically, regular sinus rhythm should then be present. However, because of increased vagal tone, the sinus node may not function normally after either synchronized or unsynchronized DC shock. Therefore, sinus bradycardia, wandering pacemaker, AV junctional rhythm, or AV junctional or ventricular escape beats often appear. They are not serious. However, if these bradyarrhythmias persist and cannot be made to disappear with atropine, underlying disease of the sinus node (sick sinus syndrome; see below), rather than a vagal effect, may exist, or premedication with digitalis or quinidine may have been excessive.

Rarely, cardiac standstill occurs after DC shock. Again, this is probably a result of hypoxia or excessive premedication with cardiac-depressant drugs such as procainamide (Pronestyl), quinidine, or propranolol (Inderal).

Sick sinus syndrome. The whimsical term sick sinus syndrome has been used with several different meanings. Lown has pointed out that about 5% to 10% of patients with atrial fibrillation who receive synchronized

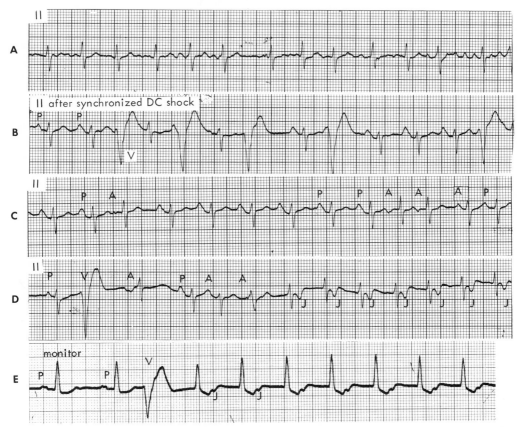

Fig. 18-4. Sick sinus syndrome. **A,** Just prior to DC shock. **B,** One minute after DC shock. Ventricular premature contractions *(V)* are present. A short run of ventricular tachycardia (not shown) developed a few moments after **B** was taken, and patient was given an IV bolus of 50 mg lidocaine. **C** and **D,** A few minutes after lidocaine had been given. **C,** Atrial premature contractions *(A)* interrupting sinus rhythm. **D,** A ventricular premature contraction *(V)* is present, as well as atrial premature contractions *(A)*, which are followed by an AV junctional tachycardia. **J,** the junctional atrial waves. **E,** Next day. Sinus rhythm is interrupted by a ventricular premature contraction *(V)* and an AV junctional tachycardia *(J)*.

DC shock do not develop sinus rhythm immediately after the cardioversion, but develop numerous abnormal atrial rhythms, including SA block, atrial standstill, multiple atrial premature contractions, or paroxysmal atrial tachycardia alternating with an AV junctional rhythm (Fig. 18-4). If sinus rhythm develops, it is only transitory, and atrial fibrillation promptly recurs.

Others have used the term to describe patients whose condition alternates between attacks of bradyarrhythmias and tachyarrhythmias (Chapter 8) or patients who show marked sinus bradycardia.

Occasionally, when synchronized DC shock is used to convert atrial flutter or paroxysmal atrial tachycardia, atrial fibrillation rather than sinus rhythm may occur. One explanation is that the DC shock occurred during the vulnerable period of the atria (just before the apex of the atrial T wave—the Ta wave—which consists of the P-R interval and a small wave that follows the P-R interval, but which is hidden in the QRS complex and the first portion of the RS-T segment).

Ventricular arrhythmias

A few ventricular premature contractions may occur immediately after the synchronized DC shock and then disappear spontaneously (Fig. 18-3). However, if they do not disappear, they must be treated promptly with an IV bolus of lidocaine or an IV lidocaine drip (Fig. 18-4).

Ventricular tachycardia and ventricular fibrillation can also occur immediately after DC shock as a result of digitalis or quinidine toxicity or hypoxia. Although these arrhythmias usually occur immediately after the DC shock, they may not appear for 8 or more hours.

Rarely, ventricular fibrillation occurs immediately after synchronized DC shock. A simple explanation for this is that the shock was not synchronized with the R wave of the ECG, but occurred during the vulnerable period, just before the apex of the T wave. This mistake can easily occur if DC shock is given to a patient with ventricular tachycardia (where the QRS complexes are wide). This can be avoided if a lead is chosen where a sharp, tall R wave is present; or, if the synchronization can be adjusted, the timing of the shock should be as close as possible to the onset of the QRS complex. If ventricular fibrillation occurs, another DC shock should be given immediately, with a setting of 400 ws.

The exact cause of these serious ventricular arrhythmias is not always certain. Digitalis toxicity is often present. Therefore, synchronized DC shock should not be given if digitalis toxicity is the cause of the tachyarrhythmia. (The only possible exception to this is the development of ventricular fibrillation due to digitalis toxicity; see Chapter 8.)

Another cause of serious abnormal ventricular rhythms after synchronized DC shock is hypokalemia. This is common in patients who have been receiving diuretics. The hypokalemia should be corrected before DC shock is given. Another factor may be the excessive use of cardiac-depressant drugs, such as propranolol, procainamide, or quinidine. Hypoxia is still another factor that produces serious ventricular arrhythmias after DC shock. Finally, many of the patients who develop ventricular arrhythmias after DC shock have serious myocardial disease, including recent or multiple myocardial infarctions.

Other complications

A mild first-degree burn of the chest beneath the paddle areas may occur. This does not require treatment.

Clinical signs of myocardial injury do not occur even after numerous DC shocks. However, elevated RS-T segments or downward T waves may develop, and the SGOT, LDH, and CPK enzyme levels may rise, due to their release from skeletal muscles.

Enlargement of the heart, with right-sided congestive heart failure, or acute pulmonary edema may occur when sinus rhythm is restored in patients who have had atrial fibrillation. One mechanism for this is that right atrial contractions may become more effective than left atrial contractions when sinus rhythm develops. As a result, more blood is pumped into the right ventricle and into the lungs than can be pumped by the left atrium into the left ventricle. Another explanation for the development of pulmonary edema after sinus rhythm is restored is that a dilated weakened left ventricle may not be able to pump the increased blood it receives from the left atrium when sinus rhythm returns. A large left ventricle and left-sided heart failure may therefore be a contraindication to cardioversion if atrial fibrillation or other atrial tachyarrhythmias are present.

Systemic or pulmonary embolizations may occur when sinus rhythm appears in patients with chronic atrial fibrillation, particularly if rheumatic heart disease is present. The incidence of this can be decreased by prior anticoagulation (see Treatment of Atrial Fibrillation with Cardioversion, above).

REFERENCES

Aberg H, Cullhead I: Direct current countershock complications, Acta Med Scand **183**:415, 1968.

Barrett JA, Hey EB Jr: Ventricular arrhythmias associated with the use of diazepam for cardioversion, JAMA **214**:1323, 1970.

Budow J, Natarajan P, Kroop IH: Pulmonary edema following direct current cardioversion for atrial arrhythmias, JAMA **218**:1803, 1971.

Castellanos A Jr, Lemberg L: Electrophysiology of pacing and cardioversion, New York, 1969, Appleton-Century-Crofts.

Cheng TO: Rapid atrial pacing in conversion of atrial flutter, Letter, Am J Cardiol **31**:287, 1973.

Editorial: Complications of direct-current countershock, JAMA **190**:465, 1964.

Engel TR, Schaal SF: The use of digitalis in the "sick sinus syndrome," Am J Cardiol **31**:129, 1973.

Fartel AB: Direct current countershock without anesthesia, JAMA **199**:939, 1967.

Ferrer MI: The sick sinus syndrome, Circulation **47**:635, 1973.

Gomaa M, et al: Pulmonary edema after direct current countershock, Chest **62**:623, 1972.

Graf WS, Etkins P: Ventricular tachycardia after synchronized direct-current countershock, JAMA **190**:470, 1964.

Green HL, et al: Clinical performance criteria—defibrillators; instrumentation study group, circulation **47**(Suppl A):359, 1973.

Grogono AW: Anaesthesia for atrial defibrillation; effect of quinidine on muscular relaxation, Lancet **2**:1039, 1963.

Leonard PF: Apparatus and appliances. IV. The capacitator and defibrillators: AC and DC, Anesth Analg **46**:247, 1967.

Lown B: Electrical reversion of cardiac arrhythmias, Br Heart J **29**:469, 1967.

Lown B, Amarasingham R, Neuman J: New method for terminating cardiac arrhythmias, JAMA **182**:548, 1962.

Lown B, Kleiger R, Wolff G: The technique of cardioversion, Am Heart J **67**:282, 1964.

Meltzer LE, Kitchell JR: Danger in cardioversion; height of R and T waves, Letter JAMA **191**:253, 1965.

Miller PH: Potential fire hazard in defibrillation, Letter, JAMA **221**:192, 1972.

Muenster JJ, Rosenburg MS, Carleton RA, and Graettinger JS: Comparison between diazepam and sodium thiopental during DC cardioversion, JAMA **199**:758, 1967.

Parsonnet V: Pacemaker failure following external defibrillation, Letter, Circulation **45**:1144, 1972.

Post M, Killip T: Application of cardiac pacing to acute myocardial infarction. In Meltzer LE, Dunning AJ, editors: Textbook of coronary care, Philadelphia, 1972, The Charles Press.

Rabbino MD, Likoff W, Dreifus LS: Complications and limitations of direct-current countershock, JAMA **190**:417, 1964.

Resnekov L: Present status of electroconversion in the management of cardiac dysrhythmias, Circulation **47**:1356, 1973.

Rosen KM, et al: Failure of rapid atrial pacing in the conversion of atrial flutter, Am J Cardiol **29**:524, 1972.

Rossi M, Lown B: The use of quinidine in cardioversion, Am J Cardiol **19**:234, 1967.

Schulman CL, et al: The "sick sinus" syndrome; clinical spectrum, Circulation **42**:(Suppl 3): 43, 1970.

Thomas TV: Cardioversion of atrial fibrillation after valve replacement, Annotation, Am Heart J **84**:840, 1972.

Woolfolk DI, et al: The effect of quinidine on electrical energy required for ventricular defibrillation, Am Heart J **72**:659, 1966.

Zoll PM, et al: Termination of ventricular fibrillation in man by externally applied electric countershock, N Engl J Med **254**:727, 1956.

19 / Cardiac monitoring systems

The mortality from acute myocardial infarction is very high the first few days after the patient is admitted to the hospital. More than 45% of the deaths occur within the first hour, and about 85% of deaths occur in the first week. Many patients die before they reach the hospital. These discouraging statistics have been improving because of new developments in coronary care, such as life support stations and cardiac care units (CCU) in hospitals.

LIFE SUPPORT STATIONS

The purpose of a life support station is to prevent death from acute myocardial infarction before the patient reaches a hospital. *Fixed* life support stations have been established at air terminals, stadiums, convention halls, and other places where many people congregate. *Mobile* life support stations are ambulances equipped with a battery-powered defibrillator, electrocardiograph with monitor, oxygen, IV infusion apparatus, and emergency drugs.

CARDIAC CARE UNIT

Most of the deaths from acute myocardial infarction within the first week of the attack result from cardiac arrhythmias, cardiogenic shock, or congestive heart failure, either alone or in combination. In the past 10 years, physicians have found that prompt, effective treatment in the hospital can significantly reduce this mortality, particularly if potentially lethal cardiac arrhythmias, such as ventricular tachycardia, ventricular fibrillation, or asystole, are promptly detected and treated. This is the

reason that CCUs with cardiac monitoring systems are now so extensively available. The major objectives of the CCU, therefore, are: (1) immediate detection and treatment of cardiac arrhythmias, particularly dangerous or life-threatening arrhythmias such as second-degree AV block, complete AV block, ventricular tachycardia, ventricular fibrillation, or cardiac asystole, and (2) immediate cardiac resuscitation.

The CCU has been helpful in decreasing mortality from acute myocardial infarction due to bradyarrhythmias and tachyarrhythmias. Unfortunately, the CCU has not been associated with a decreased mortality from other complications of acute myocardial infarction, such as cardiogenic shock or congestive heart failure. In addition, the CCU does not solve all the problems causing sudden death from acute myocardial infarction, because it has been found that 30% or more of hospital deaths from acute myocardial infarction occur after the patient has been discharged from the CCU.

Problems related to the CCU may occur because a patient may become emotionally disturbed by the extensive electronic equipment in his room, by being in a room without a window, or by witnessing or hearing cardiac catastrophes occurring to nearby patients.

Patients admitted

The following groups of patients can be admitted to the CCU.

First-priority patients include those with acute myocardial infarction or suspected acute myocardial infarction, acute pulmonary embolism or edema, cardiogenic shock, ventricular tachycardia, cardiac arrest, symptomatic AV block, or pacemaker malfunction.

Second-priority patients include those with supraventricular tachycardias, severe recurrent angina pectoris, or severe right-sided congestive heart failure, or patients after insertion of temporary or fixed-rate pacemakers.

Length of stay

In some hospitals, patients with an acute myocardial infarction are kept in the CCU only 3 days. However, it is preferable to keep patients 5 to 7 days. Patients who have had a bradyarrhythmia or tachyarrhythmia should be kept in the CCU for 5 days after the condition developed.

When the patient is moved from the CCU, he can be transferred to an intermediate coronary care unit (ICCU), where constant monitoring facilities are available, or the patient can be equipped with a radiotelemetry apparatus (see below) and transferred to a regular room until discharge.

CARDIAC MONITORING SYSTEMS

A cardiac monitoring system can be equipped with one or more of each of the following.

1. A monitor screen at the central nursing station, where the patient's ECG is visualized, and a "slave" monitor screen at the patient's bedside.

2. A direct-writing electrocardiograph at the central nursing station, which can be manually activated to record the ECG shown on the monitor screen.

3. A heart rate meter (tachometer), which determines the rate of the heartbeat by averaging the R-R interval over a given period of seconds, such as 5 to 10 sec. The heart rate meter is usually triggered by the upward slope of the QRS complex. Therefore, it does not respond to a T wave, even if the amplitude of the T is five times that of the QRS. If the QRS deflection is downward, the trigger will respond to the return of the QRS to the base line.

The heart rate meter has two alarm settings: a *high* heart rate alarm setting and a *low* heart rate alarm setting. The alarm sounds when the heart rate becomes either faster or slower than the preset values. Convenient settings are 110 beats per min (high) and 50 beats per min (low).

Theoretically, the high heart rate alarm setting can be triggered by tall spikes produced by contractions of skeletal muscles. However, the rate meters have special electronic filters to prevent this.

The low heart rate alarm setting can be falsely triggered if the electrodes do not make good contact with the skin (because of drying of the electrode paste, for example). The low heart rate alarm setting may also sound falsely if multiple premature ventricular contractions, with a small r wave, are present. It may also sound falsely if the heart rate is 70 per min but a bigeminal rhythm due to ventricular premature contractions is present and the premature contractions show very small r waves. These waves will not be sensed by the heart rate meter, which will sound because it is registering a heart rate of only 35 per min.

4. A beeper, which provides an audible signal each time the heart rate meter counts. It should be possible to vary the sound of the beeper with a volume control because the sound may be disturbing to a patient. However, the beeper should be audible at all times at the central nursing station.

5. A QRS light, which will flash every time the heart rate meter counts the QRS complex.

6. A peripheral pulse meter. The peripheral pulse can be monitored by means of a special earlobe (finger, nose, or toe) transducer. Monitoring of the peripheral pulse may be helpful because a patient may suddenly develop profound circulatory collapse and appear to be dead while the

ECG continues to remain essentially normal. A similar situation may occur in a patient with a cardiac pacemaker because the monitor may record pacemaker beats even when cardiac arrest occurs and the pacemaker is no longer stimulating the heart.

7. A memory tape loop. Some monitors have a memory tape loop that is able to record and play back on demand the ECG of the preceding 15 to 60 sec or more. In this way, the electrocardiographic events that triggered an alarm can be studied at leisure.

Electrical characteristics of cardiac monitors

When the heart beats, low-voltage and low-amperage electrical currents are produced. However, these currents may have innumerable frequencies. Therefore, several years ago the American Heart Association recommended that an acceptable electrocardiograph should be able to show a flat response (without distortion) from 0.14 to 50 cycles per second and should be able to respond to frequencies of 50 to 100 cps with a reduced response of not more than

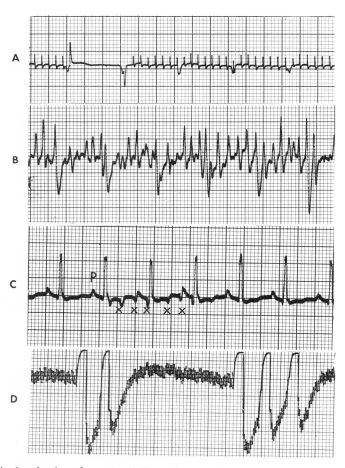

Fig. 19-1. Monitor lead artifacts. **A,** Artifacts due to electrical interference. **B,** Artifacts due to movement of patient. **C,** Artifacts (x) due to movement of patient. Monitor lead superficially resembles atrial fibrillation, but there is a normal sequence of P, QRS, and T. **D,** Artifacts due to movement of patient. Large deflections superficially resemble ventricular premature contractions. Sixty Hz (cycle) alternating current interference (fine deflections) is also present.

30%. (High fidelity electrocardiographs are able to show a flat response from 0.2 to 200 cps.)

When cardiac monitors are used, the heart currents are recorded on a cathode ray oscilloscope that is capable of displaying electrical currents or signals of an almost unlimited frequency range. However, when this happens, the cardiac monitor tracing will be distorted from "noise" (alternating current interference and other electronic signals picked up in the patient's room from lights, motors, and so on). For this reason, the frequency response of cardiac monitors is decreased to conform in a general way to the recommendations of the American Heart Association for electrocardiographs. This is done by means of electronic filters.

Electronic filters

Two types of electronic filters are used in cardiac monitors: low-frequency filters and high-frequency filters.

Low-frequency filters (high-pass filters) attenuate or block low-frequency signals. In some monitors very low frequencies, up to 0.1 to 0.2 cps, are blocked. Other monitors have switches that can block signals up to 4 cps.

The purpose of the low-frequency filters is to stabilize the base line of the ECG. Therefore, low-frequency signals, produced, for example, by breathing, slight movement of the patient, or slight slippage of the electrodes on the patient's chest, are usually blocked. Otherwise, wandering of the base line would occur. In spite of this, artifacts do occur (Fig. 19-1).

However, all low-frequency filters distort the accuracy of the ECG because as more and more filtration is introduced and the base line becomes more stable, the amplitudes of the P and T waves become smaller. In some monitors the P waves may be entirely eliminated.

Low-frequency filters can also distort the RS-T segments. An isoelectric RS-T may become elevated and may simulate the pattern of acute myocardial infarction, or it may become depressed and simulate the pattern of acute coronary insufficiency (Fig. 19-2).

In addition, the low-frequency filters can make an elevated or depressed RS-T segment appear isoelectric. The low-frequency filters may also distort and widen the QRS complexes, so that a supraventricular tachyarrhythmia may resemble a ventricular tachyarrhythmia.

High-frequency filters (low-pass filters) are used in monitors to eliminate jumpiness on the monitor scope, caused by poor electrode contact or motion of the patient. They also attenuate 60-cycle (Hz) alternating current interference that the monitor may pick up from nearby lights or motors in the patient's room. This type of interference usually occurs when the electrode paste dries and the contact of the electrodes with the patient's skin becomes poor.

In most monitors, frequency responses above 30 cps are filtered out. (Frequencies higher than this are needed to produce accurate QRS complexes, RS-T segments, and T waves. However, cardiac monitors are used primarily for observing rhythm disturbances.) Some monitors have switches that can be activated to block out high frequencies—about 200 cps.

High-frequency filters also produce distortion of the ECG. When the high-frequency components of the ECG are eliminated, the shape of the QRS complex becomes distorted because its sharp apex and nadir become blunted and rounded. In addition, notches and slurring of the QRS may disappear. The amplitude of the QRS and T may decrease, and their duration may also become prolonged.

The filters that are used in monitor lead electrocardiography may also interfere with the recording of pacemaker spikes (Fig. 19-3).

Because of these monitor artifacts, a conventional ECG must be taken on the pa-

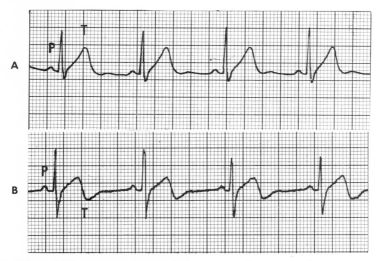

Fig. 19-2. Effect of filters on monitor lead ECGs. **A** and **B** were taken a few seconds apart. **A,** Monitor lead with a low-gain 0.2-cps filter. **B,** Effect of changing to a 4-cps filter. S wave amplitude increased, and changes in RS-T and T occurred, suggestive of pericarditis or myocardial infarction. These changes immediately disappeared when the 4-cps filter was removed.

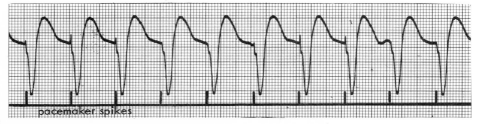

Fig. 19-3. Monitor lead ECG in a patient with a pacemaker. Timing of pacemaker spikes in this patient is shown in diagram below ECG. Pacemaker was functioning properly. However, the spikes, as recorded by monitor lead ECG, show varying sizes and are absent in some complexes. This often occurs in monitor leads and should *not* be considered a sign of pacemaker malfunction.

tient before definitive treatment is started on the basis of a monitor lead abnormality.

Monitor leads

An ideal monitor lead should resemble one of the twelve conventional leads and should clearly show all the waves and complexes of the ECG. Precordial lead V_1 is an excellent lead for recording cardiac arrhythmias. However, it requires electrodes on the patient's limbs in addition to the chest lead. Therefore, numerous bipolar chest leads have been recommended.

I believe that a modified CR_1 lead is the most practical. The positive electrode is placed in the usual position for lead V_1— on the fourth intercostal space just to the right of the sternum. The negative electrode is placed anteriorly in the hollow just below the outer end of the right clavicle. A ground electrode is placed anteriorly just below the outer end of the left clavicle (Fig. 19-4). Disposable disc electrodes should be used (see below).

Many cardiologists use a modified CL_1 lead. The positive electrode is placed in the V_1 position, but the negative electrode is placed anteriorly just below the outer end of the left clavicle. The ground electrode is placed in a similar position below the right clavicle.

I believe that this lead can cause distortion of the ECG, as compared with lead V_1 or with a modified CR_1 lead, for the following reason. When the ECG is normal, the QRST pattern will be similar regardless of whether precordial lead V_1 or a modified chest lead is taken. However, many patients who are admitted to a CCU have hypertensive or coronary artery disease and show left axis deviation. Therefore, the left arm potentials and lead aV_L will show a tall R wave. When lead CL_1 or a modified CL lead is taken, the tall R of the left arm or left shoulder will tend to be recorded as a deep S wave because the left arm or left shoulder is connected to the negative pole of the electrocardiograph. Fig. 19-5 shows an example of the distortion of lead CL_1 and modified CL_1, compared with lead V_1 and modified CR_1, in a patient who had left anterior hemiblock and right bundle branch block.

Additional monitor leads

If the monitor lead ECG shows a bizarre pattern, it may be necessary to take additional monitor leads. Preferably, the second monitor lead should show electrocardiographic events recorded from the left side of the heart. A modified lead CR_6 is satisfactory for this purpose. The positive electrode is placed on the left midaxillary line at the level of the fifth intercostal space (as for lead V_6). The negative elec-

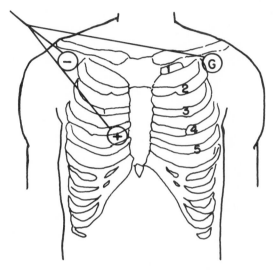

Fig. 19-4. Monitor lead, modified CR_1 (mCR_1). G, ground electrode.

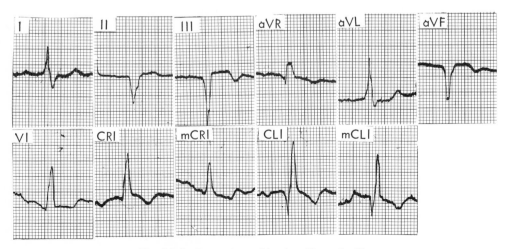

Fig. 19-5. Comparison of leads mCR_1 and mCL_1.

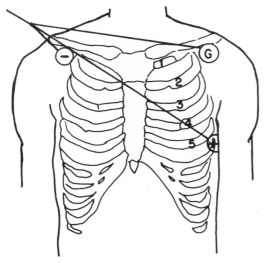

Fig. 19-6. Monitor lead mCR₆. G, ground electrode.

trode is placed anteriorly, just below the right shoulder. The ground electrode is placed anteriorly, just below the left shoulder (Fig. 19-6).

Other leads can also be used. For example, a modified lead I can be obtained by placing the positive electrode anteriorly below the left shoulder and the negative electrode below the right shoulder. A modified lead II can be obtained by placing the positive electrode on the left hip and the negative electrode anteriorly, just below the right shoulder.

Regardless of which monitor lead or leads are used, an electrocardiographic diagnosis of myocardial infarction or of any other condition involving QRS, RS-T, or T changes should *not* be made from such leads, because the patterns may appear abnormal when the ECG is normal, and vice versa. Figs. 19-2 and 19-7 illustrate this.

Size control of monitor lead electrocardiograms

The size of the electrocardiographic deflections on the monitor screen (and on

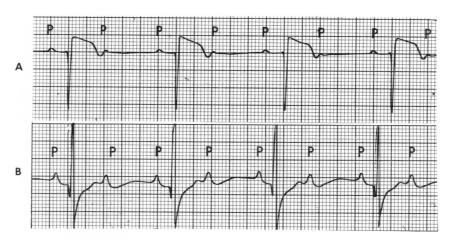

Fig. 19-7. Inadequacy of monitor leads to detect acute myocardial infarction. **A,** Q wave and abnormal RS-T elevation in a patient with an acute inferior wall myocardial infarction. A Mobitz type II AV block is also present. **B,** Few hours later when electrodes were replaced, and locations of the electrodes were shifted. Although P waves are still upward and AV block is still obvious, QRS complex and RS-T segment now do not show any pathognomonic signs of myocardial infarction.

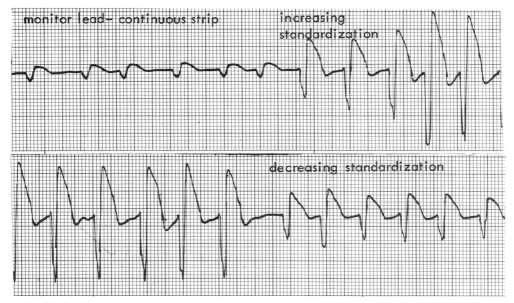

Fig. 19-8. Effect of changing size control of a monitor lead ECG. Shape and appearance of entire ECG changes greatly as standardization is increased and then decreased.

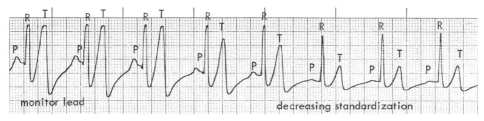

Fig. 19-9. Effect of changing size control of a monitor lead ECG. In initial portion of ECG, excessively high standardization was used. As a result, unusually large abnormal T waves, which resembled ventricular premature contractions, were recorded. When standardization was decreased, T waves resumed their normal shape.

the direct-writing electrocardiograph attached to the monitor screen) can be varied to make the ECG easily visible. The standardization should be set so that a 1-mV potential will produce a 1- or 2-cm deflection.

The standardization should be kept constant because when it varies, the ECG may appear markedly different (Figs. 19-8 and 19-9).

Polarity of monitor lead electrocardiograms

Regardless of the locations of the electrodes, the positive electrode should always be to the left, or below the negative electrode. If the polarities are changed when electrodes are reapplied to the skin, successive ECGs will show a completely reversed direction of the deflections (Figs.

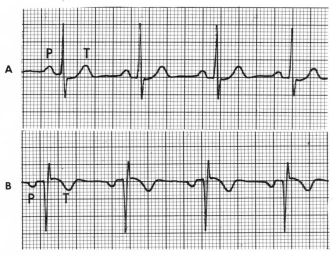

Fig. 19-10. Effect of polarity on monitor lead ECGs. **A** and **B** were taken moments apart. **B,** Reversed polarity. P, QRS, RS-T, and T of **A** and **B** are completely opposite.

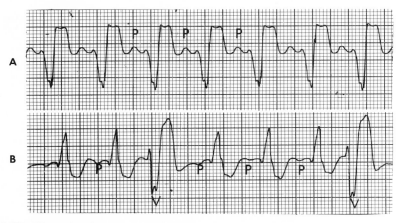

Fig. 19-11. Effect of polarity on monitor lead ECGs. **A** and **B** were taken a few hours apart. Electrodes had become loose and were changed. When they were reapplied, the polarity was reversed. **B,** Not completely opposite to **A,** because **B** shows an initial q wave, but **A** does not show an initial r wave. This discrepancy occurred because electrodes were not replaced in their identical positions. Two ventricular premature contractions (V) are also present in **B.**

19-10 and 19-11). This can be very confusing.

Electrodes used for monitor leads

It is preferable to use disposable silver–silver chloride, self-adhering disc electrodes. These electrodes are actually separated from the skin by a small built-in space that is filled with the conductive jelly. The electrodes can be left in place for several days. They allow stable ECGs to be recorded without excessive artifacts due to movement of the skeletal muscles.

When disposable electrodes are used, a drop of electrocardiographic jelly is placed in the hollow of the disc. If an excessive

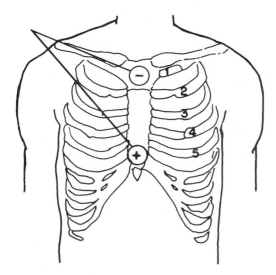

Fig. 19-12. Electrode placement for telemetry leads.

amount of jelly is used, it will spread beyond the area of the disc and prevent the disc from adhering. Electrode discs, prefilled with a conductive jelly, are also available.

The patient's skin should be prepared by drying the electrode area with a towel or gauze pad. If the skin is very oily, the electrode areas should be wiped with alcohol, and then the skin should be thoroughly dried. If the skin is very hairy, it should be shaved.

Circular metal electrodes of the type used on the extremities and chest for conventional ECGs can also be used for monitor leads. Conductive jelly is applied to the skin, and the electrodes are then taped to the skin. However, such electrodes are cumbersome and often irritate the skin when they are kept in place for more than several hours.

Needle electrodes should not be used. They are uncomfortable and can easily result in skin infection.

Radiotelemetry cardiac monitoring

Radiotelemetry is particularly valuable for postcoronary patients who no longer need to be in the CCU.

A transmitter is strapped to the patient and is attached to two electrodes on the patient's sternum, to minimize artifacts as the patient moves about. The positive electrode is placed on the lower sternum near the xiphoid process (Fig. 19-12). The negative electrode is placed on the upper sternum, over the manubrium.

Fixed-frequency quartz crystal-tuned systems, rather than regular FM broadcast bands, are used for telemetry because they eliminate cross-talk between channels and interference from other commercial broadcast sources. The characteristics of the ECGs transmitted by radiotelemetry are not as clear as with regular monitoring, but they are satisfactory. The telemetry sets are capable of picking up signals in an open area up to 300 feet. The layout of the hospital building and its type of construction determine the actual range of the telemetry. The signals may not be able to reach some areas of the hospital. Therefore, when a patient is assigned to a room outside the CCU, the telemetry set should be pretested in this room.

Dynamic electrocardiography

Continuous ECGs can be recorded over many hours with a small magnetic tape recorder (Holter apparatus), which the patient wears (dynamic electrocardiography). In this way, ECGs recorded for a full day can be scanned in a few minutes for abnormalities.

However, this apparatus can produce the following types of artifacts.

1. Pacemaker spikes may not be recorded.

2. A pseudotachycardia can be produced by a slow tape speed. This can be due to a worn-out motor or to an insufficiently charged battery. If the motor is not functioning properly, the abnormal slow tape speed will be continuous. This can be detected because a 60 beat per min calibration signal is placed on each tape. Therefore, the tape speed should be checked

when it is scanned. If it shows a calibration signal less than 58 beats per min or more than 62 beats per min, the motor is malfunctioning. If the battery is insufficiently charged, the tape will slow at the end of the recording and will be followed by a stopping of the recording.

REFERENCES

Arbeit SR, Rubin IL, Gross H.: Dangers in interpreting the electrocardiogram from the oscilloscope monitor, JAMA 211:453, 1970.

Brown KWG, et al: An intensive care center for acute myocardial infarction, Lancet 2:349, 1963.

Collins JV, et al: Basic equipment for medical intensive care units, Lancet 1:285, 1971.

Day HW: History of coronary care units, Am J Cardiol 30:405, 1972.

Gentry WD, Foster S, Haney T: Denial as a determinant of anxiety and perceived health status in the coronary care unit, Psychosom Med 34: 39, 1972.

Grace WJ: And now the ICCU, Cardiovasc Rev, 1972, p 59.

Hansmann DR, Sheppard JN: ECG-monitor artifacts, Letter, Ann Intern Med 78:621, 1973.

Helt EH, et al: Coronary care units in small hospitals, Battle Creek, Mich, 1970, WK Kellogg Foundation.

Hewlett P: Computer-assisted patient monitoring, Measuring for Med 6(2), 1972.

Killip T, Kimball JT: A survey of the coronary care unit; concepts and results, Prog Cardiovas Dis 11:45, 1968.

Margolis GJ: Postoperative psychosis on the intensive care unit, Compr Psychiatry 8:227, 1967.

Marriott HL: Constant monitoring for cardiac dysrhythmias and blocks, Mod Concepts Cardiovasc Dis 39:103, 1970.

Meltzer LE, Pinneo R, Kitchell JR: Intensive coronary care; a manual for nurses, ed 2, Philadelphia, 1970, The Charles Press.

Peterson OL: The CCU and mortality, Letter, Ann Intern Med 76:510, 1972.

Recommendations for standardization of leads and of specifications for instruments in electrocardiography and vectorcardiography, Circulation 35:583, 1967.

Thompson P, Sloman G: Sudden death in hospital after discharge from coronary care unit, Br Med J 2:136, 1971.

Wilson LM: Intensive care delirium; the effect of outside deprivation in a windowless unit, Arch Intern Med 130:225, 1972.

Yu PN, Imboden CA Jr, Fox SM III, Killip T III: Coronary care unit; a specialized intensive care unit for acute myocardial infarction, Mod Concepts Cardiovasc Dis 34:23, 1965, part 1; Mod Concepts Cardiovasc Dis 34:27, 1965, part 2.

Part three

Drugs used for cardiac emergencies

In this part the more common drugs, as well as some drugs not yet available commercially, used in the treatment of cardiac emergencies are described in terms of their pharmacological characteristics, electrocardiographic effects, absorption, indications, contraindications, side effects and toxicity, interactions with other drugs, and dosage and administration. The drugs are listed alphabetically for easy reference.

ADRENERGIC DRUGS

In 1906, Dale observed that ergot was able to reverse the pressor effects of epinephrine but that it did not reverse the stimulation of the heart produced by epinephrine. He explained this contradiction by postulating that two different neurotransmitters were liberated by the nerve endings of the adrenergic nervous system. Later, Ahlquist showed that there was only one adrenergic transmitter but two types of adrenergic receptors, which he called alpha and beta.

The alpha receptors seem to be associated with most of the usual adrenergic excitatory functions, such as vasoconstriction, stimulation of uterine and ureteral muscles and dilatation of the pupils, whereas the beta receptors are usually associated with inhibitory adrenergic functions, such as vasodilation, and inhibition of uterine and bronchial muscles.

In tissues that possess both types of receptors—for example, the blood vessels of the skeletal muscles—alpha receptor stimulation is usually excitatory, and beta receptor stimulation is usually inhibitory, although exceptions to this rule occur. In addition, when only one type of receptor is present, stimulation of the receptors may be only excitatory or only inhibitory. For example, both heart muscle and lung tissue contain only beta receptors. However, stimulation of the beta receptors of heart muscle is excitatory, resulting in a positive chronotropic effect (increase in heart rate) and a positive inotropic effect (increased force of contraction), whereas stimulation of the beta receptors of the lung is only inhibitory, resulting in relaxation of bronchial muscles.

The response of a sympathomimetic drug can often be predicted when it is known how it affects alpha or beta receptors. For example, alpha receptors respond most strongly to norepinephrine. Beta receptors respond most strongly to isoproterenol, which has little effect on alpha receptors. However, a drug may affect alpha or beta receptors in specific organs rather than generally. For example, norepinephrine stimulates the beta receptors of heart muscle but has very little effect on the beta receptors of the smooth muscles of the bronchial tree and on the blood vessels of the skeletal muscles.

REFERENCES

Ahlquist RP: A study of the adrenotropic receptors, Am J Physiol **153:**586, 1948.
Epstein SE, Braunwald E: Beta-adrenergic receptor blocking drugs; mechanisms of action and clin-

ical applications, N Engl J Med **275:**1106, 1966.

Harrison DC: Beta adrenergic blockade, Am J Cardiol **29:**432, 1972.

Innes IR, Nickerson M: Drugs acting on post-ganglionic adrenergic nerve endings and structures innervated by them (sympathomimetic drugs). In Goodman LS, Gilman A, editors: The pharmacological basis of therapeutics, ed 4, New York, 1970, The Macmillan Co.

ALDOMET ESTER. *See* Methyldopa hydrochloride.

ANSOLYSEN TARTRATE. *See* Pentolinium tartrate.

ANTIARRHYTHMIC DRUGS

The five major antiarrhythmic drugs can be divided into two groups (types) on the basis of their electrophysiological properties.

> Group I drugs, which include quinidine and procainamide (Pronestyl), decrease conduction velocity.
>
> Group II drugs, which include lidocaine (Xylocaine) and diphenylhydantoin (Dilantin), either increase or have no effect on conduction velocity.

Propranolol (Inderal) is considered a group I drug although it has some actions of group II drugs (see below).

Groups I and II drugs suppress automaticity in the His-Purkinje system in concentrations that have very little effect on the automaticity of the SA node. Therefore, any of these drugs can easily abolish a tachyarrhythmia that occurs when an ectopic pacemaker discharges (regularly or irregularly) faster than the normal pacemaker in the SA node. However, group I and group II antiarrhythmic drugs affect reentrant types of ventricular tachyarrhythmias in different ways. For example, a reentrant type of ventricular tachyarrhythmia can occur as follows. Normally, a stimulus spreads through the Purkinje network in a uniform way, as shown in Fig. 1, *A*. This is indicated by the spread of the stimulus through pathways *a* and *b*. In Fig. 1, *B*, unidirectional block is present in pathway *a*. However, the stimulus traveling down pathway *b* can penetrate the unidirectional block when it spreads through pathway *a* in a retrograde fashion. If it reaches the point of bifurcation when the Purkinje fibers are no longer refractory, it can recycle into pathway *b* again, producing a circus movement type of reentrant tachyarrhythmia.

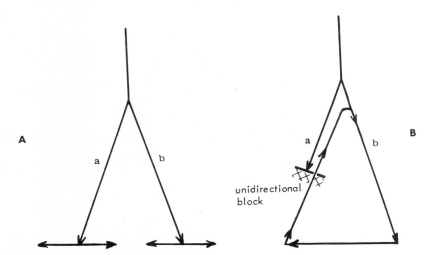

Fig. 1. Diagrams showing reentry mechanism in Purkinje fibers. **A,** Normal spread of stimulus through Purkinje fibers, *a* and *b*. **B,** How a circus type of reentry phenomenon can occur after unidirectional block.

Group I antiarrhythmic drugs (including propranolol, bretylium, and potassium salts) abolish the reentrant tachyarrhythmia by theoretically producing a bidirectional block instead of a unidirectional block.

Group II antiarrhythmic drugs abolish the reentrant tachyarrhythmia by abolishing the unidirectional block.

Groups I and II antiarrhythmic drugs can also affect reentrant tachyarrhythmias in another way; namely, by causing the effective refractory period of the Purkinje fibers and of heart muscle cells to become relatively long in relation to the action potential duration. This also occurs in two ways. Group I drugs lengthen both the effective refractory period and the action potential duration, but lengthen the effective refractory period more than the action potential duration. Group II drugs (including propranolol) shorten both the effective refractory period and the action potential duration, but the effective refractory period is shortened less than the action potential duration. The importance of this relationship is that the lengthening of the effective refractory period in relation to the action potential duration may disturb the relationship between conductivity and the refractory period in a tachyarrhythmia that has developed as a result of a reentrant pathway and thus abolish such a reentrant tachyarrhythmia.

Group I drugs (procainamide and quinidine) regularly prolong the width of the QRS complex and the Q-T interval so that these changes can be used as signs of the effect of the drug. Group II drugs do not have any significant effect on the QRS width or the Q-T interval. Propranolol has no effect on the QRS width, but decreases the Q-T interval.

Group I drugs are much more effective than group II drugs for atrial tachyarrhythmias, except, perhaps, those produced by digitalis toxicity.

Both groups I and II drugs have been used to treat ventricular tachyarrhythmias.

However, lidocaine or procainamide may be slightly more effective than quinidine for these tachyarrhythmias. However, ventricular tachycardia due to digitalis toxicity is best treated with potassium salts or with a group II drug (Chapter 8).

Group I drugs (quinidine and procainamide) are largely excreted unaltered by the kidneys. Therefore, smaller doses are needed when renal insufficiency is present. Group II drugs are metabolized primarily by the liver. Therefore, when hepatic insufficiency or congestive heart failure is present, smaller doses are needed.

Both groups of drugs can produce severe hypotension after a rapid IV injection or if an excessive amount is given IV.

Although the classification of antiarrhythmic drugs into two groups on the basis of electrophysiological changes is convenient, the changes do not completely explain all the actions of these drugs.

REFERENCES

Basset AL, Hoffman BF: Antiarrhythmic drugs; electrophysiologic actions, Ann Rev Pharmacol 11:143, 1971.

Bigger JT Jr: Antiarrhythmic drugs in ischemic heart disease, Hosp Practice 7:69, 1972.

Bigger JT Jr, Heissenbuttel RH: Clinical use of antiarrhythmic drugs, Postgrad Med 47:119, 1970.

Hayes AH Jr: The actions and clinical use of the newer antiarrhythmic drugs, Ration Drug Ther 6 (7), 1972.

Mason DT, et al: Recent advances in antiarrhythmic drugs. In Eliot RS, editor: The acute cardiac emergency, Mount Kisco, NY, 1972, Futura Publishing Co, Inc.

Morrelli HF, Melmon KL: Pharmacological basis for the clinical use of antiarrhythmic drugs, Pharmacol Phys 1:1, 1968.

Reynolds EW: Beta-blocking agents in the management of cardiac arrhythmias, Geriatrics 26: 150, 1971.

Weidmann S: Effects of calcium ions and local anesthetics on electrical properties of Purkinje fibers, J. Physiol 129:568, 1955.

Weidmann S: Membrane excitation in cardiac muscle, Circulation 24:499, 1961.

APRESOLINE. *See* Hydralazine hydrochloride.

ARAMINE BITARTRATE. *See* Metaraminol bitartrate.

ARFONAD. *See* Trimethaphan camsylate.

ATROPINE SULFATE

Atropine sulfate is a very effective parasympathetic blocking agent. It inhibits the action of acetylcholine (ACh) on structures innervated by postganglionic cholinergic nerves and on smooth muscles that respond to ACh but do not have cholinergic innervation. It therefore affects the cardiovascular system, the respiratory tract, the eye, the central nervous system, the secretory glands and the gastrointestinal tract, and other smooth muscle organs, such as the ureters and bladder.

Pharmacology

When atropine sulfate is given in therapeutic doses (0.4 to 0.8 mg), its main effect on the heart is an increased rate. When given orally, or when given parenterally in small doses, atropine may paradoxically slow the heart temporarily, possibly by stimulating vagal nuclei in the medulla. When given to a patient with sinus bradycardia, AV junctional rhythm, or first- or second-degree AV block, it may restore sinus rhythm. When given to a patient with complete AV block, its effect is variable. It may increase the ventricular rate in some patients. In other patients, it may merely stabilize the degree of AV block.

Electrocardiographic effects

When atropine is given to a person with sinus rhythm, it may produce a transient AV dissociation before sinus tachycardia occurs. With the sinus tachycardia, the amplitudes of the T waves may decrease.

When atropine is given IV in a large dose (1 mg) to a patient with the Wolff-Parkinson-White syndrome, it may restore a normal QRS width, although the P-R interval may remain short. It can also produce AV junctional rhythm, AV dissociation, or supraventricular tachycardia.

Absorption

Atropine may be given orally, subcutaneously, IM, or IV. When given IV, it begins to show an effect in a few minutes.

Its cardiovascular effects last approximately 2 hours. However other systemic effects may last 24 hours or more.

Indications

Indications are described as excellent, good, fair, or poor.

1. To counteract excessive vagal tone, as in symptomatic sinus bradycardia, AV dissociation, AV junctional rhythm, or SA block. Excellent. When ventricular premature contractions are present with the bradyarrhythmia, the atropine may not only increase the ventricular rate but may abolish the ventricular premature contractions.

2. To counteract toxic effects of digitalis or morphine, due to increased vagal tone. Excellent.

3. To increase the ventricular rate of atrial fibrillation when the ventricular rate is slow (60 per min or less). Fair.

4. First-degree AV block (prolonged P-R interval). Excellent. However, treatment is usually not needed for this condition.

5. Wenckebach type of AV block. Fair. However, treatment is not usually needed for this condition. In addition, there is a possibility that atropine may increase the *atrial* rate and in this way aggravate the degree of AV block and slow the ventricular rate.

6. Mobitz type II AV block. Same as Wenckebach type of AV block.

7. Complete AV block. Fair to poor. There may not be any response to atropine, or the ventricular rate may increase slightly. If the ventricular rate is irregular, it may become more regular. The complete AV block persists.

Contraindications

Achalasia, organic pyloric obstruction, prostatic obstruction, or glaucoma.

Side effects and toxicity

Excessive doses of atropine produce a sinus tachycardia, rarely atrial tachycardia, or atrial flutter.

When atropine is given for more than 24 hours, systemic side effects are common. Toxicity is related to the dose of atropine.

0.5 mg may cause initial slight slowing of the heart rate, decreased sweating, and dryness of the mouth.

1 mg will produce thirst, increased heart rate, mild dilatation of the pupils.

2 mg will produce palpitations, marked dryness of the mouth, dilated pupils, and some blurring of vision.

5 mg will aggravate all the above symptoms. In addition, speech is disturbed, swallowing and micturition are difficult, and there is restlessness, fatigue, and headache. The skin is hot and dry.

10 mg will produce still more marked symptoms. The skin may develop a scarlet rash (with later desquamation). There is ataxia, restlessness, and excitement. Hallucinations, delirium, and coma may occur.

Massumi and his associates have recently shown that an IV dose of 1 mg atropine given to a patient with coronary artery disease for the treatment of a bradyarrhythmia may produce ventricular premature contractions, ventricular tachycardia, or ventricular fibrillation. They therefore suggest that one should begin treatment with smaller IV doses, such as 0.3 to 0.6 mg.

Interactions with other drugs

When atropine is given to a patient during halothane anesthesia, ventricular tachyarrhythmias, including ventricular fibrillation, may occur. Conversely, when atropine and neostigmine are given during cyclopropane anesthesia, various bradyarrhythmias, including sinus arrest and death, can occur.

Dosage and administration

Orally, atropine sulfate can be given in a dose of 0.4 mg (400 μg; gr $\frac{1}{150}$) to 0.5 mg (gr $\frac{1}{120}$) every 6 hours.

Subcutaneously, IM, or IV, atropine sulfate can be given in a dose of 0.4 to 0.8 mg every 4 to 6 hours.

Preparations

Hypodermic tablets: 0.3 mg (300 μg; gr $\frac{1}{200}$), 0.4 mg (gr $\frac{1}{150}$), 0.5 mg (gr $\frac{1}{120}$), 0.6 mg (gr $\frac{1}{100}$), 1.2 mg (gr $\frac{1}{50}$).

Injection: 0.4 mg (400 μg) per 1 ml; 1-ml ampuls and 20-ml vials.

REFERENCES

Epstein SE, Redwood DR, Smith ER: Atropine and acute myocardial infarction, Circulation 45: 1273, 1972.

Gilchrist AR: Action of atropine in complete heart block, Q J Med 2:483, 1933.

Han J: Atropine and acute myocardial infarction, Letter, Circulation 47:429, 1973.

Innes IR, Nickerson M: Drugs inhibiting the action of acetylcholine on structures innervated by postganglionic parasympathetic nerves (antimuscarinic or atropinic drugs). In Goodman LS, Gilman A, editors: The pharmacological basis of therapeutics, ed 4, New York, 1970, The Macmillan Co.

Jacobson E, Adelman MH: Electrocardiographic effects of intravenous administration of neostigmine and atropine during cyclopropane anesthesia, Anesthesiology 15:407, 1954.

ATROPINE SULFATE	
Route of administration	Emergency dosage
IV	0.4 to 0.8 mg every 4 to 6 hours.
Oral	0.4 to 0.5 mg every 6 hours.

Massumi RA, et al: Ventricular fibrillation and tachycardia after intravenous atropine for treatment of bradycardias, N Engl J Med **287**:336, 1972.

Thomas M, Woodgate D: Effect of atropine on bradycardia and hypotension in acute myocardial infarction, Br Heart J **28**:409, 1966.

BRETYLIUM TOSYLATE

Bretylium tosylate is a benzyl quaternary ammonium compound. It was originally used as an antihypertensive drug because it is an adrenergic blocker and is able to block postganglionic sympathetic nerve transmission. It therefore produces a "chemical sympathectomy." However, it is no longer used for this purpose because patients rapidly develop tolerance to it.

In 1965, Leveque found that bretylium tosylate could prevent atrial fibrillation in dogs. Subsequently, other investigators found that it was effective in treating ventricular tachyarrhythmias and in preventing ventricular fibrillation.

Pharmacology

Bretylium lacks most of the electrophysiological properties associated with antiarrhythmic drugs, and its antiarrhythmic action against ventricular tachyarrhythmias may be due mostly to its effect in blocking adrenergic nerve terminals.

Bretylium selectively accumulates in sympathetic ganglia and in their postganglionic nerves. As a result, the excitability of adrenergic nerve terminals is depressed. However, catecholamine stores are not depleted. Therefore, a brief sympathomimetic effect occurs due to the release of catecholamines from sites peripheral to this adrenergic nerve blockade. (As a result, there is an initial brief tachycardia and a brief increase in blood pressure.) However, when the adrenergic blockade develops, bretylium acts like a typical ganglionic blocking agent, such as guanethidine, and hypotension and bradycardia develop.

Bretylium has a positive inotropic effect and increases the strength of cardiac contractions. However, this may be deleterious when it is given to a patient with acute myocardial infarction because it may increase the myocardial oxygen requirements more than it improves cardiac function. It also increases pulmonary artery pressure.

Absorption

Bretylium is poorly absorbed from the gastrointestinal tract but is rapidly absorbed when given IM. It can also be given IV.

Its peak effects occur in 2 to 3 hours, and its effects last approximately 6 to 8 hours.

Indications

Bretylium has been used in the following conditions.

1. To treat recurrent ventricular tachycardia when the patient has not responded to conventional drugs or to DC shock. It can also be used after DC shock to maintain sinus rhythm. It has been used in patients with ventricular tachycardia due to many conditions, such as hypokalemia and acute myocardial infarction, and after open-heart surgery.

If ventricular tachycardia is present in a patient with complete AV block, bretylium can be used after a pacemaker is inserted.

Bretylium should not be used if ventricular tachycardia is due to digitalis toxicity, because it potentiates the effects of the digitalis.

2. To prevent recurrent ventricular fibrillation. Bretylium may quickly stop ventricular fibrillation but may not completely suppress attacks of ventricular tachycardia until large doses are given.

3. Bretylium has also been used to defibrillate patients when a defibrillator was not available. Sanna and Arcidiancono (cited by Day and Bacaner) give 5 mg/kg, diluted in 50 ml 5% dextrose and water, in association with external cardiac mas-

sage and adequate ventilation of the patient. It is difficult to understand this effect of bretylium because of its slow onset of action.

4. Bretylium has also been used prophylactically in patients with acute myocardial infarction to prevent ventricular tachyarrhythmias. I prefer not to use bretylium or any antiarrhythmic agent for this purpose.

Contraindications

Digitalis-induced tachyarrhythmias.

Side effects and toxicity

Orthostatic hypotension is a result of the pharmacological action of bretylium. If the patient is kept supine, this is not usually a problem. However, if hypotension occurs while the patient is resting in bed, the condition can be controlled by small doses of a catecholamine such as levarterenol (Levophed), given IV, or a small IM dose (2 to 3 mg) of metaraminol (Aramine). (Bretylium increases the sensitivity of the body to small doses of catecholamines.) Or an infusion of plasma or blood can be given to increase the circulating blood volume.

Isoproterenol (Isuprel), which is a peripheral vasodilator, must *not* be used to overcome the hypotensive effects of bretylium.

If postural hypotension occurs, the dose of bretylium can be increased rather than decreased. When small doses of bretylium are given, peripheral vasodilation occurs without the positive inotropic effect of the bretylium. Therefore, hypotension develops. However, when a larger dose of bretylium is given, it causes a positive inotropic effect on the heart. This may increase the cardiac output sufficiently to overcome the decreased peripheral vascular resistance.

Other side effects include nausea and vomiting, particularly when bretylium is given rapidly IV. Diarrhea can also occur.

Interactions with other drugs

Bretylium should not be used with drugs that cause vasodilation. These include isoproterenol (Isuprel) (see above) and other beta adrenergic stimulating agents, or phentolamine or other alpha adrenergic blocking agents. Similarly, a drug such as chlorpromazine (Thorazine), which also has a vasodilating effect, should not be used concomitantly with bretylium.

Dosage and administration

An effective IM dose is 5 mg/kg every 6 hours. If the initial dose is ineffective, a supplementary dose of 100 mg can be given IM or IV (see below) in 1 hour.

Day and Bacaner have pointed out that this dose schedule may not be adequate. They have used an initial loading dose of 600 to 900 mg (7 to 10 mg/kg). This is followed by 200 mg every 1 or 2 hours until either the arrhythmia is controlled or until 2 gm have been injected.

An average IV dose of 5 mg/kg, diluted in 100 ml of 5% dextrose in water, is given slowly over a period of 10 to 20 min to prevent vomiting.

If renal insufficiency is present, smaller doses should be used.

Massive doses of bretylium are sometimes necessary. Day and Bacaner report on one patient who required 9 gm/24 hours to suppress recurrent ventricular fibrillation.

Toxicity does not occur until 300 mg/kg are given (a 60-fold margin of safety). Such a dose causes lethal convulsions.

Preparations

Bretylium tosylate is supplied to investigators as Bretylate (Burroughs Wellcome) in 20-ml vials containing 50 mg/ml. It is not yet available for clinical use.

REFERENCES

Allen JD, et al: The effects of bretylium on experimental cardiac dysrhythmias, Am J Cardiol 29:641, 1972.

Bacaner M: Experimental and clinical effects of bretylium tosylate on ventricular fibrillation, arrhythmias, and heart block, Geriatrics **26**:132, 1971.

Bernstein JG, Koch-Weser J: Effectiveness of bretylium tosylate against refractory ventricular arrhythmias, Circulation **45**:1024, 1972.

Cooper JA, Frieden J: Bretylium tosylate, Am Heart J **82**:703, 1971.

Day HW, Bacaner M: Use of bretylium tosylate in the management of acute myocardial infarction, Am J Cardiol **27**:177, 1971.

Kleiger RE, Shander D: Bretylium tosylate in acetylstrophanthidin-induced ventricular tachycardia, Circulation **42** (Suppl 3):174, 1970.

Leveque PE: Anti-arrhythmic action of bretylium, Nature **207**:203, 1965.

CALCIUM SALTS
Pharmacology

Calcium salts (calcium chloride or calcium gluconate) are used in cardiology particularly for cardiac standstill or after open heart surgery when epinephrine has not been able to increase the force of cardiac contractions. Calcium ions increase the contractility of the heart in a way that is still poorly understood.

Absorption

Calcium chloride should be given intracardiac or IV because it may cause tissue necrosis if given subcutaneously or IM. Calcium gluconate can be given IM to adults (not to children), but it may irritate the tissues.

Indications

Indications are described as excellent, good, fair, or poor.

1. To increase the force of cardiac contractions in ventricular standstill. Excellent. It is given intracardiac or IV.

2. To increase the force of cardiac contractions in ventricular fibrillation. Poor. However, calcium salts have been recommended when vetricular fibrillation occurs after a massive blood transfusion (and is associated with hypocalcemia due to citrated blood).

3. To counteract hypocalcemia. Excellent.

4. To counteract hyperkalemia. Good.

Contraindications

Sudden death has been reported after the IV injection of calcium chloride to patients who had been digitalized.

Side effects and toxicity

Paresthesias, hypotension, or palpitations may occur if calcium chloride (or gluconate) is given IV too rapidly. The rate of IV injection should not exceed 0.5 to 1 ml/min.

Interactions with other drugs

Digitalis. (See above.)

CALCIUM CHLORIDE or CALCIUM GLUCONATE

Route of administration	Emergency dosage
IV	For ventricular standstill, 5 to 10 ml calcium chloride (10%) intracardiac IV every 5 to 10 min until the heartbeat is restored. Calcium gluconate (10%) can be used in approximately 2 to 3 times the dose of calcium chloride. Calcium salts are not effective if ventricular fibrillation is present unless the fibrillation occurs after a massive blood transfusion.

Dosage and administration

When cardiac standstill is present, 5 to 10 ml of 10% calcium chloride solution is given intracardiac or IV. The dose can be repeated every 5 to 10 min.

A 10% solution of calcium gluconate can be used instead of calcium chloride. However, calcium gluconate contains only 9% calcium ions, whereas calcium chloride contains 27%. Therefore, the dosage of calcium gluconate is approximately 2 to 3 times that of calcium chloride.

Preparations

Calcium chloride: 10% solution; 10-ml ampuls.

Calcium gluconate: 10% solution; 10-ml ampuls.

REFERENCES

Kay JH, Blalock A: The use of calcium chloride in the treatment of cardiac arrest in patients, Surg Gynecol Obstet 93:97, 1951.

Stephenson HE Jr: Cardiac arrest and resuscitation, ed 3, St Louis, 1969, The CV Mosby Co.

CEDILANID-D. *See* Deslanoside.

CHLORPROMAZINE HYDROCHLORIDE (Thorazine)
Pharmacology

Chlorpromazine is a phenothiazine tranquilizer. It also blocks adrenergic stimuli and produces marked peripheral vasodilation and a fall in blood pressure. It has therefore been used as a vasodilator in patients with noncoronary cardiogenic shock and in those with septic shock.

It is used IV as a vasodilator and hypotensive drug. It produces an almost immediate and profound fall in blood pressure, which lasts 2 to 6 hours. When it is given IM, the maximal fall in blood pressure occurs 30 to 40 min later.

Indications

Noncoronary cardiogenic or septic shock when vasodilation is indicated to increase tissue perfusion or to overcome an increased peripheral resistance.

Contraindications

Shock due to volume depletion.

Side effects and toxicity

An excessive dose of chlorpromazine may produce severe hypotension, with the patient in the recumbent postion, or it may produce postural hypotension. This can be counteracted with levarterenol (Levophed) or phenylephrine (Neo-Synephrine), but *not* with epinephrine (see below).

Interactions with other drugs

Chlorpromazine can potentiate the effects of atropine and diphenylhydantoin, the sedative and miotic effects of morphine, and the hypotensive effects of reserpine.

Epinephrine can cause a paradoxical lowering of the blood pressure when given to a patient who has become hypotensive from chlorpromazine.

Dosage and administration

Chlorpromazine can be given as a vasodilator IV in a dose of 12.5 mg every ½ hour or hour as needed in conjunction with IV fluids to expand the circulating blood volume (p. 45). The average dose rarely exceeds 50 mg.

Preparations

Injection: 25 mg/ml in 1- and 2-ml ampuls. Chlorpromazine must be diluted to a concentration of 1 mg/ml with isotonic saline before it is given IV.

REFERENCES

American Hospital Formulary Service: Chlorpromazine hydrochloride. Category 28: 16:08.

Deep WW, et al: Physicians chart four-pronged attack on septic shock, Med World News 7:64, 1966.

Martin EW: Hazards of medication, Philadelphia, 1971, JB Lippincott Co.

Moyer JH: The pharmacology of chlorpromazine, Int Rec Med GP Clin May 1955, p 301.

Mueller HS, et al: The evaluation and treatment of cardiogenic shock, Med Times 98:137, 1970.

CORTICOSTEROIDS

Massive doses of corticosteroids, given IV to patients in shock, can cause marked vasodilation. This will overcome the excessive vasoconstriction that may be present and will allow adequate tissue perfusion.

Lillihei has used a single massive dose of either methylprednisolone (Medrol) or dexamethazone (Decadron) in patients with cardiogenic noncoronary shock in the following way. Methylprednisolone is given in a dose of 30 mg/kg body weight as a single IV bolus over a 3- to 5-min period. Methylprednisolone sodium succinate (Solu-Medrol) is supplied for injection in 1-ml vials. Each vial contains 40 mg. Since a patient requires 30 mg/kg, a 70-kg patient needs 2,100 mg (2.1 gm). This is contained in slightly more than 50 vials (50 ml).

Dexamethazone is also given in a single IV bolus over a 3- to 5-min period in a dose of 6 mg/kg body weight. Dexamethazone sodium phosphate is supplied for injection in 1- and 5-ml vials. Each ml contains 4 mg. Since a patient needs 6 mg/kg, a 70-kg patient needs 420 mg. This is contained in 105 ml.

Vasodilation after the injection of either drug follows in 2 to 4 hours.

Lillihei has not noted any side effects except flushing of the face and a fine tremor of the hands, which appear within 5 min after the injection and disappear in 5 min. However, gastrointestinal hemorrhage has been reported after large doses of corticosteroids when they are given to patients with cardiogenic shock associated with acute myocardial infarction.

REFERENCES

Lillihei RC: Pressor agents in cardiogenic shock, Am J Cardiol **23:**903, 1969.
Mueller HS, Ayres SM, et al: Evaluation and treatment of cardiogenic shock, Resident **Staff Phys,** Feb 1972, p 39.

COUMADIN SODIUM. *See* Warfarin sodium.

DESLANOSIDE (Cedilanid-D)

Deslanoside, an acetyl salt of lanatoside C, is a rapidly acting digitalis preparation, suitable for IV or IM use. Given orally, it is poorly and incompletely absorbed from the gastrointestinal tract. (Its general pharmacology is discussed under Digitalis glycosides.) When deslanoside is given IV or IM, its action starts in 5 to 10 min, reaches

DESLANOSIDE (Cedilanid-D)	
Route of administration	**Emergency dosage**
IV	8 ml (1.6 mg). It can be given undiluted as a single injection or as two injections spaced ½ to 2 hours apart.
IM	8 ml (1.6 mg) in two IM sites (4 ml in each site).
	If the patient has received digitalis in the past 2 weeks, it is preferable to start with one half of the above doses. Also, in the first 24 hours after an acute myocardial infarction, it may be preferable to use three fourths of the above doses. If the patient has azotemia or acute renal insufficiency, one third to one seventh of the above doses should be used (see Digitalis glycosides).

a peak in 1 to 2 hours, regresses in 16 to 36 hours, and is excreted in 2 to 5 days.

The maximum effect of deslanoside occurs about the same time as the maximum effect of digoxin given IV and more slowly than that of ouabain.

Dosage and administration

The recommended digitalizing dose for adults is 8 ml (1.6 mg), given either IV or IM (not subcutaneously). It can be given undiluted as a single injection or as 2 injections spaced ½ to 2 hours apart.

When it is given IM, the total dose of 8 ml (1.6 mg) should be given in two IM sites (4 ml [0.8 mg] in each site).

If the patient has received digitalis in the past 2 weeks, it is preferable to use one half of the above doses.

Maintenance therapy with an oral digitalis preparation can be started within 12 hours after the deslanoside has been given.

Preparations

Injection: 2- and 4-ml ampuls; each ml contains 0.2 mg (200 μg).

REFERENCES

See Digitalis glycosides.

DEXTRAN 40 (Rheomacrodex)

Regular dextran (dextran 75) is a polymer of dextrose. It has a large molecular weight, approximately 75,000. Low molecular weight dextran (dextran 40) has a smaller molecular weight, approximately 40,000.

Pharmacology

A solution of dextran 40 is hypertonic. Therefore, when it is infused, it increases the oncotic (osmotic) pressure of the blood, and the plasma volume rises as extracellular water enters the vascular compartment. This dilution of the plasma is associated with a decreased hematocrit value. The increased plasma volume lasts for approximately 4 to 6 hours. In addition, dextran 40 improves the microcirculation by decreasing, preventing, or reversing the aggregation of red blood cells.

Indications

Dextran 40 can be used as an adjunct in the treatment of shock because it increases the circulating blood volume. It can also be used as a priming fluid in pump oxygenators during extracorporeal circulation.

Contraindications

Renal disease, particularly if oliguria, anuria, or a low specific gravity of the urine is present. Dextran 40 is *not* contraindicated when oliguria is secondary to shock. However, if the patient shows no improvement in urinary output after the first dose, the dextran should be stopped.

Congestive heart failure or pulmonary edema. Dextran 40 may worsen the congestive heart failure, particularly if dextran 40 in saline is infused.

Dehydration. Because of its osmotic effects, dextran 40 withdraws water from the extracellular spaces.

When dextran 40 is infused, the viscosity and specific gravity of the urine will increase slightly, due to the presence of dextran molecules. However, if the patient has a diminished urinary output, these values may increase markedly. This may or may not indicate that the dextran is producing excessive dehydration, because one cannot determine from these values whether the rise in viscosity or specific gravity is due to a concentrated urine or to the presence of dextran molecules. The problem can be resolved in such patients by taking serial measurements of urine osmolality (because the urine osmolality is only slightly affected by the dextran in the urine). If clinical signs of dehydration are noted in association with a rise in urine osmolality, additional noncolloidal solutions should be given to expand the extracellular spaces.

Acute hemorrhage. The increased microcirculation produced by dextran 40 may increase bleeding.

Thrombocytopenia or hypofibrinogen-emia.

Side effects and toxicity

Severe anaphylactoid reactions, including generalized urticaria, tightness of the chest, or wheezing. In addition, hypotension, nausea, or vomiting may occur.

Abnormally high liver enzyme levels, including serum oxaloacetic transaminase (SGOT) and serum glutamic pyruvic transaminase (SGPT), may develop.

The bleeding time may become prolonged if excessive doses of dextran 40 are given, because dextran combines with fibrinogen.

Acute tubular renal failure may develop, particularly if dextran 40 is given to a patient with poor renal function.

If a patient receiving dextran 40 has blood glucose determinations taken by methods that use a high concentration of acid, the acid may hydrolyze the dextran, and falsely elevated glucose levels may be reported. Similarly, blood typing and cross-matching procedures that employ enzyme techniques may give unreliable results if the blood sample is taken after an infusion of dextran 40. Other blood typing and cross-matching procedures are not affected.

Treatment of side effects. Allergic reactions can be treated by stopping the dextran 40 and by giving an antihistamine such as diphenhydramine (Benadryl) or tripelennamine (Pyribenzamine) subcutaneously or IM, 10 to 30 mg, or by giving epinephrine hydrochloride, 0.2 to 0.5 ml of a 1:1,000 solution, or by giving 25 mg ephedrine hydrochloride subcutaneously or IM.

The infusion should be stopped if the hematocrit value falls below 30%.

If oliguria or anuria occurs as a result of dextran 40, the dextran should be stopped, and an osmotic diuretic such as mannitol (Osmitrol) should be given to increase the urinary blood flow to prevent an excessive circulating blood volume and congestive heart failure from developing.

Dosage and administration

When used as an adjunct treatment of shock to increase the circulating blood volume, the first 500 ml dextran 40 should be given rapidly with central venous pressure monitoring (p. 38). If the patient is able to tolerate the infusion, it can be continued at a slower rate. The total dosage during the first 24 hours should not exceed 20 ml/kg body weight. If dextran 40 is needed after this period, the total daily dosage should not exceed 10 ml/kg body weight, and the dextran 40 should not be given for more than 5 days.

Preparations

Injection: 10% with 5% dextrose in water; 500-ml and 1-liter bottles. 10% with isotonic sodium chloride (0.9%); 500-ml and 1-liter bottles. (Each 500 ml contains 77 mEq sodium ions.)

A solution of dextran 40 should not be used unless it is clear. The dextran 40 solution should be stored at a constant low temperature, preferably not exceeding 25° C (77° F), to prevent precipitation of dextran flakes. (If flakes develop, they can be dissolved by heating the solution at 100° C for 10 min.)

REFERENCES

American Hospital Formulary Service: Dextran 40. Category 92:00.

Loeb HS, et al: Hypovolemia in shock due to acute myocardial infarction, Circulation **40**:653, 1969.

Mason DT, et al: Cardiogenic shock in acute myocardial infarction. In Eliot RE, editor: The acute cardiac emergency, Mount Kisco, NY, 1972, Futura Publishing Co., Inc.

Michelson E: Anaphylactic reaction to dextrans, N Engl J Med **278**:552, 1968.

Pharmacia Laboratories, Inc: Rheomacrodex (dextran 40), product brochure, 1972.

DIAZOXIDE (Hyperstat)

Diazoxide is a nonsaluretic benzothiazide that has marked antihypertensive properties. It acts as an arterial vasodilator, probably by direct action on arteriolar smooth muscles. It also increases the heart rate and the cardiac output. Initially, it decreases renal blood flow, but then increases it.

Diazoxide causes a transient hyperglycemia that usually disappears in less than 12 hours. It also can cause sodium and water retention, despite its structural similarity to the thiazide diuretics.

Absorption

Diazoxide must be given IV into a peripheral vein. The maximal fall in blood pressure occurs within 1 to 5 min. The blood pressure then increases relatively rapidly in the next 10 to 30 min, and then more slowly over the following 2 to 12 hours, nearly reaching, but rarely exceeding, the preinjection level. (If the blood pressure continues to fall 30 or more min after the injection, one should suspect that it is not due to the diazoxide but to some other factor.)

Indications

Diazoxide has been used in the treatment of hypertensive emergencies, particularly hypertensive encephalopathy, hypertension associated with acute glomerulonephritis, eclampsia, or preeclampsia, hypertensive crises associated with intracranial (intracerebral or subarachnoid) hemorrhage, and malignant hypertension.

Contraindications

Pheochromocytoma, dissecting aneurysm of the aorta, hypertension secondary to coarctation of the aorta or to an arteriovenous shunt.

Congestive heart failure. When diazoxide is needed in a patient with congestive heart failure, a diuretic such as furosemide (Lasix) can be given IV in a dose of 40 mg, or ethacrynic acid (Edecrin), 50 mg IV, can be given 30 min before the diazoxide is injected. Thereafter, the diuretics can be given orally.

Angina pectoris. Diazoxide can precipitate anginal attacks and can cause typical RS-T and T changes in the ECG.

Diabetes. Diazoxide must be given cautiously to diabetic patients. Tolbutamide (Orinase) or insulin may be needed if diazoxide is used for more than 48 hours.

Sensitivity to thiazides.

Side effects

Frequent and serious adverse reactions: sodium and water retention, with the development of edema or other signs of congestive heart failure, after repeated injections of diazoxide (may be particularly serious if the patient has organic heart disease); and hyperglycemia, which often requires treatment when repeated injections of diazoxide are given to diabetic patients.

Infrequent but serious adverse reactions: hypotension, which may lead to shock; myocardial ischemia, which may lead to angina, or atrial or ventricular arrhythmias; cerebral ischemia, which may lead to cerebral thrombosis; unconsciousness, convulsions, paralysis, mental confusion; persistent elevation of the BUN or creatinine concentration after repeated injections; and hypersensitivity reactions, such as rash, leukopenia, and fever.

Other adverse reactions: anorexia, changes in taste sensation, nausea, vomiting or abdominal discomfort, constipation or diarrhea; vasodilation with flushing, generalized or localized sensations of warmth, headache (sometimes throbbing), sweating; nonanginal "tightness in the chest"; warmth or pain along the injected vein, or cellulitis without sloughing or phlebitis at the site of injection or both; bradycardia, or supraventricular tachycardia with palpitation; and dyspnea, or a choking sensation, anxiety, malaise, euphoria, parotid swelling, salivation, lacrimation, ringing in the ears, and increased nocturia.

Treatment of side effects. Severe hypotension can be corrected with levarterenol (Levophed). Local tissue irritation can be treated with hot packs to the affected area.

Interactions with other drugs

Diuretics, particularly furosemide or ethacrynic acid increase the antihypertensive effect of diazoxide and should be used concomitantly with it. (The diuretics also potentiate the hyperglycemia and hyperuricemic effects of diazoxide.)

The effect of coumarin anticoagulants is increased because diazoxide displaces coumarins from serum proteins. Therefore, smaller doses of the anticoagulant should be used.

Dosage and administration

Diazoxide is given IV, undiluted, in a bolus injection of 300 mg, as rapidly as possible (to avoid binding by serum albumin). If the patient is very light or very heavy, a dose of 5 mg/kg body weight can be used.

If no blood pressure response occurs, an additional 150 to 300 mg can be given after 30 min. Repeated injections can then be given every 4 to 24 hours as needed to keep the diastolic blood pressure under 110 mm Hg (or at a desired level). The injections should be continued until a single injection keeps the diastolic blood pressure below 110 mm Hg for more than 24 hours. The injections should not be continued for more than 4 to 5 days. In the meantime, the patient should be given oral doses of one of the antihypertensive drugs and of furosemide.

The injection should be made into a peripheral vein, particularly an anticubital vein.

The patient should remain recumbent for 30 min after each injection.

Preparations

Injection: 20-ml ampul containing 300 mg. Protect from light and freezing, and store away from heat.

REFERENCES

Bhatia SK, Frohlich ED: Hemodynamic comparison of agents useful in hypertensive emergencies, Am Heart J **85**:367, 1973.

Dunea G, Gantt CL: Diazoxide in hypertensive crisis, Lancet **2**:638, 1966.

Finnerty FA Jr, et al: Clincial evaluation of diazoxide; a new treatment for acute hypertension, Circulation **28**:203, 1963.

Miller WE, Gifford RW Jr, Humphrey DC, et al: Management of severe hypertension with intravenous injections of diazoxide, Am J Cardiol **24**:870, 1970.

Schering Corp: Hyperstat (diazoxide) IV injection, product brochure, Jan 1973.

DIGITALIS GLYCOSIDES (DIGITALIS)

Cardiotonic glycosides, such as digitalis purpurea, digitalis lanata, and strophanthus gratus, occur naturally in plants and can also be synthesized.

Pharmacology

The main pharmacological property of the digitalis glycosides is their positive inotropic effect; namely, increasing the force of myocardial contraction. In addition, they stimulate the vagus nerve and slow conduction at the SA node and the AV node.

Electrocardiographic effects

Therapeutic doses of digitalis may cause shortening of the Q-T interval, flattening or reversal of the direction of T waves associated with a scooping out effect on the RS-T segment.

Toxic doses of digitalis can cause almost any type of cardiac arrhythmia (see side effects).

Absorption, metabolism, and excretion

The oral absorption of various digitalis preparations varies. Digoxin is absorbed rapidly and almost completely; gitalin, slowly and almost completely; deslanoside, irregularly and poorly; digitoxin, slowly and practically completely; acetyldigitoxin and digitalis leaf, slowly and incompletely.

The effects of the digitalis glycosides are not directly related to their blood levels because of differences in protein binding, penetration into the myocardium, and other factors. Similarly, the fate of the glycosides is not fully known. They are cumulative in varying degrees. Ouabain is the least cumulative. This is followed in ascending order by deslanoside, digoxin, acetyldigitoxin and gitalin, and digitoxin and digitalis leaf, which are the most cumulative.

Digoxin is primarily metabolized by the kidneys. Digitoxin is primarily metabolized by the liver. Therefore, if azotemia is present, digitoxin theoretically may be of value. However, its slow excretion, compared with that of digoxin, negates this theoretical advantage.

The glycosides, except ouabain, are excreted primarily by the kidneys, but they vary widely in their rate of excretion. Digoxin and deslanoside are excreted in 2 to 3 days, gitalin and acetyldigitoxin in 7 to 12 days, digitoxin and digitalis leaf in 2 to 3 weeks.

Indications

Indications are described as excellent, good, fair, or poor.

1. Congestive heart failure. Excellent. Digitalis can be used in all forms of congestive heart failure, even when mechanical obstruction such as valvular stenosis or constrictive pericarditis is present. However, results are generally poor in high-output heart failure (AV fistula, anemia, thiamine deficiency [beriberi]); cor pulmonale; cardiac amyloidosis; acute toxic or infectious processes, including the myocarditis of diphtheria; rheumatic fever; typhoid fever; and syphilis.

2. Atrial fibrillation, to slow the ventricular rate. Excellent. In some patients with paroxysmal atrial fibrillation, digitalis may convert it to regular sinus rhythm. If hyperthyroidism is present with atrial fibrillation, large and even toxic doses of digitalis may be needed to slow the ventricular rate.

3. Atrial flutter. Excellent. Digitalis usually converts the atrial flutter to atrial fibrillation. Large doses of the drug are often needed (Chapter 6). If the digitalis is then stopped when atrial fibrillation occurs, the patient's condition usually reverts to regular sinus rhythm. Other patients may need quinidine or propranolol in conjunction with the digitalis.

4. Paroxysmal atrial tachycardia or paroxysmal AV junctional tachycardia, prophylactically, to prevent recurrent attacks. Excellent.

5. Ventricular premature contractions associated with congestive heart failure. Good. One must be certain that the premature ventricular contractions are not due to digitalis toxicity.

6. Ventricular tachycardia. Fair. Digitalis is occasionally successful in converting ventricular tachycardia to regular sinus rhythm when other antiarrhythmic drugs are not effective. However, one must be certain that the ventricular tachycardia is not due to digitalis toxicity.

7. Preoperatively, in patients undergoing open-heart surgery or thoracic surgery, to prevent tachyarrhythmias during surgery or congestive heart failure after surgery. Good to fair.

Contraindications

Idiopathic hypertrophic subaortic stenosis. Digitalis should be used with caution, if at all in these patients, because it increases the obstruction to the outflow of blood from the left ventricle.

Myxedema.

Carotid sinus sensitivity.

Second-degree AV block. Digitalis may induce complete AV block or the Adams-Stokes syndrome in such patients. However, it can be used if congestive heart failure is present with sinus bradycardia or with a stable complete AV block, and if the AV block has not been induced by the digitalis.

Cardioversion. See Chapter 18.

Side effects and toxicity

The digitalis glycosides are irritant to mucous membranes and to subcutaneous tissues. Therefore, they should be given orally (if the preparation is well absorbed),

IM, or IV. Even IM injections may be painful and may cause tenderness and local abscesses.

Toxic doses of the digitalis glycosides are approximately 60% higher than therapeutic doses. Toxicity may be precipitated by hypokalemia or by renal or hepatic insufficiency. If the BUN level is elevated, the dose of digitalis should be reduced (Table 9, p. 283).

The most common side effects are cardiovascular, gastrointestinal, neurological, or endocrine.

Cardiovascular. Digitalis can produce almost any type of arrhythmia (Chapter 8). Common arrhythmias include sinus bradycardia; prolonged P-R interval (first-degree AV block), which may progress to complete AV block; SA block; AV dissociation; AV junctional rhythm; nonparoxysmal AV junctional tachycardia; paroxysmal atrial tachycardia with AV block; bidirectional tachycardia; premature ventricular contractions; ventricular tachycardia; and ventricular fibrillation. Less commonly, atrial fibrillation or atrial flutter occurs.

Digitalis toxicity may also cause increasing congestive heart failure.

When digitalis is given IV, it may cause systemic hypertension. Therefore, it should be given slowly, and the blood pressure should be monitored if a hypertensive effect is not desired.

Gastrointestinal. Nausea and vomiting most commonly occur. Copious salivation and diarrhea may also occur. The gastrointestinal symptoms are due partly to local irritation of the mucous membranes of the stomach and also to irritation of the vomiting center in the medulla.

Neurological. Headache, confusion, disorientation, delirium, hallucinations, rarely convulsions, opisthotonos, or coma may occur. These symptoms are very serious and are partly due to the marked dehydration that is usually present because of persistent vomiting.

Blurred vision, flickering dots, or white halos around dark objects (white vision) may occur, or objects may appear yellow and green (yellow vision), or sometimes brown, red, and blue. Transient amblyopia, diplopia, scotomata, and even retrobulbar optic neuritis may develop.

Other neurological symptoms include trigeminal neuralgia or paresthesias of the extremities.

Endocrine. Unilateral or bilateral gynecomastia in males, vaginal cornification in women after menopause, and even endometrial hemorrhage may occur in women taking digitalis glycosides for a long time. These effects occur because digitalis has estrogenlike effects. An increase in urinary 17-hydroxycorticosteroids can also occur.

Hypersensitivity reactions. Thrombocytopenic purpura (particularly with digitoxin), eosinophilia associated with skin rashes that may be erythematous, macular, papular, scarlatinal, or vesicular, with or without pruritus.

Joint tenderness and drug fever may also occur.

Interactions with other drugs

Antiarrhythmic drugs such as propranolol (Inderal), procainamide (Pronestyl), or quinidine can be used simultaneously with digitalis. When propranolol is used, digitalis may be necessary to prevent congestive heart failure, which may occur from the negative inotropic effects of the propranolol. When propranolol is given with digitalis, the combined effects of both drugs may excessively slow the heart rate.

Digitalization should be done prior to the administration of procainamide or quinidine in the treatment of atrial fibrillation or atrial flutter with a rapid ventricular rate, to slow conduction through the AV node and to prevent a temporary increase in the ventricular rate that may occur when the procainamide or the quinidine slows the *atrial* rate. (When the atrial rate slows, more atrial stimuli can reach and penetrate the AV node.)

Reserpine and other rauwolfia alkaloids can potentiate the bradycardia produced by digitalis and can increase digitalis toxicity.

Sympathomimetic drugs such as ephedrine and epinephrine can produce arrhythmias in digitalized patients.

Digitalis may decrease the effect of oral doses of anticoagulants and of heparin, so that the patient may require larger doses of the anticoagulant.

IV doses of calcium salts may precipitate digitalis toxicity and even cause sudden death. (These findings have been questioned.) Hypercalcemia may also precipitate or potentiate digitalis toxicity.

Hypokalemia is often associated with digitalis toxicity, regardless of the mechanism by which it has been produced (diuretics, corticosteroids, laxatives, insulin, dialysis, antibiotics such as amphotericin B, and so on). Hyperkalemia produced by drugs such as triamterene (Dyrenium) or spironolactone (Aldactone A) or associated with acidosis may decrease the effects of digitalis.

Hypomagnesemia may also precipitate digitalis toxicity. (Hypomagnesemia usually occurs in association with hypokalemia.)

When the patient is receiving thyroid hormone or when hyperthyroidism is present, larger doses, even toxic doses, of digitalis are needed to achieve a therapeutic result.

Veratrum alkaloids may induce cardiac arrhythmias when given with digitalis.

Diphenylhydantoin may potentiate the bradycardia induced by digitalis. Diphenylhydantoin and phenylbutazone may also decrease the plasma digitalis concentration (by competing for similar enzyme systems) when given over a long period of time.

Dosage and administration

Dosage and administration are discussed for individual digitalis drugs: digoxin, deslanoside, and ouabain.

Radioimmunoassay technics are now available to determine the amount of digoxin or digitoxin in the blood and in the tissues. (There is a good correlation between blood and tissue concentrations.) A known amount of the patient's plasma or serum is added to a solution containing a known amount of radioactive digoxin (or digitoxin) and a specific antibody to digoxin (or digitoxin). The digitalis in the patient's blood competes with the radioactive digitalis for binding by the antibody. Therefore, the amount of radioactive digitalis that is bound to the antibody is a measure of the amount of digitalis in the patient's blood. (To avoid a misleadingly high value, the blood should be drawn 8 hours after a dose of digoxin or digitoxin has been given.)

Therapeutic and toxic blood levels are as follows (after Atkinson).

	Digoxin (ng/ml)	Digitoxin (ng/ml)
Therapeutic	0.8 to 1.6	14 to 26
Possibly toxic	1.6 to 3.0	26 to 39
Probably toxic	Higher than 3.0	Higher than 39

Unfortunately, a patient may have digitalis toxicity but have a normal serum digitalis concentration, whereas other patients who do not show signs of digitalis toxicity may have serum digitalis concentrations higher than those described above. There are many reasons for the overlap between therapeutic and toxic digitalis concentrations; for example, electrolyte disturbances, particularly hypokalemia, hyperkalemia, hypercalcemia, hypomagnesemia, and hyponatremia; thyroid disease; renal disease; and the severity of the underlying heart disease.

Preparations

There are many digitalis preparations available. Digoxin, deslanoside, and ouabain are rapid acting preparations and are rapidly eliminated. Digitalis leaf, digitoxin, acetyldigitoxin, and gitalin are slow-acting preparations and are slowly eliminated. Only rapid-acting digitalis preparations should be used to treat cardiac emergencies. I prefer digoxin because it can be used for both emergency and maintenance treatment. Deslanoside (Cediland-D) and ouabain are also described in this part of the book.

REFERENCES

Abelmann WH: Acute hypertensive effect of digitalis glycosides, Editorial, Chest **63**:2, 1973.

Ackerman GL, Doherty JE, Flanigan WJ: Peritoneal dialysis and hemodialysis of tritiated digoxin, Ann Intern Med **67**:718, 1967.

American Hospital Formulary Service: Cardiogenic glycosides. Category 24:04.

Atkinson AJ Jr: Clinical use of blood levels of cardiac drugs, Mod Concepts Cardiovasc Dis **42**, January, 1973.

Braunwald E, Pool PE: Mechanism of action of digitalis glycosides Mod Concepts Cardiovasc Dis **37**:129, 1968.

Chung EK: New tests and developments in digitalis therapy, Clin Trends Cardiol **1** (6), 1972.

Dick HLH, McCawley EL, Fisher WA: Reserpine-digitalis toxicity, Arch Intern Med **109**:49, 1962.

Doherty JE, Perkins WH: Studies following intramuscular tritiated digoxin in human subjects, Am J Cardiol **15**:170, 1965.

Greene R, Oliver CC: Sensitivity to propranolol after digoxin intoxication, Br Med J **2**:413, 1968.

Jelliffe RW: An improved method of digoxin therapy, Ann Intern Med **69**:703, 1968.

Jelliffe RW, Buell J, Kalaba R: Reduction of digitalis toxicity by computer-assisted glycoside dosage regimens, Ann Intern Med **77**:891, 1972.

Lewis WS, Doherty JE: Another disadvantage of intramuscular digoxin, N Engl J Med **288**:1077, 1973.

Lown B, et al: Sensitivity to digitalis drugs in acute myocardial infarction, Am J Cardiol **30**:388, 1972.

Martin EW: Hazards of medication, Philadelphia, 1971, JB Lippincott Co.

Moe GK, Farah AE: Digitalis and allied cardiac glycosides. In Goodman LS, Gilman A, editors: The pharmacological basis of therapeutics, ed 4, New York, 1970, The Macmillan Co.

Morrison J, Killip T: Serial serum digitalis levels in patients with acute myocardial infarction (Abstr), Clin Res **19**:353, 1971.

Morrison J, Killip T: Serum digitalis and arrhythmia in patients undergoing cardiopulmonary bypass, Circulation **47**:341, 1973.

Ogilvie RI, Ruedy J: An educational program in digitalis therapy, JAMA **222**:50, 1972.

Selye H: Digitoxin poisoning; prevention by spironolactone, Science **164**:842, 1969.

Shields TW, Ujiki GT: Digitalization for prevention of arrhythmias following pulmonary surgery, Surg Gynecol Obstet **126**:743, 1968.

Smith TW: Digitalis glycosides, N Engl J Med **288**:719, 1973.

Smith TW, Haber E: Digoxin intoxication; the relationship of clinical presentation to serum digoxin concentration, J Clin Invest **49**:2377, 1970.

Snyder JR, et al: Effect of digoxin on the T wave in normal individuals, Am J Cardiol **17**:781, 1966.

Vance JW: Management of patients with cor pulmonale, acute and chronic, Prog Cardiovasc Dis **9**:470, 1967.

Willman VL, Cooper T, Hanlon CR: Prophylactic and therapeutic use of digitalis in open-heart operations, Arch Surg **80**:860, 1960.

DIGOXIN (Lanoxin)

Digoxin is a rapid-acting digitalis preparation. It is almost completely absorbed orally. It can also be given parenterally (or IM or IV, but not subcutaneously).

Its general pharmacology is discussed under Digitalis glycosides.

When a single dose of 1 to 1.5 mg is given IV to an adult, effects are noted in 5 to 10 min, are maximal in 1 to 2 hours, regress in 8 to 10 hours, and disappear rapidly in approximately 2 to 3 days (although some effects may still be present up to 6 days). The half-life of an IV dose of digoxin is 33 to 46 hours.

When digoxin is given IM, its effect starts in approximately 30 min, is maximum in 4 to 6 hours, and disappears rapidly in approximately 2 to 3 days (although some effects may still be present up to 6 days). Lewis and Doherty have pointed out that when digoxin is given IM, there may be delayed absorption so that its peak serum concentration is lower and occurs slower than when it is given orally.

Following a single oral dose of 1 to 1.5 mg, effects are noted in 1 hour, are maximal in 6 hours, and disappear rapidly in approximately 2 to 3 days (although some effects may still be present up to 6 days).

Dosage

Given IV, the total digitalizing dose for an adult is 4 to 6 ml (1 to 1.5 mg). This can be given undiluted at one time. However, I prefer to give 2 to 4 ml (0.5 to 1 mg) IV, followed by 1 to 2 ml (0.25 to 0.5 mg) every 2 to 4 hours until a satisfactory response is noted or until 6 ml (1.5 mg) have been injected.

IM digitalization requires 4 to 6 ml (1 to 2 mg). Not more than 2 ml (0.5 mg) should be given IM at any one site. The injection should be made deeply into the muscles and the site firmly massaged.

Generally, a patient can be digitalized by receiving digoxin orally in a *digitalizing (loading)* dose of 0.0075 mg/lb of lean body weight (Ogilvie and Ruedy). (This assumes the absence of edema fluid or of excess fat. Therefore, if the patient is edematous or obese, a smaller digitalizing dose will be needed.) This total digitalizing dose can be given in three divided doses at 6-hour intervals.

EXAMPLE: Patient's lean weight, 150 lb.
Digitalizing dose: 150 × 0.0075 mg = 1.125 mg. This can be given in a dose of 0.375 mg every 6 hours for three doses.

However, the digitalizing dose as calculated above is only approximate. Some patients may require more than this dose. Conversely, if hypokalemia, hyponatremia, or hypercalcemia is present, a smaller digitalizing dose may be needed.

Given orally, slow digitalization can be accomplished by 0.5 to 0.75 mg daily for approximately 1 week.

The daily *maintenance* oral dose of digoxin depends on two factors: the total digitalizing dose and renal function (as determined from the BUN concentration or from the creatinine clearance) (Table 9).

EXAMPLE: Patient, lean weight 150 lb, has received 1.125 mg digoxin as a digitalizing dose. The BUN concentration is 18 mg/100 ml.
From Table 9, the daily maintenance dose of digoxin, based on a BUN concentration less than 20 mg/100 ml, is 40.2% of the digitalizing dose, or 0.402 × 1.125 = 0.4725 mg digoxin. A daily dose of 0.5 mg digoxin would therefore be satisfactory.

Again, this dose is approximate and may

have to be reduced if hypokalemia, hyponatremia, or hypercalcemia is present.

The average oral maintenance dose of digoxin is 0.25 to 0.5 mg daily. It is rarely necessary to use 0.75 mg daily for maintenance. Some patients may require as little as 0.125 mg daily, or even 0.125 mg three times a week.

If the patient has received digitalis in the past 2 weeks, it is preferable to start with one half the above parenteral or oral doses.

Patients with acute myocardial infarction may be excessively sensitive to digitalis in the first 24 hours after the attack. Therefore, if digitalis is needed, three fourths the usual digitalizing dose should be given. A similar situation is present for the first 24 hours after cardiopulmonary bypass surgery (Morrison and Killip, 1973).

If the patient has azotemia or acute renal insufficiency, one third to one seventh of the usual maintenance doses should be used (Table 9).

Digitalis dosage based on blood levels of digoxin is discussed on p. 281.

Table 9. Relationships between the daily maintenance oral dose of digoxin to the BUN concentration when the BUN concentration is stable*

BUN concentration†	Daily maintenance dose of digoxin‡
20 or less	40.2
30	33.7
40	29.1
50	25.5
60	22.6
70	20.1
80	18.1
90	16.2
100	14.4

*Modified from Jelliffe R W: Ann Intern Med **69:**703, 1968. Adjustments will be needed if the BUN concentration varies from day to day.
†Expressed as mg/100 ml.
‡Expressed as a percentage of the digitalizing dose.

DIGOXIN (Lanoxin)

Route of administration	Emergency dosage
IV	2 to 4 ml (0.5 to 1 mg), followed by 1 to 2 ml (0.25 to 0.5 mg) every 2 to 4 hours until a satisfactory response is noted or until 6 ml (1.5 mg) have been injected.
IM	4 to 6 ml (1 to 2 mg). Not more than 2 ml (0.5 mg) should be given at any one site.

If the patient has received digitalis in the past 2 weeks, it is preferable to start with one half of the above doses. Also, in the first 24 hours after an acute myocardial infarction, it is preferable to use three fourths of the above doses.

Preparations

Ampuls: 2 ml; each ml contains 0.25 mg (250 μg). The contents can be injected undiluted IV or IM.

Tablets: 0.125 mg, 0.25 mg, 0.5 mg.

REFERENCES

See Digitalis glycosides.

DILANTIN SODIUM. *See* Diphenylhydantoin sodium.

DIPHENYLHYDANTOIN (Dilantin) SODIUM

Diphenylhydantoin, whose chemical structure is similar to that of the barbiturates, was introduced about 30 years ago for the control of epileptiform seizures. In 1950, Harris and Kokernot found it effective in ventricular tachycardia occurring in acute myocardial infarction. Since then, it has been used for many other tachyarrhythmias.

Pharmacology

Diphenylhydantoin is a group II antiarrhythmic drug (see Antiarrhythmic drugs). In addition, it may decrease the cardiac output and may cause a rise in the left ventricular end-diastolic pressure. It may also cause a fall in blood pressure.

Electrocardiographic effects

The ECG usually does not show any significant changes. However, diphenylhydantoin may shorten the P-R and Q-T intervals.

Absorption

Diphenylhydantoin is absorbed orally. It can also be given IM or IV. After an oral dose, a peak blood concentration occurs in approximately 8 hours. However, the full effects of orally administered diphenylhydantoin may not develop for 6 to 9 days, and the effects may last this long after the drug is stopped.

After an IV dose, the onset of action occurs within 5 to 20 min.

A therapeutic blood concentration, regardless of how diphenylhydantoin is given, is 10 to 18 μg/ml.

Indications

Indications are described as excellent, good, fair, or poor.

The use of diphenylhydantoin in the treatment of tachyarrhythmias has not yet been approved by the Food and Drug Administration. However, it is widely used for this purpose.

1. Digitalis-induced ventricular tachycardia. Excellent.
2. Digitalis-induced supraventricular tachycardia. Excellent.
3. Ventricular tachycardia. Excellent. It has been found very effective for ventricular tachycardias of any cause, particularly digitalis-induced ventricular tachycardia and ventricular tachycardias occurring during cardiac surgery and cardiac catheterization. However, because of its possible serious side effects, it is not the drug of first choice for ventricular tachycardia.
4. Ventricular premature contractions, particularly multifocal ventricular tachycardia. Excellent.
5. Atrial premature contractions. Fair.
6. Paroxysmal atrial tachycardia. Fair.
7. Atrial flutter. Poor.
8. Atrial fibrillation (for conversion to sinus rhythm or for maintenance of sinus rhythm after conversion). Poor.
9. AV junctional premature contractions or paroxysmal AV junctional tachycardia. Poor.
10. Tachyarrhythmias associated with the Wolff-Parkinson-White syndrome. Poor.

Contraindications

Sinus bradycardia.

Tachyarrhythmias with second-degree or complete AV block. Diphenylhydantoin may inhibit the functioning pacemaker before there is any significant improvement in conduction through the AV node. This can result in ventricular standstill.

Congestive heart failure.

Hypotension.

Hypersensitivity. There is cross-sensitivity between diphenylhydantoin and phenobarbital.

Side effects and toxicity

Some of the toxic reactions observed after the IV administration of diphenylhydantoin may be due to the solvent propylene glycol.

Cardiovascular. After IV administration, hypotension, shock, respiratory depression, bradycardia, incomplete or complete AV block, asystole, or ventricular fibrillation with sudden death may occur. These toxic effects can be minimized when the diphenylhydantoin is given IV at a rate not exceeding 50 mg/min.

Repeated IV injections may decrease cardiac output and may precipitate or aggravate congestive heart failure.

Gastrointestinal. Dyspepsia, loss of taste, anorexia, nausea, vomiting, epigastric pain, hyperplasia of the gums.

Neurological and psychiatric. Cerebellar disturbances with incoordination and other signs, abducent nerve paralysis, extrapyramidal reactions, hemiplegia, facial weakness, dizziness, confusion, nightmares, inability to concentrate, depression, insomnia, apathy or nervousness, acute psychotic behavior, coma.

Ocular. Amblyopia, diplopia, transient blindness, extraocular palsy, mydriasis, ptosis, ulcers of the conjunctiva.

Skin and hypersensitivity reactions. Erythematous, scarlatinal, or morbilliform rashes, exfoliative dermatitis, Stevens-Johnson syndrome, systemic lupus erythematosus, serum sickness, lymph node hyperplasia resembling Hodgkin's disease, or infectious mononucleosis.

Hematological. Aplastic and megaloblastic anemia, leukopenia, eosinophilia, pancytopenia, thrombocytopenia.

Liver. Hepatitis, cholestasis with jaundice, increased SGOT and SGPT levels, and increased sulfobromophthalein retention.

Complete blood counts and liver and kidney function tests should be taken periodically during prolonged therapy with diphenylhydantoin.

Treatment of toxicity. There is no specific treatment for toxicity to diphenylhydantoin. One should remember that the drug is excreted slowly so that toxic reactions can continue for several days after the drug is stopped.

Peritoneal dialysis has been used for coma due to diphenylhydantoin.

Interactions with other drugs

Coumarin anticoagulants, phenylbutazone, sulfaphenazole, and diphenylhydantoin are detoxified by the same enzyme system in the liver. Therefore, if diphenylhydantoin is given with any of these drugs, the plasma concentration of each of the drugs will rise.

If the patient must have an anticoagulant, phenindione should be used instead of the coumarins because it does not interfere with diphenylhydantoin metabolism.

Phenobarbital increases the rate of metabolism of diphenylhydantoin. Therefore, larger doses of diphenylhydantoin are needed.

The hypotensive effects of diuretics and antihypertensive drugs are increased by diphenylhydantoin.

Digitalis potentiates the central nervous system effects of diphenylhydantoin, and diphenylhydantoin potentiates the AV-blocking effects of digitalis. However, diphenylhydantoin has been found to be very effective in treating digitalis-induced tachyarrhythmias.

Propranolol effects are potentiated by diphenylhydantoin.

Quinidine or procainamide effects are potentiated by diphenylhydantoin.

Tubocurarine effects are potentiated by diphenylhydantoin.

Dosage and administration

Diphenylhydantoin can be given orally or IV (or IM). Subcutaneous injections are very irritating.

Intravenous use. Before use, diphenylhydantoin must be diluted with the special solvent supplied by the manufacturer. The reconstituted clear solution may be stored at room temperature and should be discarded if haziness or precipitation develops or if the solution is not used within 4 to 6 hours after it has been prepared. The diphenylhydantoin powder dissolves slowly, requiring about 10 min, but the time can be shortened by immersing the vial in warm water after the solvent has been added. The diphenylhydantoin solution will precipitate when mixed with dextrose and water or with other acidic solutions and should therefore be injected directly into a vein. Since the solution has a pH of 12, it is very alkaline and can cause local irritation of the vein or local thrombosis. This can be avoided if it is injected through a sterile catheter inserted into the vein.

Diphenylhydantoin can be given IV undiluted at a rate of 50 mg/min for a total dose of 250 mg (approximately 5 mg/kg body weight), with continuous electrocardiographic monitoring. The injection should be stopped as soon as a therapeutic effect or signs of toxicity are noted.

If the patient shows no response to 250 mg after 20 min, an additional dose, up to 250 mg, can again be given IV (in another vein) at a rate of 50 mg/min. If there is still no response, other antiarrhythmic measures should be used.

Bigger and Heissenbuttel recommend a dose of 100 mg IV every 5 min for a total of 750 to 1,000 mg.

Intramuscular use. The dose is the same as with oral use.

Oral use. Diphenylhydantoin has also been used orally for treatment and maintenance therapy in a total daily dose of 300 to 600 mg (three to six 100-mg capsules). Therefore, one to two 100-mg capsules can be given orally every 8 hours.

Diphenylhydantoin is much less effective when given orally than when given IV or IM.

Preparations

Injection: 100-mg vials with 2-ml ampuls of special diluent; 250-mg vials with 5.2 ml ampuls of special diluent.

Oral use: capsules, 50 mg; tablets, 100 mg.

DIPHENYLHYDANTOIN (Dilantin) SODIUM	
Route of administration	Emergency dosage
IV	50 mg/min up to 250 mg. This can be repeated, if necessary, after 20 min.
IM	100 to 150 mg every 6 to 8 hours.
Oral	100 to 150 mg every 6 to 8 hours.

REFERENCES

American Hospital Formulary Service: Diphenylhydantoin. Category 28:12.

Bernstein J, Gold H, et al: Sodium diphenylhydantoin in the treatment of recurrent cardiac arrhythmias, JAMA **191**:695, 1965.

Bigger JT, Heissenbuttel RH: Clinical use of antiarrhythmic drugs, Postgrad Med **47**:119, 1970.

Bigger JT, Schmidt DH, Kutt H: The relationship between the antiarrhythmic effect and the plasma level of diphenylhydantoin sodium (Dilantin), Bull NY Acad Med **42**:1039, 1966.

Bilitch M: A manual of cardiac arrhythmias, Boston, 1971, Little, Brown and Co.

Conn RD: Diphenylhydantoin sodium in cardiac arrhythmias, N Engl J Med **272**:277, 1965.

Damato AN: Diphenylhydantoin; pharmacological and clinical use, Prog Cardiovasc Dis **12**:1, 1969.

Gellerman GL, Martinez C: Fatal ventricular fibrillation following intravenous sodium diphenylhydantoin therapy, JAMA **200**:337, 1967.

Harrah MD, Way WL, Katzang BG: The interaction of d-tubocurarine with antiarrhythmic drugs, Anesthesiology **33**:406, 1970.

Harris AS, Kokernot RH: Effects of diphenylhydantoin sodium and phenobarbital sodium upon ectopic ventricular tachycardia in acute myocardial infarction, Am J Physiol **163**:505, 1950.

Lieberson AD, et al: Effect of diphenylhydantoin on left ventricular function in patients with heart disease, Circulation **36**:692, 1967.

Louis S, Kutt H, McDowell F: The cardiocirculatory changes caused by intravenous Dilantin and its solvent, Am Heart J **74**:523, 1967.

Parke, Davis and Co: Dilantin, Steri-Vial, package insert, Feb 1972.

Voight GC: Death following intravenous sodium diphenylhydantoin (Dilantin), Johns Hopkins Med J **123**:153, 1968.

DOPAMINE

Dopamine is the immediate precursor of norepinephrine and is also a beta adrenergic stimulator of heart muscle. It increases the cardiac output by increasing the stroke volume of the heart without increasing the heart rate. It also produces vasoconstriction of the arteries of the extremities, but unlike norepinephrine it produces active dilatation of the renal and mesenteric arteries. This decreases the peripheral resistance and helps alleviate inadequate tissue perfusion through the vital splanchnic organ systems. The renal vasodilation is unusual and important because it is probably a direct effect of dopamine on the kidneys and is not blocked by either alpha or beta blocking agents.

The effects of dopamine depend on the dose used. When given in small doses, it causes an increased cardiac output and an increased renal blood flow and increased urinary sodium excretion. The heart rate does not change appreciably, and the total peripheral resistance either does not change or decreases slightly. When it is given in large doses, its alpha stimulating effect on the peripheral arteries becomes prominent, and the peripheral resistance may rise.

Indications

Dopamine has been used in the treatment of cardiogenic shock associated both with acute myocardial infarction and open-heart surgery. It appears to be most beneficial to patients with oliguria and with a low or normal total peripheral resistance. Dopamine should be used only when cardiogenic shock is *not* due to an inadequate circulating blood volume. If the patient does not respond to dopamine, levarterenol (norepinephrine, Levophed) or metaraminol (Aramine) can then be used. When further vasodilation is needed, dopamine has been used simultaneously with isoproterenol (Isuprel) or with phentolamine (Regitine).

Contraindications

Prostatic hypertrophy, thyrotoxicosis, pregnancy.

Side effects and toxicity

A sense of forceful beating of the heart, palpitations or apprehension, ventricular premature contractions, nausea, angina.

Interactions with other drugs

MAO inhibitors potentiate the action of dopamine.

Dosage and administration

Dopamine can be added to a solution of 5% dextrose in water, 5% dextrose in isotonic saline, or in $\frac{1}{6}$ molar sodium lactate solution.

Two ampuls (400 mg) can be diluted in 500 ml dextrose in water. Therefore, each ml of the diluted solution contains 800 μg. One can start with an infusion of 100 μg/min. (This is slightly less than a dose of 1.5 μg/kg/min in a 70-kg patient.) The dose can be raised, if necessary, to 3,000 μg/min (approximately 40 μg/kg/min). When a large dose such as this is given, 1,200 mg dopamine can be diluted in 500 ml dextrose in water. (Therefore, each ml of this diluted solution contains 2,400 μg.)

Holzer and associates used an average maintenance dose of 9.1 μg/kg/min in their patients who survived and an average

dose of 17 μg/kg/min in their patients who did not survive.

Dopamine has been given continuously for a period varying from several hours to 332 hours.

Preparations

Dopamine is available to investigators as Inotropin (Arnar-Stone) in 5-ml ampuls containing 200 mg dopamine hydrochloride in water with 0.1% sodium bisulfite. (The solution should not be used if discolored.) It is not yet available for clinical use.

REFERENCES

Goldberg LI: Cardiovascular and renal actions of dopamine; potential clinical applications, Pharmacol Rev **24**:1, 1972.

Goldberg LI, Talley RC, McNay JL: The potential role of dopamine in the treatment of shock, Prog Cardiovasc Dis **12**:40, 1969.

Holzer J, et al: Effectiveness of dopamine in patients with cardiogenic shock, Am J Cardiol **32**: 79, 1973.

McCannell KL, McNay JL, Meyer MB, Goldberg LI: The use of dopamine in the treatment of hypotension and shock, N Engl J Med **275**:1389, 1966.

Rosenblum R, Frieden J: Intravenous dopamine in the treatment of myocardial dysfunction after open-heart surgery, Am Heart J **83**:743, 1972.

EDECRIN. *See* Ethacrynic acid.

EDROPHONIUM (Tensilon) CHLORIDE

Edrophonium has a structure similar to that of neostigmine and is a short and rapid-acting cholinergic drug. In cardiology it is used in the treatment of paroxysmal atrial tachycardia.

Pharmacology

Edrophonium acts by inhibiting cholinesterase. It competes with acetylcholine for this enzyme and in this way allows acetylcholine to remain unmetabolized and to produce strong cholinergic effects, stimulating autonomic ganglia and cholinergic visceral receptors.

Edrophonium acts on the cardiac conduction system by potentiating the effect of acetylcholine that is normally released by the vagus nerves. As a result it produces sinus slowing and slowing of conduction through the AV node. Therefore, it is able to convert paroxysmal atrial tachycardia to regular sinus rhythm. It also decreases the cardiac output and may cause severe hypotension.

In addition to its vagotonic action on the heart, it also has a general muscarinic action that produces side effects such as salivation, perspiration, and tachypnea. It also has a direct motor end-plate action on skeletal muscle. This explains the muscle fasciculations that occur when it is given.

Absorption

It is given IV. Its effects are noted in 30 to 60 sec and last about 10 min.

Indications

The Food and Drug Administration has not yet approved edrophonium for the treatment of paroxysmal atrial tachycardia. However, it is widely used for this purpose.

Indications are described as excellent, good, fair, or poor.

1. Paroxysmal atrial tachycardia. Excellent. However, edrophonium is not the drug of first choice for the treatment of paroxysmal atrial tachycardia because of its side effects.

2. Paroxysmal AV junctional tachycardia. Same as for paroxysmal atrial tachycardia.

Contraindications

Acute myocardial infarction or any other condition in which increased parasympathetic activity is not desired. Hypersensitivity to anticholinergic drugs, mechanical intestinal obstruction, mechanical urinary tract obstruction, peptic ulcer, bronchial asthma.

Side effects

Cardiovascular. Bradycardia, hypotension, ventricular standstill, ventricular pre-

mature contractions, ventricular tachycardia.

Neurological. Dysarthria, dysphonia, dysphagia, convulsions, respiratory paralysis.

Respiratory. Laryngospasm, increased tracheobronchial secretions (bronchorrhea), bronchiolar constriction, paralysis of the muscles of respiration.

Gastrointestinal. Nausea, vomiting, increased peristalsis, abdominal cramps, diarrhea.

Skeletal muscles. Muscular weakness, muscle fasciculations.

Eye. Increased lacrimation, pupillary constriction, spasm on accommodation, diplopia, conjunctival hyperemia.

Other side effects. Urinary frequency and incontinence, diaphoresis.

Treatment of toxicity. Stop the drug.

Atropine sulfate, 0.4 to 0.8 mg, should be given IV. This can be repeated every 3 to 10 min. The total dose needed will seldom exceed 2 mg.

Obtain an open airway. Assisted respiration and oxygen may also be needed.

Interactions with other drugs

Neostigmine and other anticholinergic drugs should not be used simultaneously with edrophonium, because the combination may produce a cholinergic crisis with muscle weakness that can simulate myasthenia gravis.

Administration and dosage

Edrophonium can be given IV as follows. An IV bolus of 5 mg is given over a period of 30 to 60 sec, with constant electrocardiographic monitoring. (Some cardiologists give a 10-mg bolus as the first dose.) The injection should be stopped if sinus rhythm appears. Another 5-mg bolus can be given in 5 min if the tachyarrhythmia is still present.

To avoid hypotension, the patient *must* be in a supine position, and he should be forewarned to expect side effects such as blurred vision, lacrimation, fasciculations

EDROPHONIUM (Tensilon) CHLORIDE	
Route of administration	Emergency dosage
IV	5-mg bolus in a period of 30 to 60 sec. Repeat in 5 min, if necessary. Some cardiologists give a 10-mg IV bolus as the first dose.

of the ocular muscles, bronchorrhea, nausea, abdominal pain, or diarrhea. These side effects begin 1 to 2 min after the injection and subside in 2 to 3 min.

A syringe with 1 mg atropine *must* be available at the bedside.

If regular sinus rhythm does not appear in 3 to 4 min, carotid sinus pressure can be used to potentiate the cholinergic action of the edrophonium. If there is no response, other therapy should be used (Chapter 6).

Preparations

Injection: 10-ml vials; each ml contains 10 mg.

REFERENCES

Blumenthal MR, Kornfeld P: Edrophonium chloride for paroxysmal auricular tachycardia, JAMA **161**:1001, 1956.

Cantwell JD, Dawson JE, Fletcher GF: Supraventricular tachyarrhythmias; treatment with edrophonium, Arch Intern Med **130**:221, 1972.

Frieden J, Cooper JA, Grossman JI: Continuous infusion of edrophonium (Tensilon) in treating supraventricular arrhythmias, Am J Cardiol **27**:294, 1971.

Moss AJ, Aledort LM: Use of edrophonium (Tensilon) in the evaluation of supraventricular tachycardias, Am J Cardiol **17**:58, 1966.

Pitt B, Kurland GS: Use of edrophonium chloride (Tensilon) to detect early digitalis toxicity, Am J Cardiol **18**:557, 1966.

Roche Laboratories: Tensilon (edrophonium chloride), package insert, Aug 1970.

Spitzer S, Mason D, Lemmon WM, Moyer JH III: Use of edrophonium (Tensilon) in the evaluation of supraventricular tachycardia, Am J Med Sci **254**:477, 1967.

ETHACRYNIC ACID (Edecrin)

Ethacrynic acid is a potent diuretic, suitable for oral use. Sodium ethacrynate is its lyophilized salt suitable for IV use after dilution.

Pharmacology

Ethacrynic acid (or its sodium salt) inhibits the reabsorption of sodium ions in the ascending limb of the loop of Henle and decreases distal tubular reabsorption of sodium and chloride ions. As a result, an increased amount of sodium and chloride ions and slightly less potassium and bicarbonate ions are excreted in the urine.

Ethacrynic acid is effective even in the presence of hypochloremia and metabolic acidosis. However, it may also aggravate these metabolic disturbances.

Absorption

Following oral administration of ethacrynic acid, diuresis occurs within 30 min; a peak effect occurs in approximately 2 hours; and the diuresis lasts from 6 to 8 hours.

Following IV administration, diuresis occurs within 15 min and lasts approximately 2 hours.

IM or subcutaneous injections are painful and irritating and should not be given.

Indications

Acute pulmonary edema or congestive heart failure, acute hypertensive emergencies, edema associated with the nephrotic syndrome or with cirrhosis of the liver.

Contraindications

Anuria, oliguria, or increasing azotemia; cirrhosis of the liver, particularly if ascites is present, because hepatic coma can be precipitated; dehydration with hyponatremia due to sodium loss; metabolic alkalosis or hypokalemia.

Side effects and toxicity

Gastrointestinal. These are very common and include anorexia; nausea, vomiting; dysphagia; diarrhea that may become severe; gastrointestinal bleeding, particularly when sodium ethacrynate is given IV; and acute nonhemorrhagic pancreatitis.

Electrolyte. Disturbances of electrolyte and other blood chemistry concentrations are very common, particularly if excessive doses are given or when the drug is given to patients who are on a low sodium diet or who have cirrhosis of the liver or azotemia.

The serum sodium, potassium, and chloride concentrations may fall, and the bicarbonate (CO_2) content may rise. The BUN concentration may also rise, and tetany may develop.

The fasting blood glucose level may rise, and diabetes may be precipitated or aggravated, particularly when doses greater than 100 mg are given.

The serum uric acid concentration may rise, and an attack of gout can be precipitated.

Dehydration and a decreased circulating blood volume may also occur, with signs of hypotension or with cerebral or pulmonary thromboses, particularly in elderly debilitated patients or patients with cardiac disease or patients who are receiving sympatholytic drugs.

Side effects such as postural hypotension, headaches, weakness, muscle cramps, and thirst may be due to excessive loss of water or electrolytes or both.

In addition, when ethacrynic acid is given to uremic patients, acute hypoglycemia with convulsions may occur.

Neurological. Paresthesias, blurred vision, and confusion may occur.

Ears. Acute vertigo, reversible deafness, and tinnitus, with a sense of fullness in the ears, may occur after a rapid diuresis. Permanent deafness can occur in patients with renal insufficiency or when ethacrynic acid or its sodium salt is given concomitantly with kanamycin sulfate (Kantrex).

Other side effects. Pruritus, rash, hematuria, Henoch-Schönlein purpura (in patients with rheumatic heart disease) agranulocytosis, and thrombocytopenia may occur.

Liver. Abnormal liver function test results or jaundice may occur.

Treatment of side effects and toxicity

1. Decrease the dosage, stop the drug, or give it intermittently, such as every other day.

2. If hypokalemia occurs, gives potassium chloride orally, or give a potassium-sparing diuretic such as triamterene (Dyrenium) or spironolactone (Aldactone) concomitantly. (If this is done, potassium chloride supplements must be stopped.)

3. If hypochloremia occurs, ammonium chloride can be given orally (except in patients with cirrhosis of the liver). Potassium chloride (except if triamterene or spironolactone is also being given), arginine chloride, and L-lysine monohydrochloride are also very effective in raising the serum chloride concentration.

L-Lysine monohydrochloride can be given as a 40% solution. (Each 5 ml contains 2 gm.) From 40 to 100 ml (16 to 40 gm) daily can be given in divided doses; for example, 10 to 25 ml four times a day.

Interactions with other drugs

The effects of coumarin anticoagulants (Coumadin, Dicumarol, Panwarfin, Liquamar, Tromexan) are potentiated by ethacrynic acid, and smaller doses are needed.

Antihypertensive drugs are potentiated by ethacrynic acid.

Carbonic anhydrase inhibitors (such as Diamox) have their diuretic effects potentiated by ethacrynic acid.

When corticosteroids are given to patients receiving ethacrynic acid, a severe potassium loss may occur.

Digitalis toxicity may be precipitated if hypokalemia occurs as a result of ethacrynic acid therapy.

When given concomitantly, furosemide (Lasix) and ethacrynic acid can cause severe hypokalemia.

Mercurial or thiazide diuretics are potentiated by ethacrynic acid and can be given concomitantly or alternately.

Dosage and administration

Intravenous. A vial containing lyophilized sodium ethacrynate is dissolved in 50 ml 5% dextrose in water or in isotonic saline; this is injected slowly over a period of several minutes, either into the tubing of a running IV infusion or directly into a vein.

When the patient is heavy, a dose of 0.5 to 1.0 mg/kg body weight can be injected. However, a single IV dose should not exceed 100 mg.

If the sodium ethacrynate is added to a 5% dextrose in water solution with a pH below 5, a hazy or opalescent solution may develop. Such a solution should not be used. In addition, sodium ethacrynate should not be administered simultaneously with whole blood or blood derivatives.

If a second injection is needed, a different vein should be used to prevent local thrombosis.

The solution should be discarded after 24 hours.

Oral. The usual initial oral dose is 50 mg given as a single dose after a meal. To determine the effectiveness of this initial dose, no further dose should be given for 12 to 24 hours. If the patient has been taking diuretics, the initial dose should be 25 mg.

On the second day two doses of 50 mg are given, after meals, if necessary. The goal of oral doses of ethacrynic acid is to achieve a weight loss of approximately 1 to 2 lb a day.

On the third day 100 mg is given in the morning, and 50 to 100 mg is given following the afternoon or evening meal, depending on the response to the morning dose.

A few patients may require initial and maintenance doses as high as 200 mg twice daily. These higher doses, which should be achieved gradually, are most often needed for patients with severe refractory edema.

Preparations

Sodium ethacrynate (Edecrin, sodium lyovac). Injection: vials of lyophilized so-

ETHACRYNIC ACID (Edecrin, sodium lyovac)	
Route of administration	Emergency dosage
IV	1 vial (50 mg) dissolved in 50 ml 5% dextrose in water or in saline, given over a period of several minutes. For heavy patients, 0.5 to 1 mg/kg can be given, but the dose should not exceed 100 mg. An additional dose can be given, if necessary, after 2 hours.

dium ethacrynate; each vial contains the equivalent of 50 mg ethacrynic acid.

Ethacrynic acid (Edecrin). Tablets: 25 mg, 50 mg.

REFERENCES

American Hospital Formulary Service: Ethacrynic acid and sodium ethacrynate. Category 40:28.

Fine SL, Levy RI: Ethacrynic acid in acute pulmonary edema, N Engl J Med 273:583, 1965.

Kessler RH: The use of furosemide and ethacrynic acid in the treatment of edema Pharmacol Phy 1(9), 1967.

Martin EW: Hazards of medication, Philadelphia, 1971, JB Lippincott Co.

Merck Sharp & Dohme: Tablets Edecrin (ethacrynic acid) and lyovac sodium edecrin (sodium ethacrynate), product brochure, 1969.

Rubin AL, et al: The use of L-lysine monohydrochloride in combination with mercurial diuretics in the treatment of refractory fluid retention, Circulation 21:332, 1960.

Slone D, et al: Intravenously given ethacrynic acid and gastrointestinal bleeding, JAMA 209:1668, 1969.

FUROSEMIDE (Lasix)

Furosemide is a diuretic. Chemically it is one of the sulfonamides.

Pharmacology

The pharmacological characteristics are the same as those of ethacrynic acid.

Absorption

Furosemide is absorbed orally and can also be given IM or IV.

Following oral or IM administration, a diuretic effect occurs within 1 hour, with a peak effect in the first or second hour. The diuresis lasts from 4 to 6 or even 8 hours.

Following IV administration, diuresis starts within 5 min, with a peak effect within 30 min. The diuresis lasts approximately 2 hours.

Indications

See Ethacrynic acid.

Contraindications

Contraindications are similar to those of ethacrynic acid. In addition, it should not be given to patients who show hypersensitivity to sulfonamides. It is also contraindicated in pregnant women and nursing mothers.

Side effects and toxicity

The side effects and toxicity are similar to those of ethacrynic acid. In addition, transient deafness may occur, particularly in patients with impaired renal function or in those who are receiving other ototoxic drugs. Sudden death from cardiac arrest has been reported after either IM or IV doses of furosemide.

Treatment of side effects and toxicity. See Ethacrynic acid.

Interactions with other drugs

The interactions are similar to those of ethacrynic acid. In addition, furosemide enhances the effects of tubocurarine or other curare derivatives. Therefore, if surgery is contemplated, oral administration of furosemide should be stopped 1 week before surgery, and parenteral administration of furosemide should be stopped 2 days before surgery.

When salicylates are given concomitantly with furosemide, salicylate toxicity can occur at lower doses than usual because furosemide interferes with the renal excretion of salicylates.

Dosage and administration

Given IM, the usual dose of furosemide is 1 to 2 ampuls (20 to 40 mg).

Given IV, a similar dose of 1 to 2 ampuls (20 to 40 mg) can be given slowly over a period of 1 to 2 min.

If the diuretic response is not satisfactory, the dose can be increased (not sooner than every 2 hours) by increments of 1 ampul (20 mg) until the desired diuretic response is obtained. This effective dose should then be given once or twice

---

FUROSEMIDE (Lasix)

Route of administration	Emergency dosage
IM	1 to 2 ampuls (20 to 40 mg).
IV	1 to 2 ampuls (20 to 40 mg) given slowly over a period of 1 to 2 min.

The IM or IV dose can be increased, if necessary, not more often than every 2 hours by increments of 1 ampul (20 mg) until the desired diuretic response is obtained.

---

daily thereafter. Parenteral administration should be replaced by oral therapy as soon as possible.

Given orally, the usual dose is 1 to 2 tablets (40 to 80 mg) given as a single dose in the morning.

If the patient does not respond with a satisfactory diuresis, the dose can be increased by increments of 1 tablet (40 mg), not sooner than 6 to 8 hours after the previous dose, until a desired diuretic effect is obtained. This effective dose can then be given preferably once (or twice) daily, for example, at 8 AM (and 2 PM).

Patients with refractory edema or edema associated with renal insufficiency may require massive doses of furosemide orally or parenterally. As much as 600 mg or more furosemide has been given orally daily, and as much as 1,000 mg furosemide given IV daily has been used in such patients (Silverberg and others). However, when such large doses are given, serious electrolyte disturbances often occur.

Preparations

Injection: 2-ml ampuls; each ml contains 10 mg.

Tablets: 40 mg.

REFERENCES

Davidow M, et al: Intravenous administration of furosemide in heart failure, JAMA **200**:824, 1967.

Hoechst Pharmaceutical Co: Lasix (furosemide) injection, product brochure, 1971.

Olesen KH: A comparison of the diuretic action of mercaptomerin, ethacrynic acid and furosemide in congestive heart failure, Acta Med Scand **187**:391, 1970.

Silverberg DS, et al: Experience with high doses of furosemide in renal disease and resistant edematous states, Can Med Assoc J **103**:129, 1970.

GUANETHIDINE (Ismelin) SULFATE

Guanethidine sulfate is an oral antihypertensive drug.

Pharmacology

Guanethidine inhibits or interferes with the release of catecholamines at sympathetic nerve endings. It therefore produces only a sympathetic blockade, in contrast to ganglionic blocking agents, which produce both sympathetic and parasympathetic blockade. Because of the sympathetic blockade, the peripheral resistance and cardiac output decrease slightly so that even when the patient is supine, the blood pressure falls. In addition, guanethidine produces significant postural hypotension. It decreases renal blood flow and may cause a rise in BUN concentration if given to a patient with renal disease.

Absorption

Guanethidine is given orally, although it is only partially absorbed from the gastrointestinal tract. It may take 2 to 7 days after therapy is started before a full therapeutic lowering of the blood pressure occurs. When the drug is stopped, the blood pressure will begin to rise in 3 to 4 days, gradually reaching its pretreatment level in 1 to 3 weeks.

Indications

Malignant hypertension. It can be given in association with thiazide diuretics or hydralazine (Apresoline) or both.

Dissecting aneurysm of the aorta (in conjunction with trimethaphan and reserpine) (Chapter 13).

Contraindications

Pheochromocytoma. Guanethidine may accelerate the release of catecholamines from the pheochromocytoma.

Congestive heart failure not associated with hypertension.

Patients receiving MAO inhibitors.

Guanethidine should be used cautiously in hypertensive patients with renal disease and an increased BUN concentration; coronary insufficiency or recent myocardial infarction (within 3 months); cerebrovascular disease, especially hypertensive encephalopathy; or congestive heart failure.

It should also be used cautiously in patients with a history of peptic ulcer or ulcerative colitis.

Side effects and toxicity

Side effects due to sympathetic blockade include dizziness, weakness, lassitude, and syncope, due either to postural hypotension or hypotension on exertion.

Side effects due to unopposed parasympathetic activity include bradycardia, increased bowel movements, and diarrhea.

Cardiovascular side effects include dyspnea, fluid retention with edema, and other signs of congestive heart failure.

Other side effects include nausea, vomiting, nocturia, urinary incontinence, inhibition of ejaculation, dermatitis, loss of scalp hair, dry mouth, ptosis of the lids, blurring of vision, tenderness of the parotid glands, myalgia or muscle tremors, mental depression, nasal congestion, bronchial asthma, and a rise in the BUN concentration.

Treatment of side effects. Patients should be warned about the potential dangers of postural hypotension and syncope and should be told to sit or lie down immediately when dizziness or weakness occurs. Postural hypotension is most marked in the morning and is accentuated by hot weather, alcohol, or exercise. The patient should also be cautioned to avoid sudden or prolonged standing, or exercise, while taking the drug.

Gastrointestinal side effects can often be controlled by an anticholinergic drug such as atropine. Occasionally, guanethidine must be stopped because of persistent diarrhea.

Edema or congestive heart failure can usually be controlled by diuretics. If the edema or congestive heart failure becomes more marked, the guanethidine should be stopped.

Periodic blood counts and liver function tests should be taken if guanethidine is used for a prolonged time.

Interactions with other drugs

Reserpine and other rauwolfia preparations should be used cautiously with guanethidine because their concomitant use may cause excessive postural hypotension, bradycardia, and mental depression.

Vasopressor drugs may cause excessive hypertension because guanethidine increases the sensitivity of the body to catecholamines.

The hypotensive effect of guanethidine is decreased by amphetamines, ephedrine, methylphenidate hydrochloride (Ritalin), desipramine hydrochloride (Norpramin, Pertofrane), imipramine hydrochloride (Tofranil), protriptyline hydrochloride (Vivactil), and probably other tricyclic antidepressants, such as nortriptyline hydrochloride (Aventyl) and amitriptyline hydrochloride (Elavil).

Methylphenidate given concomitantly with guanethidine may cause ventricular tachycardia.

Digitalis given with guanethidine may excessively slow the heart rate.

Hydralazine, the thiazides, and other diuretics increase the effectiveness of guanethidine. Therefore, smaller doses of guanethidine are needed. (It is preferable to start treatment with a thiazide, for example, and then add guanethidine, rather than to start with guanethidine and later add the thiazide.)

If guanethidine is substituted for a ganglionic-blocking drug, the ganglionic blocker should be withdrawn gradually, to prevent a hypertensive reaction, because the peak effect of the guanethidine occurs slowly.

MAO inhibitors (including the antihypertensive MAO inhibitor pargyline [Eutonyl]) should not be used concomitantly with guanethidine, because the sudden release of catecholamines due to the guanethidine may precipitate a hypertensive crisis. Guanethidine should not be started for at least 1 week after an MAO inhibitor has been stopped.

Anesthetics may induce severe hypotension in patients receiving guanethidine. Therefore, if possible, guanethidine should be stopped 2 weeks before surgery is performed.

If emergency surgery is indicated, preanesthetic and anesthetic agents should be given cautiously in reduced dosage, with oxygen, atropine, and vasopressor solutions ready for immediate use. However, they should be used with extreme caution because of the possibility of increased response to vasopressor drugs, as was mentioned above.

Dosage and administration

Guanethidine can be given orally once or twice a day.

When guanethidine is given to ambulatory patients, the starting dose is 10 mg daily.

The patient's blood pressure should be checked with the patient in the supine position, after standing for 3 min,* and immediately after exercise, if possible. Dosage should be increased in ambulatory patients not more often than every 5 to 7 days.

Febrile illnesses increase the effect of guanethidine, and smaller doses may be needed.

In hospitalized patients, larger doses can be used because the patient can be watched more closely. For example, an initial oral dose is 25 to 50 mg. The dose can be increased by 25 or 50 mg daily or every other day, as indicated.

The patient must be warned about the possibility of postural hypotension (see side effects and toxicity) and must not be discharged from the hospital until the blood pressure, after the patient has been standing for 3 min, has been stabilized.

Periodic blood counts and liver function tests should be taken if guanethidine is used for a prolonged period of time.

Preparations

Tablets: 10 mg, 25 mg.

REFERENCES

American Hospital Formulary Service: Guanethidine sulfate. Category 24:08.
Ciba Pharmaceutical Co: Ismelin sulfate (guanethidine sulfate), package insert, Oct 1971.
Martin EW: Hazards of medication, Philadelphia, 1971, JB Lippincott Co.

HEPARIN SODIUM

Heparin is a naturally occurring, high molecular weight mucopolysaccharide with marked anticoagulant properties.

---

*The manufacturer recommends that the blood pressure be taken after the patient has been standing 10 min. However, I believe that this is unnecessary because the standing blood pressure will stabilize by 3 min.

Pharmacology

Heparin affects several phases of the co-agulation process and results in a prolonga-tion of the *clotting* time in vitro and in vivo. However, it does not usually affect *bleeding* time. Heparin prolongs the one-stage prothrombin time. However, valid prothrombin time determinations can be obtained if blood is drawn 3 to 4 hours after the last IV dose or 12 to 24 hours after the last subcutaneous dose of heparin.

Absorption

Heparin is inactive when given orally. Therefore, it must be given by deep sub-cutaneous injection (but not IM) or, pre-ferably, IV.

Indications

Thromboembolic disturbances. Small doses of heparin have also been used to prevent postoperative thromboembolism (see dosage and administration).

Contraindications

Active bleeding, blood dyscrasias, pa-tients with bleeding tendencies, such as pur-pura, thrombocytopenia, liver disease with hypoprothrombinemia, or hemophilia. In-tracranial hemorrhage. However, heparin can be started 48 hours after a cerebral embolus. Suppurative thrombophlebitis, ul-cerative lesions of the gastrointestinal tract, open ulcerative wounds. Ascorbic acid de-ficiency. Heparin should be used cautiously during or following surgery of the eye, brain, or spinal cord, or during continuous tube drainage of the stomach or small in-testines. It can be started 72 hours after open-heart surgery, if necessary, if excessive postoperative bleeding is not present. Shock, severe hypertension, advanced kid-ney disease, subacute bacterial endocarditis. History of hypersensitivity to heparin. Pregnancy and the immediate postpartum period. Heparin should be given cautiously to patients with a history of allergies or bronchial asthma. (A trial dose of 1,000 units can be given to such patients to deter-mine if an allergic reaction will occur.)

Side effects and toxicity

Allergic reactions or hypersensitivity may occur. Symptoms may include chills, fever, pruritus, urticaria, lacrimation, conjuncti-vitis, rhinitis, bronchospasm, arthralgia, anaphylactoid reactions, and burning of the feet. Acute reversible thrombocytopenia may also occur. Transient alopecia may be a late complication, occurring several months after treatment.

Heparin may lower the serum sodium or calcium concentration.

When given IM or subcutaneously, tis-sue irritation, hematoma, or sloughing may occur. This can be avoided by giving heparin by deep subcutaneous injection (see dosage and administration).

A rare complication of subcutaneous or IM administration of heparin is the devel-opment of arterial emboli, associated with a decrease in circulating platelets. (The platelet level returns to normal when heparin is stopped.)

Treatment of side effects and toxicity

1. If bleeding occurs, reduce the dose, or stop the heparin temporarily.

2. Protamine sulfate can also be used to counteract heparin overdosage. It neu-tralizes heparin within 5 min. One mg protamine sulfate will neutralize approx-imately 75 to 100 units of heparin. The dose of protamine sulfate should be based on the last dose of heparin that has been given. However, not more than 50 mg protamine sulfate should be given at one time. (Protamine sulfate is a weak anti-coagulant. Therefore, excessive doses may cause bleeding.)

The protamine sulfate is given IV over a period of 1 to 3 min. (It can cause side effects, including bradycardia, sudden de-creased blood pressure, dyspnea, transitory flushing of the skin, nausea, vomiting, and lassitude.)

A heparin rebound phenomenon may

occur after protamine sulfate has been injected, particularly in patients receiving extracorporeal dialysis or undergoing cardiopulmonary bypass surgery. The protamine sulfate may immediately neutralize the heparin excess in such patients, but heparin activity reappears 30 min to 18 hours later. (If this occurs, further doses of protamine sulfate should be given.)

When protamine sulfate is used to treat an overdose of subcutaneously administered heparin, repeated IV injections may be needed at 15-min intervals or longer (depending on the clotting time values).

Interactions with other drugs

Acetylsalicylic acid (aspirin) and other salicylates interfere with platelet aggregation reactions. (This is the primary way by which clotting of the blood of heparinized patients occurs.) Therefore, severe bleeding may occur if salicylates are given to patients receiving heparin.

The effect of oral anticoagulants is increased slightly by heparin. Antihistamines, digitalis, quinidine, penicillin, and tetracycline inhibit the anticoagulant effect of heparin.

Dosage and administration

In a general way, heparin dosage can be adjusted according to the prolongation of the clotting time. An attempt should be made to prolong the clotting time and maintain it between 2 and 3 times the normal value, using the Lee-White method (normal values: 6 to 17 min if glass tubes are used, 19 to 60 min if siliconized tubes are used). However, this is not always feasible or necessary.

Some patients show heparin resistance; for example, febrile patients, or those with acute myocardial infarction, early thrombophlebitis, pleurisy or peritonitis, or cancer, or patients after extensive surgical operations. Such patients may require larger than usual doses of heparin.

Elderly women (particularly those older than 60 years) frequently develop bleeding complications when heparin is given IV.

Heparin can be given in three ways.

1. Intermittent IV administration
2. Continuous IV administration
3. Deep subcutaneous administration

Clinical observations indicate that in the treatment of massive pulmonary embolism, *intermittent IV doses* of 10,000 to 15,000 units heparin should be given every 4 hours for the first critical 24 to 84 hours, without using clotting time tests (Gurewich and others). After this initial period of treatment, the dosage can be reduced or adjusted so that the clotting time is approximately 2 times normal, just before the next dose of heparin is due.

Heparin can also be given by *continuous IV infusion* in a dose of 10,000 to 40,000 units added to 1 to 2 L 5% dextrose in water. Initially, the rate of infusion should be approximately 1 ml/min. Clotting times are determined every 4 hours, and the dose is adjusted so that the clotting time does not exceed $2\frac{1}{2}$ to 3 times normal.

Heparin is strongly acidic and is therefore incompatible with solutions of numerous otner drugs, including levarterenol (Levophed), hydrocortisone sodium succinate (Solu-Cortef), and many others. However, it can be given IV in dextrose in water, sodium chloride (saline), fructose in water, Ringer's or lactated Ringer's, and $\frac{1}{6}$ molar sodium lactate solutions.

Subcutaneous injections should be made *deep* into fatty tissue. Any fat roll can be used, but abdominal fat rolls are preferable. However, the injection should not be made within 2 inches of the umbilicus.

The following "Z track" technic is satisfactory. A 26-gauge, $\frac{1}{2}$- or $\frac{5}{8}$-inch needle should be used. The skin layer of a fat roll is grasped and lifted upward. The needle is then inserted at an angle of approximately 45° to the skin surface, and the heparin solution is injected. The needle is then rapidly withdrawn and the skin simultaneously released.

The tip of the needle should not be moved during the injection, and the plunger of the syringe should not be pulled back to determine if a blood vessel has been entered. In addition, the injection site should not be massaged either before or after the injection. Subsequent injections should be made at different sites.

Deep subcutaneous injections of heparin can be given every 10 to 12 hours, using the following dose schedule, based on the patient's weight.

Patient's weight	Heparin dosage
Less than 65 kg (140 lb)	7,500 to 10,000 units
75 to 90 kg (160 to 200 lb)	15,000 to 20,000 units

When heparin is given, the patient should not receive any medication IM, to prevent bleeding at the puncture site.

Oral administration of an anticoagulant can be started at the same time heparin is started. It is given daily until the prothrombin time (tested daily) is 20 sec. Then the heparin can be stopped, but the oral doses of the anticoagulant are continued. Warfarin sodium (Coumadin, Panwarfin) is excellent for this purpose.

When heparin or anticoagulant therapy is used for thromboembolic disease, it should be given for at least 8 to 10 days. (This is the time required for a bland peripheral thrombus to adhere to the wall of a vein.) However, if the condition that predisposes to emboli is still present after this time, long-term oral anticoagulant therapy is indicated. Surgical interruption of the inferior vena cava, usually with clip compartmentation, may also be indicated in these patients.

Heparin has also been given prophylactically to prevent postoperative thromboembolic complications. Various dose schedules can be used when this is done. For example, 5,000 units aqueous sodium heparin have been given subcutaneously starting 2 hours before the operation and then continued 8 to 10 hours after the preoperative dose, in a schedule of 3 times a day, with treatment continued until the patient is fully mobile (Gallus and associates).

This type of heparin prophylaxis has been used for operations in a variety of patients (with or without cancer) undergoing surgery, including cholecystectomy, gastric surgery, large-bowel surgery, laparotomy, pancreatic surgery, repair of an abdominal aneurysm, hernia repair, thoracotomy, laminectomy, and hip replacement.

Gallus and associates found that the transfusion requirement of treated patients was increased. However, serious hemorrhage can occur even with low doses of heparin (Charnley).

Preparations

Heparin sodium. Injection: 1,000, 5,000, 7,500, 10,000, 15,000, 20,000, 40,000 units per ml; in ampuls, vials, and disposable units.

Protamine sulfate. Injection: vials containing 50 mg powdered protamine sulfate and sodium chloride, with 5-ml ampuls of sterile water. The water is added to the protamine sulfate and sodium chloride, and the contents are shaken vigorously. (Each ml contains 10 mg protamine sulfate.)

REFERENCES

American Hospital Formulary Service: Heparin sodium. Category 20:12:04.

American Hospital Formulary Service: Protamine sulfate. Category 20:12:08.

Charnley J: Prophylaxis of postoperative thromboembolism, Lancet **2**:134, 1972.

Deykin D: Current concepts; the use of heparin, N Engl J Med **280**:937, 1969.

Gallus AS, et al: Small subcutaneous doses of heparin in prevention of venous thrombosis, N Engl J Med **288**:545, 1973.

Gurewich V, et al: Some guidelines for heparin therapy of venous thromboembolic disease, JAMA **199**:116, 1967.

Organon, Inc: Liquaemin sodium (sodium heparin injection), product brochure, 1965.

Vieweg WVR, et al: Complications of intravenous heparin in elderly women, JAMA **213**:1303, 1970.

HYDRALAZINE HYDROCHLORIDE (Apresoline)

Hydralazine hydrochloride is an antihypertensive drug that acts by directly relaxing vascular smooth muscle. Hydralazine also has positive inotropic and chronotropic effects, resulting in increased cardiac output and myocardial oxygen consumption. It also increases renal and cerebral perfusion in most instances.

Absorption

Hydralazine is absorbed orally and can also be given IM or IV in urgent situations. When it is given IM, peak action occurs in 10 to 80 min and lasts 4 to 6 hours. When it is given IV, peak action occurs in 10 to 20 min. However, hydralazine is not always effective, even when given parenterally.

Indications

Hydralazine can be given parenterally for hypertensive crises, particularly with acute glomerulonephritis and toxemia of pregnancy. Because it increases cardiac output and oxygen consumption, it should not be used in dissecting aneurysm or in hypertensive crises associated with congestive heart failure or coronary artery disease.

Contraindications

Angina pectoris or coronary artery disease. Hydralazine may precipitate acute myocardial infarction in such patients. Congestive heart failure, dissecting aneurysm, mitral stenosis (hydralazine increases pulmonary artery pressure), and hypersensitivity to hydralazine are other contraindications.

Although hydralazine can be used to treat a hypertensive crisis associated with acute glomerulonephritis, it must be used cautiously in patients with hypertension and chronic renal disease.

Side effects and toxicity

Adverse reactions are usually reversible when the dosage is reduced. However, if serious side effects occur, the drug should be stopped.

Common side effects include headache,

palpitations, anorexia, nausea, vomiting, diarrhea, tachycardia, and angina pectoris.

Less frequent side effects include nasal congestion; flushing; lacrimation; conjunctivitis; peripheral neuritis with paresthesias; numbness and tingling (due to disturbance of pyridoxine metabolism); edema; dizziness; tremors; muscle cramps; psychotic reactions characterized by depression, disorientation, or anxiety; constipation; difficulty in micturition; arthralgia; dyspnea; paralytic ileus; lymphadenopathy; splenomegaly; and blood dyscrasias, including anemia, leukopenia, agranulocytosis, and purpura.

Postural hypotension or acute myocardial infarction can occur (Palmer).

When hydralazine is given for weeks or longer in doses of 400 mg or more daily, it may induce a syndrome similar to systemic lypus erythematosus, with a positive LE cell test.

Adverse reactions are usually reversible when the dosage is reduced. The peripheral neuritis can be treated with pyridoxine (vitamin B_6). If serious side effects occur, the drug should be stopped.

Interactions with other drugs

Diuretics, reserpine, and MAO inhibitors potentiate the hypotensive action of hydralazine. Therefore, smaller doses can be used. Anesthetics also potentiate the hypotensive action of hydralazine.

Hydralazine reduces the pressor effects of epinephrine or levarterenol (Levophed).

Dosage and administration

Hydralazine should be given parenterally only when it cannot be given orally.

Given IM, the usual dose is 20 to 40 mg, repeated as necessary.

When given IV, 50 to 100 mg can be dissolved in 1,000 ml 5% dextrose in water. The infusion should be given slowly and the rate adjusted according to the blood pressure response. Smaller doses may be needed when renal insufficiency is present.

The patient must be constantly supervised because the blood pressure may fall rapidly in 10 to 20 min.

Preparations

Injection: 1-ml ampuls; each ml contains 20 mg.

Tablets: 10, 25, 50, and 100 mg, for oral use.

REFERENCES

American Hospital Formulary Service: Hydralazine hydrochloride. Category 24:08.

Breslin DJ: Hypertensive crisis, Med Clin North Am **53:**351, 1969.

Ciba Pharmaceutical Co: Apresoline hydrochloride (hydralazine hydrochloride), package insert, Mar 1972.

Freis ED: Hypertensive crisis, JAMA **208:**338, 1969.

Palmer R: Extracardiac crises, Emergency Med **4:** 47, 1972.

HYPERSTAT. *See* Diazoxide.

INDERAL. *See* Propranolol hydrochloride.

ISMELIN SULFATE. *See* Guanethidine sulfate.

ISOPROTERENOL (Isuprel) HYDROCHLORIDE
Pharmacology

Isoproterenol has a chemical structure similar to that of epinephrine. It is a potent beta adrenergic stimulating agent (see Adrenergic drugs). It has almost no effect on alpha receptors. Its main circulatory effects, therefore, are on the heart and the blood vessels of the skeletal muscles and of the alimentary tract.

Isoproterenol increases the cardiac output by means of its positive inotropic and chronotropic effects, increasing the strength of cardiac contraction and increasing the discharge rate of the sinus node, the AV node, and the bundle of His. It increases the venous return to the heart and in this way also raises the cardiac output. Isoproterenol also dilates the blood vessels, mostly of the skeletal muscles, and also slightly dilates the renal and mesenteric arteries. It lowers the peripheral resistance in this way. It also relaxes smooth muscle, most

markedly in the bronchioles and gastrointestinal tract.

Electrocardiographic effects

Isoproterenol can cause minor RS-T and T changes, due to sympathetic stimulation and to the sinus tachycardia that occurs. However, it can also cause subendocardial ischemia, with characteristic RS-T changes (Chapter 9).

Absorption

Isoproterenol can be given sublingually, orally, by inhalation, subcutaneously, IM, IV, and intracardiac. Its action starts almost immediately after IV administration and lasts a few minutes. When it is given subcutaneously or IM, its action lasts 1 to 2 hours. Sublingual, oral, or rectal absorption is not uniformly reliable. When it is given sublingually, its action begins in approximately 15 to 30 min and lasts 45 min to 2 hours. When an extended-release tablet is ingested, its action starts within 30 min and lasts 6 to 8 hours. When it is given rectally, its action occurs within 30 min and lasts 2 to 4 hours.

Indications

Shock. Theoretically, isoproterenol should be most useful in treating shock associated with an increased peripheral vascular resistance (Chapter 3). However, before it is used to treat shock, it is necessary to make certain that the shock is not associated with a decreased circulating blood volume, because isoproterenol decreases the effective blood volume due to its vasodilating effects and may cause the shock to worsen. Therefore, it may be necessary to give additional IV fluids during the isoproterenol infusion. This is discussed further in Chapter 3.

Isoproterenol may not be beneficial when given to a patient with acute myocardial infarction and cardiogenic shock, because it increases the oxygen requirements of the heart. Therefore, when cardiogenic shock is associated with an increased peripheral resistance, a vasodilator drug such as phentolamine may be preferable (Chapter 3).

Isoproterenol has also been used to treat the shock of massive pulmonary embolism because it produces pulmonary vasodilation.

Cardiac arrest; see Chapter 2.

Adams-Stokes syndrome and other bradyarrhythmias. Isoproterenol has been found to be beneficial in patients with Adams-Stokes syndrome due to complete AV block, when syncopal attacks are associated with ventricular standstill, ventricular tachycardia, or even ventricular fibrillation. The isoproterenol may suppress the ventricular fibrillation by stimulating normal pacemaker activity (in contrast to epinephrine, which may precipitate ventricular fibrillation when given to a patient with complete AV block).

Isoproterenol can also be used to stimulate the heart when other bradyarrhythmias are present or in patients with carotid sinus hypersensitivity.

When a bradyarrhythmia is present with acute myocardial infarction, atropine is preferable to isoproterenol, which may increase the oxygen needs of the heart. However, an isoproterenol infusion can be used if atropine is not effective.

For emergency treatment of the Adams-Stokes syndrome, isoproterenol can be given IV, IM, or subcutaneously. For the long-term treatment of the Adams-Stokes syndrome or other bradyarrhythmias, isoproterenol can be given sublingually, orally (extended-release tablets), or rectally. However, I believe that the insertion of a cardiac pacemaker is now the treatment of choice for the Adams-Stokes syndrome.

Contraindications

When used for the Adams-Stokes syndrome, isoproterenol is contraindicated in patients with angina or hypertension. Isoproterenol is contraindicated in patients with sinus tachycardia (rate faster than 120 per min). It is also contraindicated if a tachyarrhythmia due to digitalis toxicity is present.

Side effects and toxicity

Because isoproterenol increases the cardiac output, it can precipitate angina. Excessive doses can also cause a sinus tachycardia. When the heart rate increases to 130 per min or faster, ventricular premature contractions or ventricular tachycardia may occur. In therapeutic doses it has no tendency to produce ventricular fibrillation. Severe hypertension or subendocardial myocardial infarction can also develop.

Other side effects include muscle tremor, weakness, sweating, dizziness, and nausea and vomiting. Isoproterenol may also produce hyperglycemia and hypermetabolism and must be used cautiously in diabetic and hyperthyroid patients.

Since isoproterenol decreases the peripheral resistance, the vasodilation that occurs may decrease the effective circulating blood volume. If the patient is in shock and if this decreased circulating blood volume is not corrected, the shock will become more severe (Chapter 3).

Treatment of toxicity. The effects of isoproterenol given IV are dissipated in a few minutes. Therefore, if signs of toxicity occur, the drug should be stopped. Since isoproterenol is a beta adrenergic stimulating agent, its effects can also be counteracted by propranolol, which is a beta adrenergic blocking agent.

Interactions with other drugs

Isoproterenol and epinephrine should not be given simultaneously, because they may produce too much sympathetic stimulation. However, they can be given alternately at intervals of at least 4 hours.

Isoproterenol should not be used to treat a digitalis-induced tachyarrhythmia.

Dosage and administration

The dosage of isoproterenol can easily be adjusted, using the following calculations.

If 1 mg of any substance is dissolved in 1 L of diluent, each ml contains 1 μg (1:500,000 dilution).

If 1 mg is dissolved in 500 ml of diluent, each ml contains 2 μg (1:250,000 dilution).

If 2 mg are dissolved in 500 ml of diluent, each ml contains 4 μg (1:125,000 dilution).

A convenient dilution of isoproterenol for IV use is to dissolve a 5-ml ampul (1 mg) in 500 ml dextrose and water (1:500,000 concentration). The diluted isoproterenol should be infused at a rate of 0.25 to 2.5 ml/min (0.5 to 5 μg/min) until the desired blood pressure is obtained. A pediatric microdrip bulb should be used to control the flow rate. (Microdrip bulbs are calibrated to deliver 60 or 50 drops per ml.) A high concentration of even 1:50,000 isoproterenol can be used if fluid restriction or a high dosage is needed. (A 1:50,000 dilution can be prepared by dissolving 5 ml [1 mg] isoproterenol in 100 ml 5% dextrose in water. Each ml therefore contains 10 μg.) Doses as high as 30 μg/min have been used when shock is severe (Chapter 3).

The speed of infusion should be adjusted on the basis of changes in the systemic blood pressure, heart rate, central venous pressure, urine flow, and so on (Chapter 3). If the heart rate exceeds 110 per min,

the infusion rate should be decreased or temporarily stopped.

If ventricular premature contractions occur, they can also be treated by decreasing or stopping the isoproterenol temporarily or by giving lidocaine or propranolol.

When isoproterenol is given IV to treat a bradyarrhythmia, the flow rate should be adjusted to increase and maintain the heart rate at 50 to 60 per min.

Preparations (for cardiovascular use)

Injection: 200 μg/ml (1:5,000 solution); 1-ml (0.2-mg) and 5-ml (1-mg) ampuls.

Tablets: 10 and 15 mg (Isuprel glossets), for sublingual or rectal use.

Tablets, extended release: 15 and 30 mg (Proternol) for oral use.

REFERENCES

Bing OHL, Brooks WW, Messer JV: Mechanical benefits and hazards of isoproterenol during myocardial hypoxia, Clin Res **19**:305, 1971.

Cohn JN: Treatment of shock, GP **34**:78, 1966.

Eichna LW: The treatment of cardiogenic shock. III. The use of isoproterenol in cardiogenic shock, Am Heart J **74**:848, 1967.

Kardos GG: Isoproterenol in the treatment of shock due to bacteremia with gram-negative pathogens, N Engl J Med **274**:868, 1966.

MacLean LD, Duff JH, Scott HM, and Peretz DI: Treatment of shock in man based on hemodynamic diagnosis, Surg Gynecol Obstet **120**:1, 1965.

ISOPROTERENOL (Isuprel) HYDROCHLORIDE	
Route of administration	**Emergency dosage**
Intracardiac	0.1 ml (0.02 mg) of undiluted 1:5,000 solution.
IV injection (single dose)	1 to 3 ml of a 1:50,000 dilution. (Add 1 ml of undiluted 1:5,000 solution to 9 ml 5% dextrose in water or isotonic saline.)
IV infusion	5 ml (1 mg) of 1:5,000 undiluted solution added to 500 ml 5% dextrose in water.
	In shock the usual flow is 0.25 to 2.5 ml (0.5 to 5 μg) per min.
	In bradyarrhythmias, it should be given to raise the heart rate to 50 or 60 per min.

Mueller H, Ayres SM, et al: Effect of isoproterenol, l-norepinephrine, and intraaortic counterpulsation on hemodynamics and myocardial metabolism in shock following acute myocardial infarction, Circulation 45:335, 1972.

Sharma GVRK, Kumar R, et al: "Coronary steal"; regional myocardial blood flow studies during isoproterenol infusion in acute and healing myocardial infarction, Clin Res 19:339, 1971.

Weil MH, Bradley EC: Circulatory effects of vasoactive drugs in current use for treatment of shock; a reclassification based on experimental and clinical study of their selective arterial and venous effects, Bull NY Acad Med 42:1023, 1966.

Winthrop Laboratories: Isuprel hydrochloride, package insert, Jan 1971.

ISUPREL HYDROCHLORIDE. *See* Isoproterenol hydrochloride.

LANATOSIDE C. *See* Deslanoside.

LANOXIN. *See* Digoxin.

LASIX. *See* Furosemide.

LEVARTERENOL (Levophed) BITARTRATE
Pharmacology

Levarterenol (*l*-norepinephrine) is a sympathomimetic amine with two actions on the cardiovascular system. It has a beta adrenergic stimulating effect on the heart muscle. In this way it has a positive inotropic effect. It also dilates the coronary arteries. In addition, it has an alpha adrenergic stimulating effect on the peripheral arteries and acts as a powerful vasoconstrictor of most of the vascular system, including the kidneys, brain, liver, and usually the skeletal muscles. Therefore, when levarterenol is given to a patient with acute myocardial infarction and shock, the aortic and systemic blood pressures rise, and the coronary artery flow increases. In addition, venous return increases, and the cardiac output increases. However, if excessive levarterenol is given so that the aortic blood pressure rises above 110 mm Hg, excessive vasoconstriction may occur, so that the cardiac output decreases.

Electrocardiographic effects

The most frequent effect of levarterenol is a sinus bradycardia. In addition, minor RS-T changes may occur, and the T wave amplitudes may decrease.

Absorption

Levarterenol must be given IV. Its effect begins almost immediately and lasts approximately 2 min.

Indications

There are two general indications for the use of levarterenol: (1) shock or acute hypotension occurring in acute myocardial infarction, trauma, infection, during or after spinal anesthesia, after removal of a pheochromocytoma, as a result of drug reactions, or during blood transfusions (Chapter 3), and (2) auxiliary treatment for cardiac arrest (Chapter 2).

Levarterenol (or a similar drug, such as metaraminol) is no longer considered to be the primary treatment of cardiogenic shock. Instead, it should be used as an adjunct to IV fluids (Chapter 3).

Contraindications

Levarterenol should not be given to patients who are hypotensive from an inadequate blood volume, except as an emergency measure to maintain coronary and cerebral artery perfusion until blood volume replacement therapy can be completed.

Unless life-threatening shock is also present, levarterenol should not be given to patients with peripheral or mesenteric vascular thrombosis because of the risk of increasing ischemia and extending the area of infarction.

Hyperthyroidism is also a contraindication to its use. In addition, levarterenol and other sympathomimetic amines may provoke a relapse in patients with a history of malaria.

Levarterenol is also contraindicated during cyclopropane and halothane anesthesia because these anesthetics sensitize the myocardium to the action of IV administered norepinephrine (levarterenol), epinephrine, and metaraminol (Aramine), so that an initial bradycardia may be followed by ventricular premature contractions, ventricular tachycardia, or ventricular fibrillation. Similar tachyarrhythmias may occur if levarterenol is used in patients with profound hypoxia or hypercarbia.

Side effects and toxicity

Anxiety, or headache associated with hypertension often occurs. Bradyarrhythmias due to increased vagal tone may also occur, with or without a prolonged P-R interval. AV junctional rhythm, AV dissociation, ventricular premature contractions with a bigeminal rhythm, ventricular tachycardia, and ventricular fibrillation have also been reported.

Prolonged administration of levarterenol or any other vasopressor agent may increase the peripheral resistance so much that decreased tissue perfusion and capillary stasis occur with a loss of plasma out of the vascular system into the extracellular fluid space. This will result in continued tissue hypoxia, continued hypotension, continued low cardiac output, and continued signs of shock. (In addition, a lactic acidosis may develop.) If this occurs, the circulating blood volume *must* be replaced. This can be done by giving the patient the levarterenol in dextrose and isotonic saline, rather than in dextrose and water, or by actively expanding the circulating blood volume by isotonic saline, plasma, or dextran 40.

When the circulating blood volume falls as a result of the prolonged administration or large dosage of levarterenol, the central venous pressure may become low, confirming the decreased circulating blood volume. Unfortunately, this does not always occur, because the levarterenol may cause sufficient vasoconstriction of the veins to maintain a high central venous pressure. Such patients should receive an IV fluid challenge, as described in Chapter 3.

Precautions. Levarterenol is very potent and overdosage can produce a dangerously high blood pressure. Therefore, it is desirable to check the blood pressure every 2 min from the time the infusion is started until the desired blood pressure is obtained. Then the blood pressure should be checked every 5 min as long as the infusion is continued. The rate of flow must be watched constantly, and the patient should never be left unattended while receiving levarterenol. Headache may be a symptom of hypertension due to overdosage.

Site of infusion. Levarterenol should be administered into a large vein, particularly an antecubital vein of the forearm, whenever possible, because the risk of necrosis of the underlying skin from prolonged vasoconstriction is very slight when an antecubital vein is used. Hand veins should be avoided.

The femoral vein has also been used for levarterenol infusion. However, patients with acute myocardial infarction often have peripheral vascular disease or diabetes, which increases the danger of skin necrosis if extravasation occurs. Gangrene of a lower extremity has been reported when levarterenol was given in an ankle vein. The veins of the feet should also be avoided.

Extravasation. The infusion site should be checked frequently for free flow to detect leakage and extravasation, which may cause local necrosis due to the intense vasoconstrictor action of the drug. Blanching along the course of the infused vein, sometimes without obvious extravasation, may be due to constriction of vasa vasorum, with increased permeability of the vein wall and some leakage. If this continues, a superficial slough may develop.

To prevent extravasation, the infusion site should be changed every 12 hours. In addition, the limb receiving the levarterenol infusion should be immobilized. When extravasation occurs, the area of extravasation should be infiltrated as soon as possible with 10 to 15 ml saline solution containing 5 to 10 mg phentolamine (Regitine), an alpha adrenergic blocking agent.

A syringe with a fine hypodermic needle is used, and the solution is infiltrated liberally through the area, which is easily identified by its blanched appearance and consistency.

It has also been suggested that 5 to 10 mg phentolamine should be added directly to the infusion flash to prevent sloughing even if extravasation occurs. The phentolamine may also be helpful in overcoming the shock (see Phentolamine).

Interactions with other drugs

Levarterenol can be used if metaraminol (Aramine) is not effective. Levarterenol can also be interchanged with dopamine and can be given simultaneously with isoproterenol.

An alpha adrenergic blocking drug, such as phentolamine, counteracts the hypertensive effects and the excessive vasoconstriction produced by levarterenol. Therefore, levarterenol has been used simultaneously with phentolamine to prevent excessive vasoconstriction (see Phentolamine).

Angiotensin can counteract the severe hypertension produced by levarterenol.

Anesthetics such as cyclopropane, halothane, and chloroform sensitize the myocardium to levarterenol and when used with it may produce ventricular tachycardia or ventricular fibrillation.

MAO inhibitors intensify the effects of levarterenol and may cause a severe and even lethal hypertension. Such a hypertensive reaction can be reversed by an alpha adrenergic blocking agent, such as phentolamine.

Dosage and administration

In treating shock or hypotension, levarterenol should be given IV in a 5% dextrose in water solution or 5% dextrose in saline solution (isotonic, half-isotonic, or quarter-isotonic), but not in saline alone. The dextrose prevents loss of potency due to oxidation.

When whole blood or plasma is also needed to increase volume, it should be administered separately, or if it is given simultaneously with levarterenol, a Y tube and individual flasks should be used. Levarterenol may also be given in a plasma expander such as dextran, which has antioxidant properties similar to those of dextrose. Fructose solutions may be substituted for dextrose.

Administration. In shock, the veins have a tendency to collapse. It is therefore advisable that levarterenol be administered through an IV catheter (polyethylene tubing) inserted through a suitable bore intracath needle. If the shock is mild or if the duration of therapy is likely to be short, an IV needle can be used. The polyethylene tubing or IV needle should be centrally advanced well into the vein and securely fixed with adhesive tape to prevent extravasation. A catheter tie-in should be avoided, if possible, because this promotes stasis. A microdrip bulb is needed to estimate accurately the rate of flow in drops per minute.

Average dosage. To treat shock, 1 ampul (4 ml) levarterenol bitartrate (which contains 4 mg levarternol base) should be added to 1,000 ml dilution fluid. Therefore, each ml of this dilution contains 4 μg levarterenol base.

An ampul contains a 0.2% solution of levarterenol bitartrate. This is equivalent to a 0.1% solution of levarterenol base.

One ml of a 0.1% solution contains 1 mg. Since each levarterenol ampul has 4 ml, each ampul contains 4 mg levarterenol base.

When 1 mg of a substance is dissolved in 1,000 ml, each ml of the dilution contains 1 μg. When 4 mg are dissolved in 1,000 ml, each ml of such a dilution contains 4 μg.

The response of the patient to an initial dose of 2 to 3 ml of the infusion (8 to 12 μg of the levarterenol base) should be observed. Then the flow should be adjusted to establish and maintain the desired systolic blood pressure, usually from 90 to 100 mm Hg in a previously normotensive patient (lower if hemorrhagic or hypovolemic shock is present and the deficient circulating blood volume has not yet been replaced). If the patient has been previously hypertensive, a systolic blood pressure somewhat higher than 100 mm Hg may be needed.

The average dosage required to maintain normotension when cardiogenic shock is not severe is about 0.5 to 1 ml/min (2 to 4 μg levarterenol base per min).

High dosage. Great variations occur in the dose-required to attain and maintain normotension. In all patients, the dosage of the levarterenol must be titrated according to the response of the patient. Occasionally, larger doses, up to 7 ampuls per liter, are needed. In some patients, as many as 17 ampuls (68 μg levarterenol base) have been needed daily.

Fluid intake. The degree of dilution of the levarterenol depends on the patient's fluid volume requirements. If a large volume of dextrose solution is needed at a flow rate that would cause an excessive amount of levarterenol to be given per unit of time, a more dilute solution of levarterenol than 1 ampul per liter of dextrose solution can be used. However, if the administration of a large amount of fluid is not desirable, a greater concentration of levarterenol can be given; for example, 1 ampul levarterenol in 250 or 500 ml diluent.

Duration of therapy. The levarterenol infusion should be continued until an adequate blood pressure can be maintained without it. When the patient shows signs of recovering from shock, the rate of the infusion should be gradually reduced and then stopped. It is not advisable to stop the infusion abruptly. The vein should be kept open with a dextrose drip until the danger of a hypotensive relapse has passed.

The duration of the levarterenol therapy usually varies from a few hours to a few days. Prolonged therapy of a continuous infusion for more than 6 days is rarely needed.

When prolonged therapy is needed or when massive doses of levarterenol are used and the patient remains hypotensive, one should suspect that there is blood volume depletion associated with the shock. (This may be a result of the levarterenol infusion; see side effects and toxicity.)

During cardiopulmonary resuscitation, levarterenol can be given, as it is used in treating shock, to restore and maintain an adequate blood pressure after the heart-

LEVARTERENOL (Levophed) BITARTRATE	
Route of administration	**Emergency dosage**
Intracardiac	0.5 to 0.75 ml of a 0.02% solution directly into the heart chamber. (Dilute 1 mg of standard 0.2% solution with 9 ml isotonic saline.)
IV infusion	1 ampul (4 ml) of standard 0.2% solution of levarterenol bitartrate in 1,000 ml 5% dextrose in water or dextrose in saline. (Each ml of this dilution contains 4 μg levarterenol base.)
	Average rate of infusion to raise and maintain the blood pressure to 90 to 100 mm Hg (slightly higher if the patient has been hypertensive) and to eliminate other signs of shock is 0.5 to 1 ml (2 to 4 μg levarterenol base) per min.

beat and ventilation have been restored by other means (Chapter 2).

In addition, 0.5 to 0.75 ml of a 0.02% levarterenol bitartrate solution can be given directly into the heart when the mechanism of the cardiac arrest is ventricular standstill.

A 0.02% solution of levarterenol bitartrate solution (which is equivalent to a 0.01% solution of levarterenol base) can be made by diluting 1 ml of the 0.2% levarterenol bitartrate solution with 9 ml of isotonic saline. Each ml of the resultant solution will contain the equivalent of 0.1 mg (100 μg) levarterenol base. This solution is one tenth the strength of the standard levarterenol solution prepared for IV use. It should be used only for immediate intracardiac injection.

Preparations

Injection: 4-ml ampuls; each ml contains 2 mg levarterenol *bitartrate* (0.2% solution). (This is equivalent to 1 mg levarterenol base [0.1% solution of the base]). The ampul should not be used if it shows a brown coloration or contains a precipitate.

REFERENCES

Houle DB, Weil MH, Brown EB, et al: Influence of respiratory acidosis on ECG and pressor responses to epinephrine, norepinephrine, and metaraminol, Proc Soc Exp Biol Med **94:**561, 1957.

Innes IR, Nickerson M: Sympathomimetic drugs. In Goodman LS, Gilman A, editors: The pharmacological basis of therapeutics, ed 4, New York, 1970, The Macmillan Co.

Schmutzer KL, Rashke E, Maloney JV Jr: Intravenous l-norepinephrine as as cause of reduced plasma volume, Surgery **50:**452, 1961.

Winthrop Laboratories: Levophed Bitartrate, package insert, May 1971.

Zaimis E: Vasopressor drugs and catecholamines, Anesthesiology **29:**732, 1968.

Zucker G: Use of phentolamine to prevent necrosis due to levarterenol, JAMA **163:**1477, 1957.

LEVOPHED BITARTRATE. *See* Levarterenol bitartrate.

LIDOCAINE (Xylocaine) HYDROCHLORIDE (Lignocaine)

Lidocaine hydrochloride, an aminoacyl amide, is a local anesthetic. It also has powerful antiarrhythmic effects, particularly against ventricular tachyarrhythmias.

Pharmacology

Lidocaine is a group II antiarrhythmic drug (see Antiarrhythmic drugs). In addition, it may cause a fall in blood pressure, may decrease the force of cardiac contraction, may raise the left ventricular end-diastolic pressure, and may decrease the cardiac output.

Lidocaine also affects the central nervous system. In small doses it has sedative, central analgesic, and anticonvulsive effects. However, higher doses can cause convulsions and respiratory arrest. In anesthetized patients, very large doses of lidocaine will increase the neuromuscular blocking effect of succinylcholine.

Electrocardiographic effects

Lidocaine may shorten the P-R or Q-T interval.

Absorption

Although lidocaine is absorbed orally, it may produce unpleasant side effects and is therefore given IV or IM.

When lidocaine is given IV as a bolus injection, a peak plasma concentration is obtained within 10 sec to 3 min. Its duration of action is 10 to 20 min. However, recent studies have shown that this is the result of the drug's rapid distribution through the body and that its metabolic half-life is approximately 2 hours. Therefore, when closely spaced doses are given or when large doses are given by continuous IV infusion, toxicity may result.

When given by way of a continuous infusion in a therapeutic dose, lidocaine may not become effective for 10 to 20 min after the start of the infusion.

A lidocaine blood concentration of approximately 1 to 2.3 μg/ml is needed to suppress ventricular arrhythmias. Such a concentration can be achieved if an initial IV bolus of 1.5 mg/kg body weight is given (100 mg for a 70-kg patient) and is followed by an infusion of 50 μg/kg/min (3.5 mg/min for a 70-kg patient). (See also dosage and administration.) Toxicity will occur if the lidocaine blood concentration rises above 5 μg/ml.

When lidocaine is given IM, a peak plasma concentration is obtained in 30 to 45 min. The plasma concentration then falls to approximately half the peak value approximately 2 hours after the IM injection.

Indications

Indications are described as excellent, good, fair, or poor.

1. Ventricular premature contractions, particularly occurring more frequently than 5 per min or occurring in groups of 2 or more, or multifocal, or occurring at the apex of the T wave, in acutely ill patients, such as those with acute myocardial infarction, or during the cardiac manipulation of cardiac catheterization, or cardiac surgery. Excellent.

2. Ventricular tachycardia. Excellent.

3. Ventricular tachyarrhythmias due to digitalis toxicity or after synchronized DC shock. Excellent.

4. Cardiac arrest due to ventricular fibrillation (auxiliary treatment). Excellent.

5. Atrial tachyarrhythmias. Poor.

6. Acute myocardial infarction, prophylactically to prevent ventricular premature contractions or ventricular tachycardia. It has not been shown that lidocaine or any other antiarrhythmic drug given prophylactically this way to prevent ventricular tachyarrhythmias that may appear, but that have not yet appeared, has resulted in a decreased mortality. I therefore do not recommend it for this purpose at this time.

Contraindications

1. Hypersensitivity to local anesthetics of the amide type.

2. The Adams-Stokes syndrome or severe degrees of SA, AV, or intraventricular block.

3. Sinus bradycardia with ventricular (or nodal) escape beats. If lidocaine is given in an attempt to eliminate escape beats, it may precipitate more frequent and more serious ventricular arrhythmias unless the patient's heart rate has been accelerated by means of isoproterenol or electrical pacing prior to the use of lidocaine.

4. Atrial fibrillation with aberrant QRS complexes in the ECG. When this tachycardia is mistakenly diagnosed as a "ventricular" tachycardia and lidocaine is given, it may increase conduction through the AV node and produce a very rapid ventricular rate.

5. Liver disease. Lidocaine should be used cautiously, if at all, in patients with severe liver disease because accumulation may occur and may lead to toxic reactions, since it is metabolized in the liver. However, no exact statement can be made about the degree of liver impairment that completely contraindicates the use of lidocaine. If lidocaine is urgently needed in a patient with liver disease, small IV bolus injections, rather than a continuous infusion, should be used.

6. Congestive heart failure. There is a reduced volume of distribution of lidocaine in the body. Therefore, smaller doses are required.

7. Renal disease, hypovolemia, or shock. Decreased renal excretion of lidocaine may occur. Therefore, it must be given cautiously to such patients.

Side effects and toxicity

Side effects are usually dose related and occur when more than 200 or 300 mg are given within 1 hour.

Local thrombophlebitis may occur at the site of the infusion.

Neurological. Dizziness or lightheadedness; apprehension or euphoria; drowsiness; tinnitus or decreased hearing; blurred or double vision; difficulty in breathing, speaking, or swallowing; vomiting; sensations of heat, cold, or numbness; muscle twitching or tremors; focal or generalized convulsions; unconsciousness; respiratory depression and respiratory arrest.

Cardiovascular. The cardiovascular system is usually not affected. However, excessive doses can produce hypotension, shock, bradycardia, complete AV block, SA block, and cardiac arrest.

Treatment of toxicity

1. If a severe reaction occurs, stop the lidocaine immediately.

2. Start emergency resuscitative procedures, and give the emergency drugs necessary to manage the toxic reaction.

3. If a convulsion occurs, a small dose of an ultra–short-acting barbiturate, such as 0.1 to 0.2 gm sodium thiopental (Pentothal) or 5 to 10 mg diazepam (Valium) can be given IV.

4. If the patient is under anesthesia, a short-acting muscle relaxant can be used.

Interactions with other drugs

Cross-sensitivity between lidocaine and procainamide or between lidocaine and quinidine is rare but can occur. When lidocaine and procainamide are given simultaneously, they increase the sensitivity of the central nervous system and may produce restlessness, visual hallucinations, and other symptoms.

Lidocaine prolongs the effects of muscle relaxants such as decamethonium, succinylcholine, and tubocurarine.

Dosage and administration

Although lidocaine can be given orally, it is recommended only for IV (or IM) use at the present time.

Lidocaine can be given in the following ways.

1. IV bolus injections

2. Continuous IV infusion

3. IM injections

4. Orally

IV bolus injections. Initially, it is usually given, undiluted, IV as a bolus injection. The usual adult bolus dose is 50 to 100 mg, given at a rate of 25 to 50 mg/min (to enable a slow circulation to carry the lidocaine to its site of action).

If necessary, a second bolus can be given 5 min after the first injection is completed. Not more than 200 to 300 mg should be given during a 1-hour period.

Continuous IV infusion. It is often necessary to continue lidocaine therapy after it has been given by IV bolus to prevent a recurrence of the ventricular premature beats or the ventricular tachycardia. It can be given as an IV infusion as follows.

An IV infusion solution can be prepared by adding 2 gm lidocaine (a 50-ml container) to 450 ml 5% dextrose in water. This provides a solution that contains 4 mg lidocaine per ml. The infusion can be given at a rate of 1 to 4 mg/min. (This is equivalent to 20 to 50 μg/kg body weight for an average 70-kg adult.) Larger doses will cause toxicity.

The dose can be titrated, using a microdrip bulb, as follows.

15 drops/min	provides	1 mg/min
30 drops/min	provides	2 mg/min
45 drops/min	provides	3 mg/min
60 drops/min	provides	4 mg/min

This assumes that the microdrip bulb is calibrated to deliver 1 ml with each 60 drops. Some microdrip bulbs are calibrated to deliver 1 ml with each 50 drops. In such a case, the above relations would be 12½, 25, 37½, and 50 drops/min.

It is often possible to stop the infusion in 24 hours. However, patients with acute myocardial infarction may need the lidocaine for several days. At this time an antiarrhythmic drug such as procainamide or quinidine can be given orally for maintenance therapy. (Harrison and Alderman describe a case in which lidocaine was needed for 6 weeks.)

Caution: IV lidocaine infusions must be given under constant electrocardiographic monitoring to avoid toxicity. The IV infusion should be stopped as soon as the patient's basic cardiac rhythm appears to be stable or as soon as signs of toxicity appear. It is mandatory to have emergency resuscitative equipment and drugs immediately available to manage possible adverse reactions.

IM injections. Lidocaine can also be given IM in a dose of 200 to 300 mg. This may be of value when a patient with acute myocardial infarction and ventricular premature contractions is seen at home and is to be transported to the hospital.

Oral use. Lidocaine has been given orally in a dose of 500 mg (two 250-mg capsules), with food. A therapeutic plasma concentration occurs within 30 to 90 min and may last for 5 hours. (If given to a fasting patient, its effect lasts only 2 hours.) However, oral preparations of lidocaine are still not available for clinical use.

Preparations

Lidocaine (Xylocaine) hydrochloride is supplied for antiarrhythmic use as a 2% solution (without preservatives) in the following forms.

1. In 5-ml ampuls or prefilled syringes; each ml contains 20 mg. These are used for direct IV bolus injection.

2. In 25- or 50-ml ampuls, or vials; each ml contains 40 mg. These are used for preparing a solution for IV infusion, not for direct injection.

Preparations of lidocaine intended for use as a local anesthetic contain epinephrine and should *not* be used for treating tachyarrhythmias.

REFERENCES

Astra Pharmaceutical Products, Inc: Xylocaine hydrochloride 2%, package insert, May 1970.

Bellet S, Roman L, et al: Intramuscular lidocaine in the therapy of ventricular arrhythmias, Am J Cardiol **27:**291, 1971.

Cheng TO, Wadhwa K: Sinus standstill following intravenous lidocaine administration, JAMA **223:**790, 1973.

Crampton RS, Oriscello RG: Petit and grand mal convulsions during lidocaine hydrochloride treatment of ventricular tachycardia, JAMA **204:**201, 1968.

Gianelly R, von der Groeben JO, Spivack AP, Harrison DC: Effect of lidocaine on ventricular arrhythmias in patients with coronary heart disease, N Engl J Med **277:**1215, 1967.

Harrison DC, Alderman EL: The use of lidocaine and procaine amide in the treatment and prevention of arrhythmias associated with myocardial infarction. In Meltzer LE, Dunning AJ, editors: Textbook of coronary care, Philadelphia, 1972, The Charles Press.

LIDOCAINE (Xylocaine) HYDROCHLORIDE	
Route of administration	**Emergency dosage**
IV bolus	Given undiluted in a dose of 50 to 100 mg (1 to 2 mg/kg body weight) at a rate of 25 to 50 mg/min. If necessary, a second IV bolus can be given 5 min after the first bolus injection is finished.
Continuous IV infusion	2 gm (50 ml) added to 450 ml 5% dextrose in water, given at a rate of 1 to 4 mg (15 to 60 microdrops) per min, using a drip bulb that delivers 60 drops per ml.

Hartel G, Karhunen P: Lidocaine and ventricular arrhythmia, letter to the Editor, N Engl J Med **278**:798, 1968.

Hayes AH Jr: The actions and clinical use of the newer antiarrhythmic drugs, Ration Drug Ther **6**(7), 1972.

Ilyas M, Owens D, Kvasnicka G: Delirium induced by a combination of antiarrhythmic drugs, Lancet **2**:1368, 1969.

Jeresaty RM, Kahn AH, Landry AB Jr: Sinoatrial arrest due to lidocaine in a patient receiving quinidine, Chest **61**:683, 1972.

Lichstein E, Chadda KD, Gupta PK: Atrioventricular block with lidocaine therapy, Am J Cardiol **31**:277, 1973.

Lown B, Vassaux C: Lidocaine in myocardial infarction, Am Heart J **76**:586, 1968.

Malach M, Kostis JB, Fischetti JL: Lidocaine for ventricular arrhythmias in acute myocardial infarction, Am J Med Sci **257**:52, 1969.

Marriott HJL, Bieza CF: Alarming ventricular acceleration after lidocaine administration, Chest **61**:682, 1972.

Parkinson PI, Margolin L, Dickson DSP: Oral lignocaine; its absorption and effectiveness in ventricular arrhythmia control, Br Med J **2**:29, 1970.

Scott DB, Jebson PJ, et al: Plasma levels of lignocaine after IM injection, Lancet **2**:1209, 1968.

Selden R, et al: Systemic use of lidocaine, letter to the Editor, N Engl J Med **278**:626, 1968.

Thomson PD, et al: Lidocaine pharmacokinetics in advanced heart failure, liver disease, and renal failure in humans, Ann Intern Med **78**:499, 1973.

MAGNESIUM SULFATE

Pharmacology

In cardiology, magnesium sulfate has been used parenterally to treat atrial and ventricular tachyarrhythmias (but not atrial fibrillation). However, it is not generally effective and should be used only when a tachyarrhythmia is associated with hypomagnesemia. (Hypomagnesemia may occur as a result of the malabsorption syndrome, excessive diuresis, or chronic alcoholism, or with other conditions that produce hypokalemia. The normal serum magnesium concentration is 1.5 to 2.4 mEq/L, or 1.8 to 2.9 mg/100 ml.)

The effectiveness of magnesium sulfate may be due partly to the fact that it prevents the loss of intracellular potassium from heart muscle cells by decreasing the permeability of cell membranes to potassium. Magnesium deficiency is therefore associated with a secondary loss of potassium ions from the body.

The electrocardiographic changes of hypomagnesemia are similar to those of hypokalemia, and the electrocardiographic changes associated with hypermagnesemia are similar to those of hyperkalemia. (See also side effects and toxicity.)

There is some evidence that hypomagnesemia predisposes to digitalis toxicity.

Absorption

Magnesium sulfate is absorbed orally. However, in the treatment of tachyarrhythmias, it should be given IV or IM.

Indications

Tachyarrhythmias associated with magnesium deficiency.

Contraindications

Conditions associated with hypermagnesemia, such as uremia.

Side effects and toxicity

Magnesium is a cardiac and central nervous system depressant. When given IM, it produces a fall in blood pressure and can cause cardiac arrest. It can produce ventricular premature contractions or ventricular tachycardia. Toxic electrocardiographic signs include a prolonged P-R interval and a widened QRS interval.

Central nervous system signs include lassitude, coma, and particularly respiratory depression.

Other side effects include a generalized sensation of heat, perspiration, weakness, dizziness, and nausea.

Treatment of toxicity. Calcium salts rapidly counteract the central nervous system depressant effects of magnesium. Therefore, an ampul (10 ml of 10%) of calcium gluconate should be immediately available for IV injection when magnesium sulfate is used.

Interactions with other drugs

Calcium salts; see above.

Magnesium sulfate potentiates the neuro-blocking action of procainamide (Pronestyl).

Dosage and administration

Ten to 20 ml of a 20% solution of magnesium sulfate can be given IV slowly at a rate of 1 ml/min, with electrocardiographic monitoring.

Magnesium sulfate can also be given IM as a 50% solution in a dose of 2 gm (4 ml) every 6 to 8 hours for several days.

One should remember that even when magnesium sulfate is given to a patient with magnesium deficiency, the symptoms and signs may not be completely relieved for several days.

Preparations

Injection: 100 mg/ml (10%), 20-ml ampuls; 250 mg/ml (25%), 1- and 10-ml ampuls; 500 mg/ml (50%), 2-, 5-, and 10-ml ampuls. A 20% solution of magnesium sulfate can be prepared by diluting the contents of two 2-ml ampuls of 50% magnesium sulfate with 6 ml distilled water.

REFERENCES

American Hospital Formulary Service: Magnesium sulfate. Category 28:12.

Bellet S: Clinical disorders of the heart beat, ed 3, Philadelphia, 1971, Lea & Febiger.

Chadda KD, Lichstein E, Gupta P: Hypomagnesemia and refractory cardiac arrhythmia in a nondigitalized patient, Am J Cardiol 31:98, 1973.

Enselberg CD, Simmons HG, Minta AA: Effects of magnesium upon cardiac arrhythmias, Am Heart J 39:703, 1950.

Goldberger E: Heart disease, ed 2, Philadelphia, 1955, Lea & Febiger.

Goldberger E: A primer of water, electrolyte and acid-base syndromes, ed 4, Philadelphia, 1970, Lea & Febiger.

Neff MS, et al: Magnesium sulfate in digitalis toxicity, Am J Cardiol 29:377, 1972.

Seller RH: The role of magnesium in digitalis toxicity, Am Heart J 82:551, 1971.

Seller RH, Moyer JH: Magnesium and digitalis toxicity, Heart Bull 18:32, 1969.

METARAMINOL (Aramine) BITARTRATE
Pharmacology

Metaraminol is a sympathomimetic amine whose pharmacological actions are similar to those of levarterenol. Metaraminol increases blood pressure mainly by means of peripheral vasoconstriction (including the renal and cerebral arteries). It also has a direct positive inotropic effect.

In animals, there is some evidence that metaraminol also acts by releasing norepinephrine from nerve endings. Therefore, theoretically, it may not be effective if hypotension or shock is due to a catecholamine-depleting drug, such as reserpine. However, clinically, it has been found to be effective in such conditions (Fletcher).

The major difference between metaraminol and levarterenol is the slower onset and longer duration of metaraminol. Following an IV injection, a pressor effect appears in 1 to 2 min, is maximum in 5 min, and lasts for 20 to 25 min. After IM or subcutaneous administration, a pressor response is observed in 5 to 12 min, is maximum in about 30 min, and lasts about 50 min.

When an IV infusion of metaraminol is given, the blood pressure rises gradually over a period of 10 to 15 min. Therefore, one should wait at least 10 min before further increasing a dose of metaraminol because a maximal effect is not immediately apparent.

In addition, when a metaraminol infusion is stopped, one should observe the patient carefully for about 20 min as the effect of the drug wears off, so that if the blood pressure falls too much, the metaraminol can be restarted.

Indications and contraindications

See Levarterenol.

Side effects

The vasoconstrictor effect of metaraminol is less than that of levarterenol, so that there is less danger of tissue necrosis if extravasation occurs. However, an abscess may form after IM or subcutaneous injection. The preferred vein is an antecubital vein of the forearm.

Similarly, large doses or prolonged administration of metaraminol may cause excessive vasoconstriction, a decreased circulating blood volume, a decreased cardiac output, and continued shock, just as may occur with levarterenol. This must be treated with isotonic saline, plasma, or dextran 40 (see Levarterenol).

Interactions with other drugs

See Levarterenol.

Dosage and administration

In an emergency, metaraminol can be injected undiluted IV in a dose of 0.05 to 0.5 ml (0.5 to 5 mg), or it can be given IM (or subcutaneously) undiluted in a dose of 0.2 to 1 ml (2 to 10 mg).

The usual method of administration is by means of a continuous IV infusion. The metaraminol is diluted in either isotonic saline or dextrose in water solution.

The usual dilution is 2.5 to 10 ml (25 to 100 mg) in 500 ml isotonic saline or 5%

dextrose in water solution. Higher concentrations of metaraminol, up to 100 mg in 100 ml dilution fluid, can also be used.

> When 25 mg metaraminol is dissolved in 500 ml fluid, each ml of this dilution contains 0.05 mg metaraminol.
>
> When 100 mg metaraminol is dissolved in 500 ml fluid, each ml of this dilution contains 0.2 mg metaraminol.
>
> When 100 mg metaraminol is dissolved in 100 ml fluid, each ml of this dilution contains 1.0 mg metaraminol.

The rate of infusion is adjusted to maintain the blood pressure at a desired level (see Levarterenol). This will require from 0.05 to 1 mg metaraminol per min.

If the patient needs more saline or dextrose solution at a rate of flow that would cause an excessive amount of metaraminol to be given per unit of time, the metaraminol can be added to more than 500 ml infusion fluid. Conversely, the desired dose of metaraminol can be added to less than 500 ml infusion fluid, if desired.

When metaraminol is used as a hypertensive drug to stop a paroxysmal atrial tachycardia, a smaller volume can be used; for example, 10 to 20 mg can be added to 50 ml 5% dextrose in water, given by slow IV drip to raise the blood pressure 20 to 30 mm Hg (but not exceeding 160 mm Hg), to produce slowing of the heart (Chapter 6).

METARAMINOL (Aramine) BITARTRATE	
Route of administration	**Emergency dosage**
IV, single dose	0.05 to 0.5 ml (0.5 to 5 mg) undiluted.
IM (or subcutaneously), single dose	0.2 to 1 ml (2 to 10 mg) undiluted.
Continuous IV infusion	1.5 to 10 ml (15 to 100 mg) in 500 ml 5% dextrose in water or isotonic saline, to raise and maintain the blood pressure to 90 to 100 mm Hg (slightly higher if the patient has been hypertensive) and to eliminate other signs of shock.

Preparations

Injection: 1-ml ampuls and 10-ml vials; each ml contains 10 mg metaraminol bitartrate.

REFERENCES

Catenacci AJ, DiPalma JR, et al: Serious arrhythmias with vasopressors during halothane anesthesia in man, JAMA **183**:662, 1963.

Fletcher GF: Hypotensive reactions after small doses of reserpine given parenterally, N Engl J Med **268**:309, 1963.

Mills LC, Steppacher R: Hemodynamic effects of vasopressor agents in hemorrhagic shock, Am J Cardiol **12**:614, 1963.

Mills LC, Voudoukis IJ: Treatment of shock with sympathomimetic drugs; use of metaraminol and comparison with other vasopressor agents, Arch Intern Med **106**:816, 1960.

METHOXAMINE HYDROCHLORIDE (Vasoxyl)

Methoxamine hydrochloride is a sympathomimetic amine with pharmacological properties similar to those of phenylephrine, but without producing cardiac irritability. When given IV, it produces a pressor effect almost immediately. The effect lasts for approximately 1 hour.

Methoxamine, like phenylephrine, has been used to counteract the hypotensive effect of spinal anesthesia and surgery, and as a hypertensive agent to produce reflex bradycardia in patients with paroxysmal atrial tachycardia.

Side effects and toxicity

See Phenylephrine hydrochloride.

Contraindications

Hyperthyroidism, hypertension.

Dosage and administration

A dose of 5 to 10 mg is given slowly IV, with continuous blood pressure and electrocardiographic monitoring. The blood pressure should be raised 20 to 30 mm Hg (but not above 160 mm Hg).

Preparations

1-ml ampuls: each ml contains 20 mg methoxamine hydrochloride.

10-ml vials: each ml contains 10 mg methoxamine hydrochloride.

REFERENCES

Berger AJ, Rackliffe RL: Treatment of paroxysmal supraventricular tachycardia with methoxamine, JAMA **152**:1132, 1953.

Chotkowski LA, et al: Methoxamine hydrochloride in the treatment of paroxysmal supraventricular tachycardia, N Engl J Med **250**:674, 1954.

Durham JR: Severe reaction to methoxamine hydrochloride, JAMA **167**:1835, 1958.

METHYLDOPATE (Aldomet Ester) HYDROCHLORIDE

Methyldopa is a hypotensive drug whose chemical structure is similar to that of the catecholamines, although it is not a catecholamine. Methyldopate is the ethyl ester of the hydrochloride salt of methyldopa It is suitable for IV use.

Pharmacology

The antihypertensive mechanism of methyldopa is not known. It probably lowers the blood pressure indirectly by decreasing the synthesis of catecholamines, possibly by way of a false neurotransmitter. Blood pressure is reduced when the patient is in the supine position as well as in the standing position. After IV administration, there is a slight decrease in cardiac output, but renal blood flow is maintained, so that methyldopa can be used in the presence of renal insufficiency.

After IV administration, it has an onset of action in 4 to 6 hours, and a duration of action of 10 to 16 hours. When the drug is stopped, the blood pressure usually returns to its original level within 48 hours.

Methyldopa is partially metabolized by the liver and kidneys. It is excreted, primarily in the urine, mostly unchanged.

Indications

Hypertension where there is no immediate need for blood pressure reduction (because of its slow onset of action). Not all patients respond adequately to methyldopa, and some patients may develop a paradoxical rise in blood pressure after it is given IV. It has been chiefly recommended for use in hypertension associated with acute or chronic glomerulonephritis because of its ability to maintain renal blood flow.

Contraindications

Active hepatic disease, such as acute hepatitis or active cirrhosis; pheochromocytoma. It is also contraindicated in patients known to be sensitive to it.

Side effects and toxicity

Sedation is the most usual early side effect. It occurs within the first 48 to 72 hours. Other transient side effects include asthenia, headache, or vertigo, which may be due to postural hypotension. If this occurs, the dosage should be reduced. Postural hypotension occurs more frequently when given to patients with decreased renal function. Therefore, in such patients, smaller doses should be used. Paradoxical hypertension can also occur when it is given IV.

Sodium retention with weight gain and edema may occur. This can usually be controlled with a thiazide diuretic. However, if the edema does not recede or if other signs of congestive heart failure occur, the methyldopa should be stopped. Methyldopa can also aggravate angina pectoris.

When methyldopa is given orally over a long period of time, numerous other side effects, including drug fever, a positive reaction to Coombs' test, with or without hemolytic anemia, may occur.

Abnormal liver function test results, including elevated SGOT and alkaline phosphatase levels, associated with liver biopsy evidence of focal hepatic necrosis, may occur when the drug is used for 10 or more days. Therefore, liver function tests should be routinely taken on patients receiving methyldopa and the drug stopped if enzyme changes occur.

Methyldopa is excreted in the urine, where it may cause falsely increased urinary catecholamine values. It may also cause falsely elevated creatinine values in the blood (when the test is done by the alkaline picrate method) or falsely elevated serum uric acid values (when the test is done by the phosphotungstate method). A true increased serum sodium concentration may also occur.

Interactions with other drugs

Guanethidine and the thiazide diuretics increase the hypotensive effects of methyldopa.

Dosage and administration

Methyldopate hydrochloride is given by IV infusion. The desired dose of the drug is added to 100 ml 5% dextrose in water. The infusion is then given over a period of 30 to 60 min.

The usual adult IV dosage is 250 to 500 mg every 6 hours. The maximum dosage is 1 gm every 6 hours. However, when renal insufficiency is present, smaller doses are needed.

When the blood pressure has been lowered, the patient can be given oral methyldopa therapy at the same dose.

Preparations

Injection: 5-ml ampuls; each ml contains 50 mg.

Methyldopa is also available in 250-mg tablets for oral use.

REFERENCES

AMA drug evaluations, 1971, Methyldopate hydrochloride.
American Hospital Formulary Service: Methyldopa, methyldopate hydrochloride. Category 24:08.
Gifford RW Jr: The hypertensive crisis, In Clinician; managing medical emergencies, Chicago, 1972, GD Searle & Co.
Merck Sharp & Dohme: Injection, Aldomet Ester HCl (methyldopate HCl), brochure, Dec 1971.

NEO-SYNEPHRINE HYDROCHLORIDE. *See* Phenylephrine hydrochloride.

OUABAIN (G-Strophanthin)

Ouabain is a digitalis glycoside obtained from the seeds of the *Strophanthus gratus* or from the wood of *Acocanthera schimperi*. It is the most potent pure digitalis glycoside. It is not absorbed from the gastrointestinal tract and is given IV.

Its general pharmacology is discussed under Digitalis glycosides.

Following the IV administration of a single dose of 0.5 mg, effects are noticeable in 3 to 10 min, are maximal in ½ to 2 hours, regress in 8 to 12 hours, and disappear in 1 to 3 days. Ouabain therefore acts more rapidly and its effects disappear more quickly than digoxin or deslanoside.

Dosage and administration

IM injections are painful and are not recommended.

The adult digitalizing dose of ouabain is 1 mg. It must be given by slow IV injection in divided doses, starting with 0.25 to 0.5 mg (250 to 500 μg). After this, additional IV injections of 100 μg can be given hourly until a desired therapeutic response has occurred or toxic signs appear.

Oral digitalis therapy can be started even after the initial dose of ouabain. For example, one fourth to one half the average digitalizing dose can be given after the initial dose of ouabain. Maintenance oral digitalis therapy can then be continued the next day. Maintenance oral doses of digitalis can also be started after the patient has been digitalized with ouabain.

Ouabain should not be used if the patient has had digitalis in the previous 2 weeks.

I believe that the very rapid action of ouabain is a disadvantage rather than an advantage because serious and even lethal toxic reactions can occur very quickly. For this reason, I give either digoxin or deslanoside IV.

Preparations

Ampuls: 1 and 2 mg; each ml contains 0.25 mg (250 μg).

REFERENCES

See Digitalis glycosides.

PENTOLINIUM (Ansolysen) TARTRATE

Pentolinium tartrate, a quaternary amine, is a ganglionic blocking drug. Such drugs block the transmission of impulses through both the sympathetic and parasympathetic ganglia of the autonomic nervous system. Blockade of the sympathetic stimuli decrease the blood pressure by decreasing vasomotor tone. As a result, peripheral resistance is decreased. The decreased vasomotor tone results in venous pooling in the lower extremities with decreased venous return and consequent decreased cardiac output.

Absorption

Pentolinium is usually given either subcutaneously or IM. It is irregularly absorbed after oral administration. When given IV, it is ionized slowly, and its effects are inconstant. Therefore, IV administration is not recommended.

After subcutaneous or IM injection, its action starts in 30 to 60 min, reaches a peak within 2 hours, and lasts for 4 to 8 hours.

Indications

Hypertensive emergencies, particularly those associated with acute hypertensive encephalopathy, acute pulmonary edema, intracranial (intracerebral or subarachnoid) hemorrhage, acute dissecting aneurysm, malignant hypertension.

Contraindications

Organic pyloric stenosis. Should be used cautiously with bleeding peptic ulcer.

Recent myocardial infarction or recent cerebral thrombosis. However, after a period of 6 weeks, pentolinium can be given, but hypotension should be avoided.

Severe renal disease with a BUN concentration of 80 mg/100 ml or higher.

Side effects and toxicity

The side effects are actually direct pharmacological actions of the pentolinium and are related to the dosage and to the susceptibility of individual patients. Most of the side effects (except postural hypotension) are related to blockade of the parasympathetic ganglia and can be counteracted by parasympathomimetic drugs.

Postural hypotension and syncope can occur if the blood pressure is reduced too rapidly or too greatly. Postural hypotension is most likely to occur if the patient stands suddenly or stands motionless. Postural hypotension is more frequent after parenteral than after oral administration of pentolinium.

Visual. Blurring of vision is due to partial paralysis of accommodation. (This can be prevented by using a parasympathetic-stimulating drug, such as 2.5 to 5 mg pilocarpine nitrate with each dose of pentolinium.) Fixed pupils can also occur. This should not be misinterpreted as a sign of intracranial bleeding.

Gastrointestinal. Dryness of the mouth is common. Constipation, paralytic ileus, vomiting, or diarrhea can occur as a result of blockade of the autonomic nervous system. Constipation is most common. The patient must have a daily bowel movement. A cathartic of the saline or irritating type, such as milk of magnesia, cascara sagrada, and phenolphthalein, should be used. Bulk laxatives should *not* be used. Pilocarpine nitrate (see above) can also be used to prevent constipation.

If diarrhea occurs, it can be controlled with kaolin and pectin mixtures.

Dryness of the mouth is common, especially at first. It can be controlled by pilocarpine nitrate (see above). Vomiting can also occur.

Genitourinary. Decreased libido and delayed orgasm may occur. Elderly patients with prostatic enlargement may develop urinary retention or delayed bladder emptying. If the patient is comatose, an indwelling catheter should be inserted into the bladder.

Treatment of side effects. It may be necessary to decrease the dosage or stop the drug temporarily if side effects become severe. Pilocarpine nitrate (see above) can be used to prevent ocular or gastrointestinal side effects.

If the blood pressure falls too low, the foot of the bed can be elevated. If this is not effective, the patient can be given isotonic saline IV or, if necessary, a very small dose of levarterenol (Levophed) IV (because patients receiving pentolinium or other ganglionic blocking agents are very sensitive to it).

Interactions with other drugs

Pentolinium potentiates the pressor effect of levarterenol and other sympathicomimetic drugs because patients with sympathetic blockade are very sensitive to norepinephrine (Levophed). It also potentiates the hypotensive effects of reserpine, spironolactone (Aldactone), the thiazides, and ethacrynic acid (Edecrin).

The hypotensive effect of pentolinium is increased by MAO inhibitors.

Other antihypertensive drugs can be used concomitantly with pentolinium. For example, reserpine can be given IM alternately or simultaneously with pentolinium. In this way, smaller than usual doses of both drugs will be effective and have lessened side effects. For example, after small initial doses of both drugs, 1 mg pentolinium can be given subcutaneously or IM alternately or simultaneously with 2 mg reserpine given IM whenever the diastolic blood pressure exceeds a desired level, such as 130 mm Hg.

Dosage and administration

Pentolinium should be given subcutaneously or IM when used to treat a hypertensive emergency. The injections should be made in the distal part of an extremity, so that a tourniquet can be applied above the injection site if the patient develops hypotension or syncope.

The first subcutaneous dose should be

1 mg (or less) because hypertensive patients with uremia or intracranial complications may be extremely sensitive to the drug. The blood pressure should be taken at least every 10 min for at least 60 min, or until the maximum fall in blood pressure occurs.

The patient should be kept in a sitting position in bed, if possible, and the blood pressure should be measured with the patient sitting or with his legs dangling, because pentolinium produces its blood pressure effects by means of postural hypotension. A fall in blood pressure may not be observed if the reading is taken with the patient lying. However, the patient should be warned to rise slowly to a sitting or standing position and to lie down immediately when a feeling of weakness or giddiness occurs.

After an initial dose of 1 mg, a dose of 2 mg can be given subcutaneously in 4 hours. If the diastolic pressure remains high after 4 to 6 hours, the next dose can be 4 mg; this can be followed by a dose of 6 mg in 4 to 6 hours.

Dose increments should not be given more often than every 4 to 6 hours to prevent a cumulative effect. A single effective dose will usually range between 2.5 and 10 mg.

Once the effective single dose is found, it can be repeated every 6 to 8 hours, as needed, or more frequently if the diastolic blood pressure rises beyond a desired level (for example, 120 mm Hg).

Severe side effects, such as urinary retention, obstipation, or even paralytic ileus usually develop within a few days and necessitate stopping the drug.

Preparations

Injection: 10-ml vials; each ml contains 10 mg.

Tablets are also available for oral use.

REFERENCES

American Hospital Formulary Service: Pentolinium tartrate. Category 24:08.

Breslin DJ: Hypertensive crisis, Med Clin North Am 53:351, 1969.

Wyeth Laboratories: Ansolysen Tartrate (pentolinium tartrate), product brochure, Aug 1971.

PHENTOLAMINE (Regitine) MYSELATE
Pharmacology

Phentolamine is an alpha adrenergic blocking drug (see Adrenergic drugs). It also has direct positive inotropic and

PENTOLINIUM (Ansolysen) TARTRATE	
Route of administration	Emergency dosage
Subcutaneous (or IM)	Initial dose 1 mg (or less). Take blood pressure with patient sitting or legs dangling, at least every 10 min, for at least 60 min or until the maximum blood pressure fall occurs. Then increase dose by 2-mg increments (even to 10 mg) every 4 to 6 hours, until desired blood pressure fall occurs. Maintain this dose every 6 to 8 hours, or more frequently, if necessary. (Average maintenance dose is 2.5 to 10 mg.) If blood pressure falls too low, elevate the foot of the bed, give isotonic saline intravenously, or if necessary, very small doses of levarterenol (Levophed) intravenously (because patients receiving pentolinium or other ganglionic blocking agents are very sensitive to it).

chronotropic effects on heart muscle and has a direct vasodilator effect on the smooth muscle of blood vessel walls. As a result, the blood pressure falls. It also has a histaminelike action on the gastrointestinal tract.

Absorption

Phentolamine myselate is given parenterally. Phentolamine hydrochloride can be given orally but is much less effective than parenteral administration of phentolamine myselate.

Indications

1. Prevention or control of hypertensive crises that may occur in a patient with a pheochromocytoma as a result of stress or manipulation during preoperative preparation and surgical excision.
2. Acute hypertensive crisis in a patient taking an MAO inhibitor (Chapter 12).
3. Prevention of sloughing of the skin if a levarterenol (Levophed) infusion extravasates.
4. Treatment of shock when excessive vasoconstriction (excessive afterload) is present when the central venous pressure is high (20 cm water or higher). It can be used either alone or in combination with levarterenol or metaraminol (p. 42).
5. Diagnosis of pheochromocytoma (Regitine-blocking test).

Contraindications

Gastritis, peptic ulcer.

Side effects and toxicity

When phentolamine is given parenterally, it can cause sinus tachycardia or a tachyarrhythmia associated with anginal pain, weakness, dizziness, or flushing. In addition, severe hypotension that may lead to shock or acute myocardial infarction may develop.

The histaminelike action of phentolamine may cause nasal stuffiness and gastrointestinal distress, including nausea, vomiting, intestinal cramps, or diarrhea.

Treatment of side effects. Severe hypotension and shock can be counteracted with an infusion of levarterenol. Epinephrine, which may cause a paradoxical fall in blood pressure, should *not* be used.

Interactions with other drugs

Levarterenol or metaraminol can be used concomitantly with phentolamine in the treatment of shock (p. 42).

Propranolol can be given during the surgical treatment of a pheochromocytoma (if used simultaneously with phentolamine) to diminish the risk of excessive hypertension.

Digitalis should not be given following any untoward reaction to phentolamine until the patient has fully recovered from the reaction.

Epinephrine is contraindicated if shock occurs due to phentolamine, because it may produce a paradoxical hypotension.

The hypertension produced by an MAO inhibitor can be counteracted by phentolamine.

Dosage and administration

Dosage and administration are described on p. 42.

Preparations

Phentolamine (Regitine) myselate. Injection: ampuls, each containing 5 mg phentolamine myselate in lyophilized form and accompanied by a 1-ml ampul of distilled water for dilution.

Phentolamine hydrochloride. Tablets: 50 mg.

REFERENCES

American Hospital Formulary Service: Phentolamine myselate (Regitine Myselate). Category 24:08.

Bradley EC: Results with phentolamine (Regitine) in the treatment of selected patients with shock, Calif Med **103**:314, 1965.

Ciba Pharmaceutical Co: Regitine (Phentolamine), brochure, May 1971.

Corday E, Swan HJC, editors: Myocardial infarction, Baltimore, 1973, The Williams & Wilkins Co.

Gould L: Phentolamine, Am Heart J 78:276, 1969.

Kones RJ, Phillips JH: Newer inotropic agents for cardiogenic shock, South Med J 65:329, 1972.

Majid PA, Sharma B, Taylor SH: Phentolamine for vasodilator treatment of severe heart failure, Lancet 2:719, 1971.

Martin EW: Harzards of medication, Philadelphia, 1971, JB Lippincott Co.

Shubin H, Weil MH: The treatment of shock complicating acute myocardial infarction, Prog Cardiovasc Dis 10:30, 1967.

PHENYLEPHRINE (Neo-Synephrine) HYDROCHLORIDE

Pharmacology

Phenylephrine is a sympathomimetic amine. Its structure is similar to that of epinephrine. It has pharmacological actions similar to those of epinephrine, but it has less effect on the heart than epinephrine. Its effects occur within 1 min after IV injection and last from 7 to 10 min.

Indications

Paroxysmal atrial tachycardia. Because phenylephrine has pressor effects, it has been used to overcome the acute hypotension that may develop during spinal anesthesia. It has also been used to treat paroxysmal atrial tachycardia by causing hypertension. In this way it stimulates vagal fibers in the carotid sinus and aortic arch and causes slowing of the heart. However, it is not a drug of first choice in the treatment of paroxysmal atrial tachycardia (Chapter 6).

Contraindications

Hyperthyroidism, hypertension, coronary artery disease.

Side effects and toxicity

Tingling of the extremities and coolness of the skin due to cutaneous vasoconstriction and piloerection usually occur. The patient may develop a strong urge to urinate. (Therefore, the bladder should be emptied before the injection is given.) Anxiety, palpitations, a sense of fullness in the head, substernal pressure, ventricular premature contractions, or ventricular tachycardia may also occur. Excessive bradycardia and cardiac arrest may also develop.

Interactions with other drugs

Phenylephrine should not be given to a patient who is receiving halothane anesthesia, because the combination may induce tachyarrhythmias. Similarly, phenylephrine should not be given if the patient has been taking an MAO inhibitor, such as Eutonyl, Nardil, Niamid, or Parnate, 10 days to 2 weeks previously, because the combination of the two drugs can cause an acute hypertensive crisis with cerebral hemorrhage, convulsions, coma, and even death.

Dosage and administration

In the treatment of paroxysmal atrial tachycardia, 0.5 mg (0.25 ml of the 0.2% solution) is injected rapidly (within 20 to 30 sec). The phenylephrine can be diluted with 1 to 10 ml sterile isotonic saline and placed in a tuberculin syringe so that it can be conveniently injected.

If the tachycardia is present when the blood pressure has returned to its preinjection level (in approximately 10 min), a larger dose, exceeding the original dose by 0.1 to 0.2 mg, can be given IV. The exact dose depends on the rise in blood pressure that has occurred. (The systolic blood pressure should rise 20 to 30 mm Hg, but should not exceed 160 mm Hg.) The total dose should not exceed 1 mg.

Preparations

Injection: 2-ml ampuls (0.2% solution); each ml contains 2 mg phenylephrine hydrochloride.

REFERENCES

Bernstein H: Treatment of paroxysmal supraventricular tachycardia with Neo-Synephrine, NY State J Med 56:2570, 1956.

Martin EW, Hazards of medication, Philadelphia, 1971, JB Lippincott Co.

Youmans WB, Goodman MJ, Gould J: Neosynephrine in treatment of paroxysmal supraventricular tachycardia, Am Heart J **37:**359, 1949.

PROCAINAMIDE (Pronestyl) HYDROCHLORIDE

Procainamide hydrochloride is the amide analog of procaine hydrochloride. It is also structurally similar to lidocaine. Although it also has anesthetic actions, it is used as an antiarrhythmic agent.

Pharmacology

Procainamide is a group I antiarrhythmic drug (see Antiarrhythmic drugs). Its actions are very similar to those of quinidine. It may produce systemic hypotension, partially by way of peripheral vasodilation. It decreases the force of cardiac contractions and causes a rise in left ventricular end-diastolic pressure. It also decreases the cardiac output and may also decrease pulmonary artery pressure.

Electrocardiographic effects

Widening of the QRS width and prolongation of the Q-T interval occur most frequently. Less regularly, the P-R interval is prolonged. The T waves may show decreased amplitudes and occasionally inversion.

Absorption

Procainamide is well absorbed from the gastrointestinal tract. It can also be given IM and, in an emergency, IV.

When procainamide is given orally, its effects appear within ½ hour. A peak plasma concentration occurs in approximately 1 hour; then the plasma concentration falls to one half in 2½ to 5 hours.

When procainamide is given IM, a maximum effect occurs in 15 to 60 min. The plasma concentration then falls slowly over a period of 6 to 8 hours.

When it is given IV, its action begins almost immediately. A peak plasma concentration occurs in a few minutes and then falls slowly at a rate of 10 to 20% per hour.

An effective plasma concentration of procainamide (given by any route) is 4 to 8 μg/ml (4 to 8 mg/L).

Indications

Indications are described as excellent, good, fair, or poor.

Procainamide is not necessarily the drug of first choice, even when it is known to be effective, because of its side effects.

Procainamide, like quinidine, can be used to treat atrial or ventricular tachyarrhythmias but is usually more effective in the treatment of ventricular tachyarrhythmias. It is effective in the following conditions.

1. Ventricular premature contractions. Excellent.

2. Ventricular tachycardia. Excellent. Procainamide is effective against ventricular tachycardia due to any cause. It has been found very helpful when ventricular tachycardia occurs during anesthesia, especially when cyclopropane is used.

If procainamide slows the ventricular rate of a ventricular tachycardia significantly, without regular sinus rhythm developing, it should be stopped because of the danger of cardiac arrest.

3. Atrial premature contractions. Good.

4. Paroxysmal atrial tachycardia. Good.

5. Atrial fibrillation, for conversion to sinus rhythm (after the patient has been digitalized). Fair. It is most effective when the atrial fibrillation is of short duration.

The patient should be digitalized prior to using procainamide to convert atrial fibrillation (or atrial flutter) to sinus rhythm because the procainamide may increase conduction through the AV node and produce a temporary increase in the ventricular rate. This possibility is lessened by prior digitalization.

When regular sinus rhythm develops after procainamide is given to a patient with chronic atrial fibrillation, forceful atrial contractions may develop and may dislodge a small mural thrombus from the left (or right) atrial wall, resulting in embolization. (The use of anticoagulants to prevent such embolization is discussed on p. 250.)

6. Atrial fibrillation converted to sinus rhythm, for maintenance of sinus rhythm. Fair.

7. Atrial flutter, for conversion to sinus rhythm (after the patient has been digitalized). Fair.

8. Atrial flutter converted to sinus rhythm, for maintenance of sinus rhythm. Fair.

9. AV junctional premature contractions. Good.

10. AV junctional paroxysmal tachycardia. Good.

11. Digitalis-induced supraventricular tachycardia. Good (if AV block is not present).

12. Digitalis-induced ventricular tachycardia. Good. However, procainamide may cause additional depression of conduction and may produce ventricular asystole or ventricular fibrillation. Therefore, a drug such as lidocaine or diphenylhydantoin is preferable.

Procainamide is also indicated for any condition where quinidine is indicated but the patient is unable to tolerate it.

Prophylactic use. Procainamide has been used prophylactically in acute myocardial infarction and before surgery, especially thoracic surgery, to prevent ventricular premature contractions, ventricular tachycardia, or ventricular fibrillation. I do not believe that it should be used prophylactically for a tachyarrhythmia that has *not* occurred, because it is not always effective and may be associated with serious toxicity (see below). In addition, if ventricular fibrillation occurs, it is more difficult to defibrillate the patient if procainamide has been given.

Contraindications

Second-degree or complete AV block, myasthenia gravis, hypersensitivity reac-

tions. Cross-sensitization to procaine and related drugs may also occur.

Shock. However, if the shock is due to a ventricular tachycardia, and other therapeutic measures are not effective, procainamide can be used with a vasopressor agent.

Side effects and toxicity

Procainamide can cause serious and even lethal side effects.

Cardiovascular. Severe hypotension and shock may occur, particularly when procainamide is given IV. The drug should be temporarily stopped if the systolic blood pressure falls 15 mm Hg or more. Procainamide may also potentiate the hypotensive effects of diuretics and other hypotensive drugs.

Bradycardia, incomplete or complete AV block, asystole, ventricular premature contractions, ventricular tachycardia, or ventricular fibrillation may also occur.

If the QRS interval widens beyond 25% to 50% or if it exceeds 0.13 to 0.14 sec, the procainamide should be temporarily stopped, because either sign may be a precursor of ventricular tachycardia or ventricular fibrillation. When the QRS width decreases, the drug can be slowly started again.

Gastrointestinal. Anorexia, a bitter taste, nausea, vomiting, abdominal pain, and diarrhea.

Neurological and psychiatric. Confusion, malaise, mental depression, even hallucinations and other psychotic behavior, giddiness, muscle weakness, paresthesias, nocturnal hyperhidrosis, convulsions.

Hypersensitivity reactions. These are common, particularly if procainamide is used chronically. Drug fever, serum sickness, urticaria, pruritus, bronchial asthma, and a syndrome resembling systemic lupus erythematosus with a positive LE cell test, polyarthralgia, arthritis, pleuritic pain, pleural effusion, and pericarditis may develop. (When procainamide is given for a prolonged period, periodic blood counts and LE cell tests should be taken.)

Hematological. Agranulocytosis, leukopenia, leukocytosis, bone marrow plasmacytosis with resultant anemia, thrombocytopenia or a Coombs'-positive hemolytic anemia, hypergammaglobulinemia, and increased sedimentation rate.

Liver. Hepatomegaly with or without abnormal liver function test results, including elevated serum levels of glutamic oxaloacetic pyruvic transaminase, lactic dehydrogenase, and increased cephalin flocculation reaction, and increased sulfobromophthalein retention.

Treatment of toxicity. The procainamide should be stopped.

Hypotension can be treated with vasopressor agents, if necessary.

Marked widening of the QRS complexes with slowing of the heart rate can be treated by IV administration of sodium bicarbonate.

Systemic lupus erythematosus usually regresses when the procainamide is stopped. However, if lupus erythematosus develops in a patient with a life-threatening tachyarrhythmia that is not controllable by any other antiarrhythmic drug, the procainamide can be continued concomitantly with corticosteroids.

Interactions with other drugs

Procainamide can be used in combination with lidocaine, propranolol, or quinidine. When this is done, smaller doses of each drug is needed. Lidocaine and procainamide have a synergistic effect on the central nervous system and may produce restlessness or noisy behavior with visual hallucinations.

Procainamide can be used in combination with digitalis, particularly in the treatment of paroxysmal atrial fibrillation or atrial flutter (see indications). It must be used cautiously in treating digitalis-induced tachyarrhythmias (see indications).

Because of the hypotensive effects of procainamide, it must be used cautiously with diuretics and hypotensive drugs (see pharmacology).

Pressor agents can be used to overcome the hypotensive effects of procainamide (see dosage and administration).

Anticholinergic drugs are potentiated because procainamide has similar anticholinergic properties. Procainamide may also antagonize the depolarizing effects of acetylcholine. Therefore, it should be used cautiously in patients with muscular weakness, and it is contraindicated in myasthenia gravis.

Procainamide may potentiate the neuromuscular-blocking actions of antibiotics such as bacitracin, colistimethate, dihydrostreptomycin, gentamycin, gramicidin, kanamycin, neomycin, polymyxin B, streptomycin, and viomycin. The combined effects of these antibiotics and procainamide may produce serious respiratory depression.

The interaction of procainamide with muscle relaxants and magnesium salts is the same as with antibiotics.

Dosage and administration

Oral use. An initial dose of 0.5 to 1 gm can be given, followed by 0.25 to 0.5 gm every 4 to 6 hours. The total daily oral dose should not exceed 4 gm. (Oral doses as large as 5 to 10 gm daily have been given. However, such large doses can produce serious toxic effects.)

Koch-Weser and Klein have recently pointed out that a drug must be given at intervals not greater than its biologic half-life. Since the biological half-life of procainamide averages $3\frac{1}{2}$ hours and may be as short as 2.6 hours, they believe that the usual 4- to 6-hour schedules do not raise the plasma procainamide concentration adequately. They therefore suggest that procainamide be given orally every 3 hours, in a daily dose of 50 mg/kg body weight (3.5 gm daily for a 70-kg patient). They suggest that a priming dose two times the maintenance dose be used. For example,

glucose level and can precipitate hypoglycemia. It must therefore be given cautiously to patients who have attacks of spontaneous hypoglycemia or to diabetic patients who receive insulin or hypoglycemic drugs. Propranolol may prolong the hypoglycemia caused by insulin and may prevent the usual signs of hypoglycemia—tachycardia, sweating, wide pulse pressure —from appearing.

Propranolol may occasionally raise the blood urea nitrogen level and can raise the levels of serum glutamic oxaloacetic and pyruvic transaminases, alkaline phosphatase, lactice dehydrogenase, and bilirubin.

Hematological. A transient elevation of the white blood cell count may occur. In addition, propranolol can cause thrombocytopenic and nonthrombocytopenic purpura.

Treatment of toxicity. The propranolol should be stopped, or the dose should be reduced. In addition, the following can be done.

For bradycardia: atropine, 0.4 to 0.8 mg IV. If there is no response, a slow IV infusion of isoproterenol (Isuprel) can be given.

For congestive heart failure: digitalization and diuretics.

For hypotension: preferably epinephrine, or levarterenol.

For bronchospasm: isoproterenol (by inhalation) and aminophylline.

Interactions with other drugs

Propranolol can be used concomitantly with antiarrhythmic drugs such as quinidine and procainamide. When this is done, smaller doses of each drug are needed.

Propranolol can also be used with digitalis, which may be necessary to prevent the excessive negative inotropic effects of propranolol.

Propranolol must be used cautiously in patients who are receiving a drug such as reserpine, which has a catecholamine-depleting action. The combination of these two drugs may cause excessive reduction of the sympathetic nervous system activity.

Propranolol may also potentiate the action of central nervous system depressants, such as narcotics, analgesics, barbiturates and other sedatives, anesthetics, or alcohol.

Anesthetics, such as ether or chloroform, which are myocardial depressants, should not be used in a patient who is receiving propranolol.

Dosage and administration

Propranolol can be given orally or IV. The oral route of administration is preferred.

Oral use. Tachyarrhythmias: 10 to 30

PROPRANOLOL HYDROCHLORIDE (Inderal)

Route of administration	Emergency dosage
IV injection	1 to 3 ml (1 to 3 mg) at a rate of 1 mg/min, with electrocardiographic monitoring. A second dose can be given after 2 or more min, if necessary. Additional IV doses should not be repeated more than every 4 hours, and oral therapy should be started as soon as possible.
Oral	10 to 30 mg, three or four times a day, before meals and at bedtime.

mg, three or four times a day, *before* meals and at bedtime.

Intravenous use. The usual dose is 1 to 3 mg IV, with electrocardiographic monitoring. The rate of administration should not exceed 1 mg (1 ml) per min. Sufficient time should be allowed to enable a slow circulation to carry the propranolol to the site of action. As soon as a change in the heart rate or rhythm occurs, the propranolol should be stopped until its full effect is noted.

Depending on the response, a second IV dose may be repeated after 2 or more min. Additional doses should not be repeated more than every 4 hours. Therapy with oral dosage is advisable as soon as possible.

Preparations

Tablets: 10 and 40 mg.
Injection: 1-ml ampuls; each ml contains 1 mg.

REFERENCES

Donoso E, et al: Effects of propranolol on patients with complete heart block and implanted pacemakers, Circulation 36:534, 1967.

Dreifus LS, Lim HF, et al: Propranolol and quinidine in the management of ventricular tachycardia, JAMA 204:736, 1968.

Fors WJ Jr, Vanderark CR, Reynolds EW Jr: Evaluation of propranolol and quinidine in the treatment of quinidine-resistant arrhythmias, Am J Cardiol 27:190, 1971.

Frohlich ED: Beta adrenergic blockade in the circulatory regulation of hyperkinetic states, Am J Cardiol 27:195, 1971.

Greenleaf DJ, Koch-Weser J: Adverse reactions to propranolol in hospitalized medical patients, Am Heart J 86:478, 1973.

Harrison DC: Beta adrenergic blockade, 1972, Am J Cardiol 29:432, 1972.

Kotler MN, Berman J, Rubenstein AH: Hypoglycemia precipitated by propranolol, Lancet 2:1389, 1966.

Lemberg L, Castellanos A Jr, Azucena GA: The use of propranolol in arrhythmias complicating acute myocardial infarction, Am Heart J 80:479, 1970.

Lucchesi BR, Whitsitt LS: Pharmacology of beta-adrenergic blocking agents, Prog Cardiovasc Dis 11:410, 1969.

Matloff JM, Wolfson S, et al: Control of postcardiac surgical tachycardias with propranolol, Circulation 38(Suppl 2), 1968.

McNeill RS, Ingram CG: Effect of propranolol on ventilatory function, Am J Cardiol 18:473, 1966.

Reveno WS, Rosenbaum H: Propranolol hypoglycemia, Lancet 1:920, 1968.

Reynolds EW Jr, Vanderark CR: Treatment of quinidine-resistant arrhythmias with the combined use of quinidine and propranolol, Circulation 36(Suppl 2):221, 1967.

Rothfeld EL, et al: Management of persistently recurring ventricular fibrillation with propranolol hydrochloride, JAMA 204:546, 1968.

Sloman JG, Robinson JS, McLean KH: Propranolol (Inderal) in persistent ventricular fibrillation, Br Med J 1:895, 1965.

Smith JE, et al: Studies of the effect of beta adrenergic blockade on abnormal RS-T segments and T wave changes, Aerospace Med 41:190, 1970.

Stephen SA: Unwanted effects of propranolol, Am J Cardiol 18:463, 1966.

Taylor RR, Halliday EJ: Beta adrenergic blockade in the treatment of exercise-induced paroxysmal ventricular tachycardia, Circulation 32:778, 1965.

Turner JRB: Propranolol in the treatment of digitalis-induced and digitalis-resistant tachycardia, Am J Cardiol 18:450, 1966.

Warner WA, Andersen TW: Beta adrenergic blocking agents and anesthesia, South Med J. 61:233, 1968.

Watt DA: Sensitivity to propranolol after digoxin intoxication, Br Med J 4:413, 1968.

QUINIDINE

Quinidine is one of the natural alkaloids found in cinchona bark. It is the dextro-isomer of quinine. Although it has antipyretic and other properties of quinine, it is used as an antiarrhythmic drug. It is available as the sulfate, gluconate, or polygalacturonate salt.

Pharmacology

Quinidine is a group I antiarrhythmic drug (see Antiarrhythmic drugs) and is very similar to procainamide in its actions.

Quinidine also has a vagal blocking action. It blocks the cardiac slowing produced by vagal stimulation and by cholinergic drugs. This is an important action of quinidine, particularly when it is used to treat atrial fibrillation or atrial flutter (see indications).

Quinidine does not have much effect on the force of myocardial contraction when therapeutic doses are given to normal subjects. However, it has a beta adrenergic blocking effect on heart muscle and acts as a myocardial depressant when given to patients with severe heart disease, to patients with tachyarrhythmias associated with hypotension, and to elderly patients.

Quinidine also has an alpha adrenergic blocking effect (see Adrenergic drugs) on the peripheral blood vessels, decreasing systemic and pulmonary artery blood pressures. In addition, the peripheral arteries may not respond to sympathetic stimulation or to an alpha adrenergic stimulating drug, such as levarterenol. This can be serious if quinidine has caused severe hypotension.

Electrocardiographic effects

The electrocardiographic changes due to quinidine are related to its electrophysiological effects. Slowing of conduction through the AV node is associated with prolongation of the P-R interval. Prolongation of the action potential duration of the ventricular muscle is associated with widening of the QRS complex and prolongation of the Q-T interval. In addition, flattening, notching, or reversal of the direction of the T waves, associated with sagging of the RS-T segments and prominent U waves, may also occur. The P waves may become widened and notched.

Many of the electrocardiographic changes are related to the pharmacological activity of quinidine. However, a QRS interval widened more than 25% to 50% above its control value is a sign of toxicity. Quinidine should therefore be withheld when the QRS interval widens to 0.12 to 0.13 sec. In addition, quinidine must be given very cautiously to patients with bundle branch block or intraventricular conduction disturbances (except when the Wolff-Parkinson-White syndrome is present).

Other electrocardiographic signs of quinidine toxicity include slowing of the atrial rate, which may lead to atrial standstill; slowing of the ventricular rate, with the development of a slow idioventricular rhythm; or cardiac arrest. In other patients, ventricular premature beats, ventricular tachycardia, or ventricular fibrillation may occur.

Absorption

Quinidine salts are well absorbed from the gastrointestinal tract. Quinidine polygalacturonate is absorbed more slowly than quinidine sulfate or gluconate.

When a single dose of quinidine is given *orally*, a peak plasma concentration occurs in 1 to 3 hours. The duration of action is at least 6 to 8 hours. Significant amounts of quinidine are present in the plasma at the end of 12 hours, but very little is present after 24 hours.

When a single dose of quinidine is given *IM*, cardiac effects start in 5 to 15 min. A peak concentration occurs in 30 to 90 min, and then slowly falls.

When a single dose of quinidine is given IV, a peak plasma concentration is obtained more rapidly.

When congestive heart failure or renal insufficiency is present, the urinary excretion of quinidine is slowed. Therefore, smaller doses are needed in these patients. In addition, the excretion of quinidine is delayed when the urine is alkaline, and is accelerated when the urine is acid.

If hypokalemia is present, it may completely nullify the antiarrhythmic effects of quinidine. Conversely, hyperkalemia may enhance the development of quinidine toxicity.

Relation between plasma quinidine concentrations and therapeutic effects of quinidine

The maximum effect of quinidine on the heart does not occur until 4 to 6 hours after it is given. At this time, the plasma quinidine concentration is decreasing. However, it is not possible to measure the quinidine concentration in heart muscle. Therefore, its pharmacological effects must be noted indirectly from either its plasma concentration, electrocardiographic changes, or clinical signs.

In a general way, a plasma quinidine concentration of less than 2 mg/L is not associated with any antiarrhythmic effect. A therapeutic effect appears with a quinidine plasma concentration of 4 to 8 mg/L. Toxic effects are noted when the quinidine plasma concentration is greater than 10 mg/L.

Indications

Indications are described as excellent, good, fair, or poor.

The indications for quinidine and procainamide are similar. There is evidence that quinidine may be slightly more effective than procainamide for supraventricular tachyarrhythmias and that procainamide may be slightly more effective than quinidine for ventricular tachyarrhythmias. However, because of the many toxic side effects of procainamide, quinidine may be the preferable drug, particularly for long-term use.

1. Atrial premature contractions. Excellent.

2. Paroxysmal atrial tachycardia. Excellent.

3. Atrial fibrillation (after digitalization), for conversion to sinus rhythm. Excellent.

When quinidine is given to a patient with atrial fibrillation, it often produces transient atrial flutter before sinus rhythm appears because quinidine decreases the rate at which the atria fibrillate. When the fibrillatory rate reaches approximately 300/ min, atrial flutter appears. (If the atrial flutter persists when quinidine is given, the quinidine should be stopped.)

In addition, when quinidine is given to a patient with atrial fibrillation (or atrial flutter), its vagal blocking effect may improve the conduction of stimuli through the AV node. Therefore, when the rate at which the atria fibrillate (or flutter) decreases because of the quinidine, more stimuli may be able to penetrate the AV node, causing a transient increase in the ventricular rate. This can be prevented by digitalizing the patient prior to giving quinidine.

4. Atrial fibrillation, for maintenance of sinus rhythm, after conversion. Excellent.

5. Paroxysmal atrial fibrillation associated with the Wolff-Parkinson-White syndrome. Excellent.

6. Atrial flutter (after digitalization), for conversion to sinus rhythm. Fair. (Also see atrial fibrillation, above.)

7. AV junctional premature contractions. Good.

8. AV junctional paroxysmal tachycardia. Good.

9. Ventricular premature contractions. Good to excellent.

10. Ventricular tachycardia. Good to excellent.

11. Digitalis-induced supraventricular tachycardia. Fair.

12. Digitalis-induced ventricular tachycardia. Fair. However, quinidine may depress the conduction system, resulting in ventricular fibrillation or cardiac standstill. Therefore, diphenylhydantoin (Dilantin) or lidocaine (Xylocaine) is preferable in these patients.

Contraindications

Ventricular fibrillation. Quinidine decreases the amplitude of the ventricular fibrillation waves, and increased electrical energy is needed to defibrillate the patient.

Second-degree or complete AV block, previous serious side effects or toxicity to quinidine or to other cinchona derivatives, tachyarrhythmias occurring during surgery, myasthenia gravis or patients with muscular weakness or respiratory distress.

Side effects and toxicity

Periodic blood counts, ECGs, and tests of kidney and liver function should be taken when quinidine is used for long-term therapy.

Cinchonism is the most common side effect. It consists of nausea, vomiting, diarrhea, dizziness or headache, and tinnitus. It is not usually necessary to stop the quinidine if these symptoms appear, unless they are very disturbing to the patient. If the quinidine is stopped and then started at a lower dosage, the patient may be able to tolerate even larger doses than those that previously caused the symptoms. There is no relation between the plasma quinidine concentration and the development of signs of cinchonism.

Cardiovascular. Bradycardia, congestive heart failure, hypotension or shock, incomplete or complete AV block, cardiac standstill in diastole, ventricular premature contractions, ventricular tachycardia, ventricular fibrillation, atrial flutter.

Syncope is a very serious side effect. It is usually due to transient ventricular fibrillation and may result in sudden death.

Peripheral embolism may occur in patients with chronic atrial fibrillation that is converted to sinus rhythm by quinidine or synchronized DC shock, because the forceful atrial contractions that result may cause a small thrombus in the right or left atrial appendage to break off. For this reason, prior anticoagulation (p. 250) has been used in these patients.

Gastrointestinal. Anorexia, bitter taste, salivation, nausea, vomiting, diarrhea, abdominal pain, an urge to defecate. These gastrointestinal side effects can be minimized by giving the quinidine with food or by using a different preparation. Paregoric can be used to control the abdominal cramps and diarrhea.

Hematological. Thrombocytopenic purpura, hypoplastic or hemolytic anemia, leukopenia, agranulocytosis.

Respiratory. Bronchial asthma, dyspnea, cyanosis, respiratory paralysis.

Neurological. Apprehension, excitement, confusion, headache, tinnitus, cold sweat.

Visual. Blurred vision, photophobia, diplopia, disturbed color perception, mydriasis, scotoma, night blindness, and even constricted visual fields may occur.

Dermatological and hypersensitivity reactions. Urticaria or flushing, exofoliative dermatitis, maculopapular or scarlatinal rashes, drug fever.

Treatment of toxicity. Stop the quinidine.

If marked widening of the QRS complex (more than 50% or 0.14 sec or more) or frequent ventricular premature contractions are present, lidocaine or IV doses of sodium bicarbonate can be given. If ventricular tachycardia occurs, DC shock can be given. However, if ventricular fibrillation occurs as a result of quinidine toxicity, DC shock will not be effective, but the other measures just mentioned can be used.

Sodium bicarbonate may also be of value when a bradyarrhythmia with widened QRS complexes occurs as a result of quinidine toxicity. Molar sodium lactate has also been used for quinidine or procainamide toxicity. However, it has the same pharmacological actions as sodium bicarbonate. Neither drug should be used if hypokalemia or alkalosis is present, and it should be stopped if it causes the appearance or increased frequency of ventricular premature contractions.

Severe hypotension or shock can be treated with levarterenol (Levophed) or a similar vasopressor drug.

Interactions with other drugs

Digitalis: see indications.

Procainamide: quinidine can be used in combination with procainamide in treating tachyarrhythmias. Smaller doses of each drug should be used.

Propranolol: see Procainamide.

Quinidine may antagonize the action of

neostigmine (Prostigmine) or edrophonium chloride (Tensilon) and the depolarizing effects of acetylcholine.

Quinidine may potentiate or be potentiated, by the neuromuscular-blocking effects and respiratory depressant effects of both depolarizing and nondepolarizing muscle relaxants, such as dimethyl tubocurarine (Metubine, Mecostrin), tubocurarine (Tubarine), decamethonium bromide (Syncurine), succinylcholine (Anectine, Sucostrin, Sux-cert), gallamine triethiodide (Flaxedil); by antibiotics that also have a neuromuscular-blocking effect, such as kanamycin, neomycin, and streptomycin; and possibly by magnesium salts. The patient may therefore develop muscle weakness or apnea when quinidine is used with any of the above drugs.

Anticholinergic drugs may potentiate the action of quinidine or may be potentiated by it.

Anticoagulants, such as coumarin, may be potentiated by quinidine, and smaller doses may be needed. Frequent prothrombin time tests should be taken to regulate the dosage of the anticoagulant.

Rauwolfia alkaloids, or veratrum alkaloids must be used cautiously when quinidine is given because cardiac arrhythmias can occur.

Quinidine may increase the hypotensive effect of diuretics such as the thiazides, furosemide, ethacrynic acid, and other antihypertensive drugs.

Dosage and administration

Quinidine should be given orally if possible. In an emergency, quinidine can be given IM. Quinidine should not be given IV, because IV preparations of procainamide are now available. Extended release tablets should be used only for maintenance and for prolonged therapy. Regardless of the route of administration, the effects of quinidine should be checked with the ECG or with plasma quinidine concentrations.

Oral use. In order to determine possible idiosyncracy to quinidine, a test dose of 200 mg quinidine sulfate, or 330 mg quinidine gluconate, or 275 mg quinidine polygalacturonate is given by mouth. A therapeutic dose can then be started in 2 hours if no signs of idiosyncracy develop (see side effects and toxicity). (This does not indicate that the patient may not later develop side effects or toxicity when therapeutic doses of quinidine are given.)

Quinidine sulfate. A widely used oral dose schedule of quinidine sulfate is 200 to 300 mg (0.2 to 0.3 gm) every 3 or 4 hours for 1 to 3 days. The quinidine dose is omitted at night to permit sleep. If sinus rhythm does not reappear, each individual dose may be increased to 400 mg, given every 3 or 4 hours. This can be continued for another 1 to 3 days.

It may be necessary to give higher doses, but if the total daily dose exceeds 4 gm, there is great danger of toxicity. If the daily dose exceeds 2 gm, an ECG should be taken before each successive dose. The quinidine should be stopped if excessive widening of the QRS occurs (see electrocardiographic effects).

An average maintenance dose of quinidine sulfate is 200 to 300 mg (0.2 to 0.3 gm) three or four times a day. Unfortunately, many patients require a maintenance dose that is almost as large as the dose needed to stop the tachyarrhythmia.

Maintenance therapy can be continued for a few weeks or longer or indefinitely, depending on the frequency and type of tachyarrhythmia.

Extended-release tablets of quinine sulfate can be given in a maintenance dose of 2 tablets (approximately 600 mg) every 8 to 12 hours.

Quinidine gluconate. Orally, the average initial dose of quinidine gluconate is 1 to 2 tablets (330 to 660 mg) every 8 to 12 hours. (Each tablet is equivalent to 200 mg quinidine sulfate.) Some patients may require the dose every 6 hours.

The average maintenance dose ranges from 1 tablet every 12 hours to 2 tablets every 6 hours.

Quinidine polygalacturonate. The usual recommended adult oral dose is 1 to 3 tablets (275 to 825 mg) every 3 to 4 hours for 4 doses. (Each 275-mg tablet is equivalent to 200 mg quinidine sulfate. Three tablets given for 4 doses equal a total of 12 tablets, equivalent to 2.4 gm of quinidine sulfate.) The manufacturer recommends that if the tachyarrhythmia persists after the fourth dose is given, the dosage can be increased by increments of ½ to 1 tablet (137.5 to 275 mg) for another 4 doses, before increasing the dose further. However, such large doses of quinidine may produce serious toxicity.

The recommended maintenance dose of quinidine polygalacturonate is 1 tablet (275 mg) two or three times a day.

Intramuscular use. Quinidine gluconate can be given IM if the patient cannot take quinidine orally. A test dose of 1 ml (80 mg) can be given. If signs of idiosyncrasy do not appear in 30 min, a dose of 5 ml (400 mg) can then be given IM every 2 to 4 hours as necessary. Not more than 2 to 2.4 gm should be given in a 24-hour period.

Intravenous use. Quinidine gluconate can also be given IV, when diluted. However, it is rarely if ever used now because IV preparations of procainamide are available.

Preparations

Quinidine sulfate. Capsules: 100, 200, 325 mg.

Extended-release tablets (Quinidex extentabs—Robins): 300 mg.

Tablets: 100, 130, 200, 325 mg, scored.

Quinidine gluconate. Extended-release

QUINIDINE

Route of administration	Dosage
Oral	Quinidine sulfate Test dose: 0.2 gm (200 mg). Therapeutic dose (after 2 hours): 0.2 to 0.3 gm every 3 to 4 hours. Quinidine gluconate Test dose: 330 mg. Therapeutic dose: 1 to 2 tablets (330 to 660 mg) every 8 to 12 hours. Quinidine polygalacturonate Test dose: 275 mg. Therapeutic dose: 1 to 3 tablets (275 to 825 mg) every 3 to 4 hours. Higher doses of each of the quinidine preparations may be necessary; see text.
IM	Quinidine gluconate Test dose: 1 ml (80 mg). Therapeutic dose (after 30 min): 5 ml (400) every 2 to 4 hours up to a total of 2.0 to 2.4 gm in 24 hours.
IV	Not used.

tablets (Quinaglute—Cooper): 330 mg; each tablet is equivalent to 206 mg quinidine sulfate.

Injection: 10-ml vials; each ml contains 80 mg quinidine gluconate (equivalent to 60 mg quinidine sulfate). The solution should be used only if clear and colorless.

Quinidine polygalacturonate. Tablets: 275 mg, scored (Cardioguin—Purdue Frederick); each tablet is equivalent to 200 mg quinidine sulfate.

REFERENCES

AMA Drug Evaluations, 1971, quinidine sulfate.

Barzel US: Quinidine sulfate induced hypoplastic anemia and agranulocytosis; JAMA **201**:325, 1967.

Browning RJ: Fever secondary to ingestion of quinidine, Proc Staff Meet Mayo Clin **35**:111, 1960.

Cheng TO: Atrial flutter during quinidine therapy of atrial fibrillation, Am Heart J **52**:273, 1956.

Conn HL Jr: Mechanisms of quinidine action. LS Dreifus, Likoff W, editors: In Mechanisms and cardiac arrhythmias, New York, 1966, Grune & Stratton.

Cooper Laboratories: Quinagulate Dura Tabs, brochure, Mar 1968.

Gerhardt RE, et al: Quinidine excretion in aciduria and alkaluria, Ann Intern Med **71**:927, 1969.

Goldman MJ: Combined quinidine and procaine amide treatment of chronic atrial fibrillation, Am Heart J **54**:742, 1957.

Heissenbuttel RH, Bigger JT: The effect of oral quinidine on intraventricular conduction in man; correlation of plasma quinidine with changes in QRS duration, Am Heart J **80**:453, 1970.

Hillestand L, Storstein O: Conversion of chronic atrial fibrillation to sinus rhythm with combined propranolol and quinidine treatment, Am Heart J **77**:137, 1969.

Kaplinsky E, et al: Quinidine syncope; report of a case successfully treated with lidocaine, Chest **62**:764, 1972.

Koch-Weser J: Quinidine-induced hypoprothrombinemic hemorrhage in patients on chronic warfarin therapy, Ann Intern Med **68**:511, 1968.

Lindsay J Jr: Quinidine and countershock; a reappraisal, Annotations, Am Heart J **85**:141, 1973.

Linenthal HA, Coll PM: A-V block due to quinidine and procaine amide, Circulation **40**(Suppl 6):129, 1969.

Moe, GK, Abildskov JA: Antiarrhythmic drugs. In Goodman LS, Gilman A, editors: The pharma-cological basis of therapeutics, ed 4, New York, 1971, The Macmillan Co.

Nickel SN, Thibaudeau Y: Quinidine intoxication treated by isoproterenol (Isuprel), Can Med Assoc J **85**:81, 1961.

Oravetz J, Slodki SJ: Recurrent ventricular fibrillation precipitated by quinidine, Arch Intern Med **122**:63, 1968.

Purdue Frederick Co: Cardioquin tablets, brochure, Feb 1971.

Romanucci D, et al: Quinidine polygalacturonate in the treatment of cardiac arrhythmias, Am J Clin Res **1**:77, 1970.

Rossi M, Lown B: The use of quinidine in cardioversion, Am J Cardiol **19**:234, 1967.

Schen RJ, Rabinowitz M: Thrombocytopenic purpura due to quinidine, Br Med J **2**:1502, 1958.

Selzer A, Wray HW: Quinidine syncope, Paroxysmal ventricular fibrillation occurring during treatment of chronic atrial arrhythmias, Circulation **30**:17, 1964.

Shaftel N, Halpern A: The clinical study of quinidine polygalacturonate, Am J Med Sc **236**:184, 1958.

Sokolow M, Perloff DB: The clinical pharmacology and use of quinidine in heart disease, Prog Cardiovasc Dis **3**:316, 1961.

Thomson GW: Quinidine as a cause of sudden death, Circulation **14**:757, 1956.

Wagner GS, McIntosh HD: The use of drugs in achieving successful D-C cardioversion, Prog Cardiovasc Dis **11**:431, 1969.

Wanatabe Y, Dreifus LS: Antagonism and synergism of potassium, quinidine, and antiarrhythmic agents, Am J Cardiol **12**:702, 1963.

Wanatabe Y, Dreifus LS: Interactions of quinidine and potassium on atrioventricular transmission, Circ Res **20**:434, 1967.

Wasserman F, et al: Successful treatment of quinidine and procaine amide intoxication, N Engl J Med **259**:797, 1958.

Wetherbee DG, Holzman D, Brown MG: Ventricular tachycardia following administration of quinidine, Am Heart J **43**:1, 1952.

Woolfolk DJ, et al: The effect of quinidine on electrical energy required for ventricular defibrillation, Am Heart J **72**:659, 1966.

RESERPINE (Serpasil)

Reserpine is a pure crystalline alkaloid derived from the plant *Rauwolfia serpentina*. It is the most potent and the most generally used of the rauwolfia alkaloids.

Pharmacology

Reserpine acts as an antihypertensive drug by depleting nerve stores of catecholamines (epinephrine and norepinephrine), thus blocking catecholamine-mediated vaso-constriction. It also has sedative and tran-quilizing properties, due to depletion of serotinin and catecholamines from the brain.

Reserpine generally does not decrease renal blood flow. However, because it de-pletes the myocardial catecholamines, it can decrease the cardiac output.

Absorption

Reserpine is absorbed from the gastro-intestinal tract; it can also be given IM or IV. However, there is no advantage of giv-ing it IV.

When reserpine is given IM, an effect occurs in 1 to 3 hours; a peak effect occurs in 2 to 5 hours; and its effect lasts 4 to 8 hours.

Indications

Hypertensive emergencies, particularly acute dissecting aneurysm of the aorta (in conjunction with trimethaphan and guan-ethidine; see Chapter 13), eclampsia and preeclampsia, hypertensive crises associated with acute or chronic glomerulonephritis, and accelerated (malignant) hypertension. It can also be used in hypertensive enceph-alopathy or hypertensive crises associated with intracranial (intracerebral or sub-arachnoid) hemorrhage. However, in these latter conditions, its sedative effects may make an assessment of the patient's condi-tion more difficult.

Contraindications

Digitalis toxicity, history of mental de-pression, presence or history of ulcerative colitis, peptic ulcer, or bronchial asthma. Patients undergoing surgery should stop taking reserpine 2 weeks prior to the sur-gery, to prevent hypotension during anes-thesia. Pregnant patients, because the drug passes the placental barrier and can also interfere with uterine contractions.

Side effects and toxicity

Neurological. Mental depression (which may lead to suicide), drowsiness or para-doxical nervousness or anxiety, headache, nightmares (which may be an early sign of mental depression), rarely atypical Parkin-sonism, catatonia, central nervous system sensitization manifested by dull sensorium, deafness, glaucoma, uveitis, and optic atrophy.

Cardiovascular. Anginal-like syndrome, premature contractions especially when reserpine is used with digitalis, bradycar-dia, weight gain due to sodium retention.

Gastrointestinal. Increased salivation, in-creased gastric secretions, nausea, vomiting, diarrhea, increased appetite.

Dermatological and hypersensitivity re-actions. Pruritus, skin rashes, dryness of the mouth, thrombocytopenic purpura, bronchial asthma.

Other side effects. Nasal congestion, epi-staxis, conjunctival congestion, impotence or decreased libido, weight gain due to in-creased appetite, flushing of the skin.

Treatment of toxicity. Stop the drug. Severe hypotension and shock due to reserpine can be treated with a sympatho-mimetic drug such as methamphetamine hydrochloride (5 to 15 mg can be given IV for the emergency treatment of hypotensive shock).

Interactions with other drugs

Reserpine increases digitalis toxicity, and digitalis enhances the effect of reserpine on the heart. Therefore, ventricular tachyar-rhythmias, or bradycardia may occur when both drugs are given simultaneously.

Antihypertensive drugs, such as the thi-azides, furosemide (Lasix), ethacrynic acid (Edecrin), hydralazine (Apresoline), meca-mylamine (Inversine), and pentolinium (Ansolysen), increase the hypotensive action of reserpine. Therefore, smaller doses of each drug may be needed.

Guanethidine (Ismelin) potentiates the hypotensive effect of reserpine and may also produce bradycardia and mental depression.

Anesthetics are potentiated by reserpine. Therefore, reserpine should be stopped 2 weeks prior to surgery.

MAO inhibitors interact with reserpine and may produce serious side effects, such as sudden hypertension or suicidal depressive reactions. Reserpine should not be used for at least 1 week after the patient has stopped taking an MAO inhibitor (even the antihypertensive MAO inhibitor pargyline [Eutonyl]).

Quinidine may cause cardiac arrhythmias when given with reserpine.

Propranolol may produce excessive sedation when given with reserpine.

Dosage and administration

Reserpine should be given IM for hypertensive emergencies. An initial test dose of 0.25 mg should be given IM because some patients may respond with an excessive drop in blood pressure, particularly if the patient has been taking other antihypertensive drugs or if the patient has an intracranial hemorrhage. Other patients may also respond initially to the usual therapeutic dose of reserpine with a drop in blood pressure and shock. Such patients show an unusual combination of hypertension associated with excessive vasoconstriction due to hypovolemia. If such a paradoxical drop in blood pressure occurs after reserpine has been given IM, the patient should be treated with IV fluids or a pressor agent, such as metaraminol (Aramine), to raise the blood pressure (Chapter 3).

Because an excessive hypotensive effect does not occur after 5 hours, the usual IM dose of 2.5 mg can be given every 6 to 8 hours. When more than 4 or 5 mg is given, the therapeutic effect does not increase, but the patient will become increasingly somnolent. To prevent overdosage, reserpine should never be given more frequently than every 3 hours. Similarly, the blood pressure should be checked before each injection.

Routine orders for IM administration of reserpine should not be written. Instead, specific instructions, such as "2.5 mg reserpine, IM, when systolic blood pressure rises to 190 mm Hg or diastolic blood pressure rises to 130 mm Hg," should be given. (The actual dose will depend on the patient's responses to previous doses.)

When reserpine is given IM, the blood pressure should respond within 8 to 12 hours. If no effect is noted by then, a more potent antihypertensive drug, such as pentolinium (Ansolysen), should be given subcutaneously or IM. (The two drugs can also be used simultaneously or alternately.)

IM doses of reserpine should be stopped

RESERPINE (Serpasil)	
Route of administration	Emergency dosage
IM	Initial test dose of 0.25 mg is given. If excessive hypotension does not develop in 1 to 2 hours, the usual dose of 2.5 mg is given every 6 to 8 hours, depending on the lowering of the blood pressure. Doses higher than 5.0 mg will merely produce excessive side effects. Similarly, injections should not be made more frequently than every 3 hours, to prevent excessive hypotension or other side effects.

as soon as possible, and therapy should be continued with oral medication (including oral doses of reserpine), because when it is given IM for several days, the patient may become very depressed, comatose, or may develop severe parkinsonism-like symptoms.

Preparations

Injection: 2 ml ampuls (each ml contains 2.5 mg); 10-ml vials (each ml contains 5 [or 2.5] mg).

Tablets: 0.1, 0.25, 0.5 mg, and stronger strengths are also available for oral use.

REFERENCES

American Hospital Formulary Service: The rauwolfia alkaloids. Category 24:08.

Breslin DJ: Hypertensive crisis, Med Clin North Am **53**:351, 1969.

Ciba Pharmaceutical Co: Serpasil (reserpine), product brochure, Mar 1972.

Cohn JN: Paroxysmal hypertension and hypovolemia, N Engl J Med **275**:643, 1966.

Freis ED: Hypertensive crisis, JAMA **208**:338, 1969.

Martin EW: Hazards of medication, Philadelphia, 1971, JB Lippincott Co.

SERPASIL. *See* Reserpine.

SODIUM BICARBONATE
Pharmacology

Sodium bicarbonate given IV is a very effective alkalinizing drug.

Sodium lactate has also been used as an alkalinizing drug. Sodium lactate is a racemic salt, consisting of levo and dextro forms. The levo form is metabolized in the body into sodium bicarbonate. The dextro form is converted into glycogen. However, when shock, liver disease, or right-sided congestive heart failure is present, the metabolism of lactic acid is impaired. Therefore, sodium bicarbonate is preferable to sodium lactate (8.4 gm sodium bicarbonate is equivalent to 100 ml molar sodium lactate).

Indications

Sodium bicarbonate is given IV to counteract the severe metabolic acidosis that occurs in cardiac arrest. It can also be used to counteract hyperkalemia or quinidine or procainamide toxicity when the QRS widens and AV block occurs.

Contraindications

Metabolic or respiratory alkalosis, congestive heart failure, hypokalemia, or hypocalcemia.

Side effects and toxicity

The IV infusion of a large amount of sodium bicarbonate may cause a metabolic alkalosis or congestive heart failure. The patient should be monitored with periodic pH determinations. If a metabolic alkalosis occurs, the sodium bicarbonate infusion should be stopped, and an infusion of isotonic saline should be given. If tetany develops, calcium gluconate may also be helpful.

Dosage and administration

It is difficult to determine the dose of sodium bicarbonate needed to overcome a metabolic acidosis. Numerous formulas have been devised, but none is accurate. The following are general statements.

1. 150 ml (3 ampuls) of the 7.5% sodium bicarbonate solution will raise the pH approximately 0.05 to 0.1 unit. The pH should be raised above 7.30.

2. The following formula can be used to determine the dose of sodium bicarbonate if the CO_2 content of the arterial blood is known.

Bicarbonate dose (mEq) = body weight (kg) $\times$ (27 $-$ CO_2 content [mEq/L]) $\times$ 0.2.

This assumes that the extracellular fluid volume is 20% of the body weight and that the normal CO_2 content is 27 mEq/L.

EXAMPLE: Patient's weight, 70 kg; CO_2 content, 12 mEq/L

Bicarbonate dose needed = 70 $\times$ (27 $-$ 12) $\times$ 0.2
= 70 $\times$ (15) $\times$ 0.2
= 210 mEq sodium bicarbonate needed.

This is equivalent to approximately five

50-ml vials of 7.5% sodium bicarbonate solution.

Actually, when acidosis occurs, the excessive hydrogen ions must be buffered intracellularly as well as extracellularly. Therefore, the above formula produces only approximately one half the buffering needed to bring the CO_2 content to normal. However, the use of the formula is clinically satisfactory because the CO_2 content should be raised to approximately 20 mEq/L but *not* to a normal value of 27 (or 28) mEq/L, for the following reason.

When a metabolic acidosis is present, a compensatory respiratory alkalosis develops. Both the metabolic acidosis and the respiratory alkalosis produce a low CO_2 content. Therefore, the measured CO_2 content in such a patient represents the combined effects of an acidosis (metabolic) and an alkalosis (respiratory). If enough sodium bicarbonate is given to control the metabolic acidosis and raise the CO_2 content to normal, a severe alkalosis may develop because the compensatory respiratory alkalosis often persists after the metabolic acidosis disappears. (Patients in shock may also show a *primary* respiratory alkalosis due to the hyperventilation that is present.)

3. When cardiac arrest occurs, sodium bicarbonate can be given IV in one of two ways.

Two 50-ml ampuls of 7.5% sodium bicarbonate should be immediately injected as a priming dose into the IV tubing of the infusion bottle. Then one 50-ml ampul should be given IV every 5 min until the circulation has been restored. (Larger doses may be necessary; p. 23.)

Sodium bicarbonate can also be given IV as a 1.5% solution. A priming dose of 100 ml should be given as quickly as possible. Then the solution should be given rapidly at a rate of 10 ml/min (approximately 150 drops per min, using a regular drip bulb).

4. When quinidine or procainamide toxicity is present, one 50-ml ampul can be injected slowly, with electrocardiographic monitoring. The dose can be repeated every 5 min if improvement in the ECG is noted (decrease in the width of the QRS complexes or return of sinus rhythm). However, if ventricular premature contractions appear or become more frequent, the sodium bicarbonate infusion should be stopped.

Preparations

Injection: 50-ml vials (7.5%); each 50-ml vial contains 3.75 gm sodium bicarbonate (44.64 mEq sodium ions and 44.64 mEq bicarbonate ions). A 1.5% solution of sodium bicarbonate can be prepared by di-

SODIUM BICARBONATE	
Route of administration	Emergency dosage
IV, undiluted 7.5% solution	For cardiac arrest: two 50-ml ampuls, injected into the tubing of an IV infusion immediately; then 1 ampul (50 ml) every 5 min until the circulation is restored. (Larger doses may be necessary; p. 23.)
IV, continuous 1.5% solution	For cardiac arrest: 100 ml as quickly as possible, as a priming dose; then 10 ml/min (approximately 150 drops per min, using a regular drip bulb).

luting one 50-ml vial of the 7.5% solution with 200 ml sterile water, isotonic saline, or 5% dextrose in water solution.

REFERENCES

American Hospital Formulary Service: Sodium bicarbonate. Category 40:08.

Bellet S: Clinical disorders of the heart beat, ed 3, Philadelphia, 1971, Lea & Febiger.

Bellet S, Wasserman F: Indications and contraindications for the use of molar sodium lactate, Circulation **15**:591, 1957.

SODIUM NITROPRUSSIDE

Pharmacology

Sodium nitroprusside produces hypotension by directly relaxing the smooth muscles of the arterioles. It does not directly affect the cardiac output or the heart rate. It is given IV and acts within 1 to 2 min. Its effects last 5 to 10 min.

Indications

Acute hypertensive emergencies, such as acute hypertensive encephalopathy, hypertensive emergencies associated with acute glomerulonephritis, intracranial (intracerebral or subarachnoid) hemorrhage, pheochromocytoma.

Contraindications

Cerebrovascular disease or coronary artery disease.

Side effects and toxicity

When the blood pressure falls, the patient may become apprehensive, agitated, and nauseated. Retching, sweating, and muscular twitching may occur. These symptoms abate quickly when the rate of infusion is slowed or temporarily stopped. Skin rash, mental confusion, or psychotic behavior may also develop.

Dosage and administration

Sodium nitroprusside solution is not available commercially and must be prepared by the hospital pharmacy. Details of its preparation and use can be found in the articles of Fairbairn, Gifford, Page, and Sheps.

Usually, 5 ml of stock solution (which contains 50 mg sodium nitroprusside) is added to 1 L 5% dextrose in water. The infusion is started at a rate of 10 drops per min (using a microdrip bulb). The flow can then be increased, if necessary, by 5 drops per min at intervals of 2 to 3 min.

When it is necessary to decrease the volume of fluid given, the concentration of the sodium nitroprusside can be increased to 120 or even 240 mg/L (Fairbairn).

The undiluted stock solution can be kept for 4 weeks in the stoppered amber bottles in the refrigerator.

When the diluted solution is infused continually, a fresh solution must be prepared every 12 hours because it loses its stability after this time.

Although sodium nitroprusside is used for the emergency treatment of acute hypertensive emergencies, Sheps has used it continuously in some patients for 3 to 4 weeks, without ill effects.

The sodium nitroprusside infusion must be monitored constantly because there is a narrow margin between the dose causing hypotension or maintaining hypertension. Therefore, the patient should be treated in the CCU. The blood pressure should be checked every $\frac{1}{2}$ min when the infusion is first started. Later, it can be checked every 5 min.

When sodium nitroprusside is used, it is preferable to have an IV infusion containing any appropriate solution, such as dextrose in water, inserted into a vein so that a patent vein is available if it is necessary to stop the sodium nitroprusside infusion temporarily (see Trimethaphan camsylate).

Sodium nitroprusside is converted to thiocyanate. If the infusion is continued longer than 72 hours, the blood thiocyanate level should be determined every other day; and if the thiocyanate concentration exceeds 12 mg/100 ml, the infusion should be stopped to avoid toxicity.

REFERENCES

Fairbairn JF II: Drug management of hypertensive emergencies. In Brest AN, Moyer JH, editors: Cardiovascular drug therapy, Eleventh Hahnemann Symposium, New York, 1965, Grune & Stratton.

Gifford RW Jr: The management of emergencies associated with essential hypertension. In Cyclopedia of medicine, surgery, specialties, vol 4, Philadelphia, 1964, FA Davis Co.

Page IH, Corcoran AC, et al: Cardiovascular actions of sodium nitroprusside in animals and hypertensive patients, Circulation 11:188, 1955.

Sheps SG: Hypertensive crisis, Postgrad Med **49**: 95, 1971.

TENSILON CHLORIDE. *See* Edrophonium chloride.

TRIMETHAPHAN CAMSYLATE (Arfonad)

Trimethaphan camsylate is a nonquaternary ammonium compound. It is used to lower the blood pressure very rapidly.

Pharmacology

Trimethaphan camsylate is a ganglionic blocking agent. It inhibits transmission of nerve impulses through both the sympathetic and parasympathetic ganglia. It also has a direct peripheral vasodilator effect, which also lowers the blood pressure. In addition, it liberates histamine.

Absorption

It is given IV. Its effects appear almost immediately and last for 10 to 20 min.

Indications

Hypertensive emergencies, particularly acute dissecting aneurysm of the aorta, hypertension associated with acute pulmonary edema, acute hypertensive encephalopathy, hypertension with intracerebral or subarachnoid hemorrhage. It has also been used to achieve controlled hypotension, particularly during neurosurgery.

Contraindications

It is contraindicated in patients in whom hypotension may be dangerous; for example, uncorrected anemia, hypovolemia, shock, asphyxia, or uncorrected respiratory insufficiency. It should be used with extreme caution in patients with arteriosclerosis, cardiac disease, hepatic or renal disease, degenerative disease of the central nervous system, Addison's disease, or diabetes, in patients who are receiving corticosteroids, in pregnant women (because it may seriously injure the fetus), and in allergic patients (because trimethaphan releases histamine).

Side effects and toxicity

It has a specific effect on the pupils and causes pupillary dilatation, which should not be considered a sign of either the depth of anesthesia (if used during surgery) or anoxia. (If the pupils become dilated and nonresponsive to light, a further increase of the dose of trimethaphan will not lower the blood pressure further.)

Other side effects are tachycardia, respiratory depression, or excessive hypotension.

Trimethaphan can be used for only 12 to 48 hours because after this time its release of histamine may cause problems in allergic patients.

Treatment of side effects. If excessive hypotension develops, the trimethaphan infusion should be stopped, and the foot of the bed or operating table should be raised. In addition, an infusion of phenylephrine (Neo-Synephrine) hydrochloride should be immediately available (20 to 30 mg dissolved in 500 ml 5% dextrose in water). (Mephentermine [Wyamine] sulfate can also be used as a pressor agent.) Levarterenol (Levophed) should be used only if the patient does not respond to phenylephrine (or to mephentermine).

When trimethaphan is used during surgery, the patient should have a Foley catheter inserted because the sudden cessation of urine also indicates that serious hypotension has developed.

Interactions with other drugs

Procainamide and other cardiac-depressant drugs potentiate the action of trimethaphan. Other drug interactions are similar to those of pentolinium.

Dosage and administration

Trimethaphan must always be diluted and given IV. The solution should be freshly prepared and any unused portion discarded. In addition, it must be used only by physicians trained in its use. To avoid coronary or cerebral anoxia, it is also important that the patient be adequately oxygenated when trimethaphan is given. Cardiopulmonary resuscitation supplies and equipment must be immediately available.

When trimethaphan is infused, it is preferable to have an IV infusion containing an appropriate solution, such as dextrose in water, inserted into a vein, so that a patent vein is always available if it is necessary to stop the trimethaphan infusion temporarily. This is done by using two infusion bottles. The infusion containing dextrose in water is connected to a suitable vein. The needle from the infusion bottle containing the trimethaphan is then inserted directly behind the IV needle into the tubing of the first infusion bottle (Fig. 2). In this way, the trimethaphan infusion can be stopped or started when desired because a patent vein is always available. When the trimethaphan solution is infused, the tubing of the dextrose in water solution is clamped, and vice versa. (A hemostat can be used to clamp the tubing of the trimethaphan solution to make certain that it flows only when desired.)

A 0.1% (1 mg/ml) concentration of trimethaphan in 5% dextrose in water solution should be used. This is obtained by adding one 10-ml ampul of trimethaphan (which contains 500 mg) to 500 ml 5%

dextrose in water. Therefore, each ml of the diluted solution contains 1 mg.

An IV drip of trimethaphan is started at an average rate of 60 drops (4 ml) per min (using a regular drip bulb). This is equivalent to a flow rate of 4 mg/min. After the first 60 drips have been infused, the flow should be stopped for approximately 1 min to observe the extent of the fall of the blood pressure. The rate of administration is then adjusted to maintain the desired level of hypotension. It may vary from 4 drops per min to rates exceeding 100 drops per min.

Since individual patients vary markedly in their response to trimethaphan, the blood pressure must be taken in the opposite arm every 30 sec at first. The hypotensive effect of trimethaphan can be increased by elevating the head of the bed 35° to 45°, to obtain postural hypotension.

The trimethaphan infusion solution must not be used for any other drug.

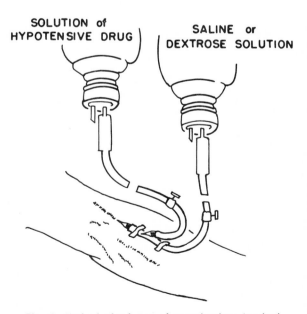

SOLUTION of HYPOTENSIVE DRUG

SALINE or DEXTROSE SOLUTION

Fig. 2. Method of infusion of trimethaphan (method after Gifford).

Preparations

Injection: 10-ml ampuls; each ml contains 50 mg; therefore, the ampul contains 500 mg.

REFERENCES

Freis ED: Hypertensive crisis, JAMA **208**:338, 1969.

Gifford RW Jr: The management of emergencies associated with essential hypertension. In Cyclopedia of medicine, surgery, specialties, vol 4, Philadelphia, 1964, FA Davis Co.

Messer JV: Management of emergencies. XIII. Acute cardiac decompensation, N Engl J Med **274**:1491, 1966.

Roche Laboratories: Arfonad (trimethaphan camsylate) ampuls, package insert, Sept 1971.

Sheps SG: Hypertensive crisis, Postgrad Med **49**:95, 1971.

Smiley RH, et al: Successful treatment of a fulminant hypertensive crisis after bilateral carotid sinus denervation, Am J Surg **114**:784, 1967.

Wheat MW Jr, Palmer RF: Dissecting aneurysms of the aorta, Curr Prob Surg, July 1971.

THORAZINE. *See* Chlorpromazine hydrochloride.

VASOXYL. *See* Methoxamine hydrochloride.

WARFARIN (Coumadin) SODIUM (Panwarfin)

Warfarin sodium and warfarin potassium (Athrombin-K) are coumarin anticoagulants.

Pharmacology

Warfarin inhibits the action of vitamin K in the liver and in this way interferes with the synthesis of four plasma procoagulants: factor IX (plasma thromboplastin component, or Christmas factor), factor VII (serum prothrombin conversion accelerator, or the stable factor), factor X, (Stuart), and factor II (prothrombin). As a result, warfarin has anticoagulant activity.

When warfarin is given, factor VII disappears more rapidly than the other factors. Disappearance of factor VII is associated with bleeding. However, protection against intravascular thrombi is associated with disappearance of factors IX and X. These observations indicate that the use of a "loading dose" technic of giving warfarin may produce bleeding, but may not give protection against thrombi formation, and that it is preferable to start warfarin treatment by giving a small dose (10 mg) daily until the prothrombin time reaches a therapeutic level (see dosage and administration).

Absorption

Warfarin is absorbed from the gastrointestinal tract. It can also be given parenterally, but there is no advantage in giving it this way. After oral (or parenteral) administration, its effect starts in approximately 12 hours, reaches a peak in approximately 36 hours, and lasts approximately 2 to 5 days.

Indications

Treatment of pulmonary embolism and deep venous thrombosis. Prevention of systemic emboli from the heart, as in mitral valvular disease with atrial fibrillation, myocardiopathies, ventricular aneurysms, and after artificial heart valve implants (some of the newer valves do not require postoperative or long-term anticoagulant therapy). Warfarin can be started on the third postoperative day if excessive postoperative bleeding or an abnormally prolonged prothrombin time is not present. Prevention of thromboemboli in patients with acute myocardial infarction, after surgery for a fractured hip, and so on.

Contraindications

Active or suspected bleeding from any source, including the gastrointestinal tract and the genitourinary tract; bleeding from the respiratory tract (unless the hemoptysis is due to pulmonary embolism or mitral stenosis); patients with a hemorrhagic tendency; dissecting aneurysm of the aorta; generalized pericarditis complicating acute myocardial infarction; postmyocardial infarction syndrome; severe hypertension (when the diastolic blood pressure is higher

than 110 mm Hg); subacute bacterial endocarditis; injury to the brain or spinal cord;
prior to elective surgery, particularly surgery of the central nervous system, eyes,
lungs, or prostate gland; late pregnancy, or
threatened or incomplete abortion.

Warfarin should be given cautiously to
patients with liver or kidney disease because
its metabolism and excretion may be impaired.

Warfarin must be given cautiously in the
following conditions, which can be associated with an increased prothrombin time
response: visceral carcinoma (particularly
pancreatic), collagen diseases, congestive
heart failure, infective hepatitis, jaundice,
diarrhea, febrile illness, prolonged hot
weather, poor nutrition, steatorrhea, vitamin K deficiency, and radiotherapy.

Side effects and toxicity

Hemorrhage is the usual side effect. It is
usually due to overdosage, but it may also
indicate the presence of an occult source of
bleeding (such as a peptic ulcer or neoplasm).

Other side effects include drug rash or
fever, nausea, vomiting, diarrhea, and
jaundice.

Hematological side effects include leukopenia or leukemoid reactions, and thrombocytopenia.

Hemorrhage into the skin or fatty tissue
with massive necrosis of the breast, thigh,
hip, or leg tissue may occur. (This may
be due to an allergic vasculitis.)

Treatment of side effects and toxicity.
If slight bleeding occurs, warfarin should
be stopped temporarily, and phytonadione
(vitamin K_1 Mephyton) should be given in
a dose of 5 to 10 mg (1 to 2 tablets) orally.
This will lower the prothrombin time to
a therapeutic range in approximately 12
hours.

If severe bleeding occurs, 5 to 25 mg
(rarely 50 mg) phytonadione should be
given IV slowly (at a rate not exceeding
10 mg/min). In addition, a transfusion of
whole blood may be needed. (If liver disease is present, large doses of phytonadione
are contraindicated. Therefore, if the prothrombin time does not reach normal in
48 hours, the phytonadione should be
stopped.)

Necrosis of the skin or fatty tissues requires the use of heparin.

Interactions with other drugs

Warfarin is affected by numerous drugs.

Drugs that potentiate warfarin action*
Allopurinol (Zyloprim)
Chloral hydrate†
Chlorpropamide (Diabinese)
Cinchophen
Clofibrate (Atromid S)
Dextran
Dextrothyroxine
Diazoxide (Hyperstat)
Disulfiram
Diuretics†
Ethacrynic acid (Edecrin)
Hepatotoxic drugs
Indomethacin (Indocin)
Inhalational anesthetics
Mefenamic acid (Ponstel)
Methylphenidate (Ritalin)
Monamine oxidase inhibitors
Nalidixic acid (NegGram)
Oxyphenbutazone (Tandearil)
Phenylbutazone (Butazolidin)
Phenyramidol
Quinidine and quinine
Salicylates (in excess of 1 gm a day)
Sulfinpyrazone (Anturane)
Sulfonamides (long-acting)
Thyroid drugs
Tolbutamide (Orinase)
Triclofos sodium
Drugs that inhibit warfarin action‡
Adrenocorticosteroids
Alcohol†
Antacids
Antihistamines
Barbiturates
Chloral hydrate†
Chlordiazepoxide (Librium)
Cholestyramine
Diuretics†

---

*Therefore, smaller warfarin doses are needed.
†Increased and decreased prothrombin time re-
sponses have been reported.
‡Therefore, larger warfarin doses are needed.

Drugs that inhibit warfarin action—cont'd
Ethchlorvynol (Placidyl)
Glutethemide (Doriden)
Griseofulvin (Fulvicin)
Haloperidol (Haldol)
Meprobamate (Equinal, Miltown)
Oral contraceptives
Vitamin C (ascorbic acid)

Warfarin, on the other hand, increases the effects of diphenylhydantoin, insulin, and the sulfonylureas.

Dosage and administration

Numerous dose schedules for warfarin have been described, including the use of an initial "loading dose." However, it is preferable to place the patient immediately on a daily smaller dose of 10 mg until the prothrombin time (tested daily) approaches 20 sec (see pharmacology). The dose of warfarin is then adjusted to reach and maintain a prothrombin time between $1\frac{1}{2}$ and $2\frac{1}{2}$ times the control value. (A control value of below 12 sec or above 15 sec suggests that the thromboplastin used in the test is faulty and is resulting in incorrect prothrombin time values.)

If the situation is urgent, the patient should be given heparin simultaneously with the warfarin (see Heparin).

The usual maintenance dose is 5 to 10 mg daily. Many patients require varying daily doses; for example, 5 mg alternating with 7 or 7.5 mg; or 7.5 mg daily for 3 days, with no warfarin the fourth day; and so on.

Preparations

Tablets: 2, 2.5, 5, 7.5, 10, and 25 mg.

REFERENCES

American Hospital Formulary Service: Warfarin sodium. Category 20:12:04.
American Hospital Formulary Service: Phytonadione. Category 88:24.
Deykin D: Warfarin therapy, N Engl J Med **283:** 691, 1970.
Endo Laboratories, Inc: Coumadin (sodium warfarin), product brochure, Sept 1972.
Koch-Weser J, Sellers EM: Drug interactions with coumarin anticoagulants, N Engl J Med **285:** 547, 1971.
Martin EW: Hazards of medication, Philadelphia, 1971, JB Lippincott Co.
Merck Sharp & Dhome: Aquamephyton, Mephyton, product brochure, 1962.

XYLOCAINE HYDROCHLORIDE. *See* Lidocaine hydrochloride.

Index

*Main discussions of drugs are indicated by boldface numbers.

347